Human African Trypanosomiasis (Sleeping Sickness)

Human African Trypanosomiasis (Sleeping Sickness)

The Road to Elimination Revisited—Achievements and Remaining Challenges

Special Issue Editor

Christian Burri

MDPI • Basel • Beijing • Wuhan • Barcelona • Belgrade • Manchester • Tokyo • Cluj • Tianjin

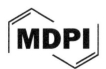

Special Issue Editor
Christian Burri
Swiss Tropical & Public Health Institute
Switzerland

Editorial Office
MDPI
St. Alban-Anlage 66
4052 Basel, Switzerland

This is a reprint of articles from the Special Issue published online in the open access journal *Tropical Medicine and Infectious Disease* (ISSN 2414-6366) (available at: https://www.mdpi.com/ journal/tropicalmed/special issues/HAT).

–

For citation purposes, cite each article independently as indicated on the article page online and as indicated below:

LastName, A.A.; LastName, B.B.; LastName, C.C. Article Title. *Journal Name* **Year**, *Article Number, Page Range.*

ISBN 978-3-03928-963-9 (Pbk)
ISBN 978-3-03928-964-6 (PDF)

Cover image courtesy of Swiss Tropical & Public Health Institute.
Trypanosoma brucei; F. Brand, Swiss TPH; Picture taken with the transmission electron microscope at the Center for Cellular Imaging and NanoAnalytics, University of Basel, Switzerland

Contents

About the Special Issue Editor

Christian Burri PhD, is the Deputy Head of the Department of Medicine and the Head of the Medicines Implementation Research Unit at the Swiss TPH, and Professor of Pharmacy & Clinical Pharmacology at the Department of Pharmaceutical Sciences, University of Basel. For almost 25 years, he has been involved in the management and conduct of clinical trials on drugs and vaccines against neglected tropical and poverty-related diseases, mainly in low income countries. In 2018, he handed over this service-oriented responsibility and founded a research group studying the implementation of medicines in resource-low settings in the two main fields of interests of access and pharmacoepidemiology. Throughout his training and professional career, he has had the privilege of becoming involved in most aspects of drug research and development, including gene cloning and parasite cultivation, drug screening, pharmacology and toxicology, lead selection, the conducting of clinical trials of Phases I–III, quality management, ethical and regulatory tasks, but also in various aspects of public health and the implementation of new interventions. Despite his involvement on a broad range of topics and contribution to various diseases, the original and continued passion of Prof. Burri is sleeping sickness (human African trypanosomiasis), where he has significantly contributed to improvement of the treatment. Prof. Burri has been trained as a pharmacist at the University of Bern, Switzerland, holds a PhD in medical parasitology from the University of Basel, and conducted postdoctoral training in molecular pharmacology at the Johns Hopkins University, Baltimore. He has held a Diploma in Pharmaceutical Medicine of the Swiss Association of Pharmaceutical Professionals (SwAPP) since 2000.

Preface to "Human African Trypanosomiasis (HAT, Sleeping Sickness)"

Human African trypanosomiasis (HAT; sleeping sickness) is a parasitic disease with a long and prominent history. For over half a century, major efforts and investments were made toward combating this disease, and it was driven back by the Colonial forces in sub-Saharan Africa from over 100,000 cases per year at the turn of the 19th century to 4435 cases by 1964. Although the interventions used were overly complex, the diagnostic tools were poor, and the drugs dreadful, an impressive decrease in case numbers could be achieved. After independence, national research organizations were created, but in the 1980s, other health priorities emerged, and the available funds for HAT were reduced, and awareness and surveillance of the disease decreased. Consequently, in 1998, almost 40,000 cases were reported with over 300,000 estimated but undiagnosed and, therefore, untreated. In response, there were additional efforts made by the World Health Organization (WHO) and many partners to reverse this trend. Since 2000, the number of new HAT cases reported dropped by 95%. The WHO added HAT to its neglected tropical diseases road map in 2012 and targeted its elimination as a public health problem by 2020 and interruption of transmission (zero cases) by 2030.

To win the "end game" against this massively stigmatized disease that is often shrouded in beliefs and evil spirits, the human factor will play a key role. We need to understand whether patients are willing to accept HAT as a diagnosis in areas where the disease was believed to have been eliminated. Will the physicians of the younger generation, who have never seen a case, still have HAT on their minds and be able and willing to diagnose such a scary disease? Will patients accept the new treatments and treatment approaches that we scientists believe to be superior? What happens to patients in a remote area who get a positive result from a screening test?

In this Special Issue, room is given to these key research questions about the understanding of the communities' beliefs, needs, and approaches. The topic of long-term infection and animal reservoir is also touched upon; these questions are of high interest and may have a lasting impact on the approach to disease selection. This issue also summarizes approaches to the successes in disease control from several angles. The review articles summarize the contribution of partners, the development of new drug classes, and treatment breakthroughs and the research articles portray the potential future treatment portfolio, which is more promising than ever. The success of drug development goes beyond the new substances: It is shown that the clinical trials themselves had a positive effect on the reduction of patient numbers and on the quality of treatment. The efficiency of product development partnerships goes way beyond HAT, as similar approaches are used in other diseases and may be a successful model for future drug development.

Christian Burri
Special Issue Editor

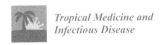

Tropical Medicine and Infectious Disease

Editorial

Sleeping Sickness at the Crossroads

Christian Burri [1,2]

[1] Swiss Tropical and Public Health Institute, Socinstrasse 57, 4002 Basel, Switzerland;
    christian.burri@swisstph.ch
[2] University of Basel, Petersplatz 1, 4001 Basel, Switzerland

Received: 3 April 2020; Accepted: 7 April 2020; Published: 8 April 2020

1. A Disease with Historical Dimension

Human African trypanosomiasis (HAT; sleeping sickness) is a disease with truly historic dimensions. Its maximum possible distribution corresponds to the range of tsetse flies, which covers an area of eight million km^2 between 14° North and 20° South latitude on the African continent. Trypanosomes are very ancient parasites, which emerged around 380 million years ago and today are ubiquitous. Some salivarian forms began to transmit to mammals when tsetse flies emerged some 35 million years ago. The relatively late arrival of humans may explain why African game animals are tolerant towards most species of trypanosomes, but humans and most domestic animals are susceptible to certain species. Accounts of encounters with cachectic and sleep-affected people and the death of important authorities were already reported by Arabian travellers in the 12th to 14th century [1].

HAT likely had a limited impact on the local population until the slave traders and later the colonial forces arrived in Africa. The tsetse belt was extremely thinly populated (< 6 persons/km^2) and people lived in very small, dispersed villages. Tsetse infested areas were avoided due to the annoyance by the flies and tales of witchcraft, the bush around the villages was cleared for protection against game animals and in some cultures there was an awareness about the danger of the tsetse flies to cattle [2].

From the beginning of the times of colonization onwards, HAT has had a tremendous impact on populations and societies, and the disease is very closely tied to the development of Africa. HAT hampered the colonization of the continent, since, unlike the Conquistadors in Latin America, all invaders in Africa faced dramatic logistical problems caused by the fact that horses are highly susceptible to trypanosomes [3]. The impact on trade (particularly slave trade) was recognized very early on. In 1792, the British physician Thomas Winterbottom described a disease in Sierra Leone he depicted as 'negro lethargy'. He observed that slave shippers rejected those with swelling of the posterior cervical lymph nodes—a sign associated with HAT that is still known as Winterbottom's sign. Therefore, it is not difficult to understand the manifold early attempts to control the disease. However, it was only in 1895 when Sir David Bruce reported that the tsetse fly was linked to cattle trypanosomiasis, and Dutton in 1902 (West Africa) and Castellani 1903 (East Africa) detected the causative agents of African sleeping sickness [4].

These findings coincided with the first reported major epidemic in East Africa in 1900, which devastated the Busoga focus at the Kenya–Uganda border and left about half a million people dead. The responsible subspecies is not entirely clear until today. It was earlier described to be *T. b. gambiense*, however, at that time, the more likely East African subspecies, *T. b. rhodesiense*, had not yet been described; clinically the descriptions rather support the hypothesis that the latter pathogen was responsible [4]. HAT had a similar impact on the population in the Belgian Congo, e.g., along the Mpoko river: in 1917, 79,000 people were counted in a census, in 1919, only 1,200 people were still in the area. The colonial powers were horrified by the speed at which their working force was dying. They ordered the displacement of the population from the shores of Lake Victoria and infected people were isolated in sleeping sickness camps. Similar actions were taken in the Belgian Congo [3]. These activities marked the start of incredible efforts of the colonial powers to control the disease, but particularly also of the vertical approach towards disease control, with special programs run in parallel with the public health system—which is now one of the challenges in the elimination "end game" with very few patients remaining requiring an integrated public health approach.

The detection of the causative agent, the mode of transmission and the first documented major epidemics coincided with the advent of modern pharmacology. It is, therefore, no surprise that there was an interest to find drugs against this disease. In 1908, the colonial powers, in a joint conference, decided to give drug development a high priority and in course, several molecules were developed.

2. The First Turning Point and a Colossal Failure

The history of the oldest drug still in use against HAT, suramin, is described in the context of the history in the article of Madeja et al., Not only is the drug still manufactured, but also the continued support of Bayer since the year 2000 is a major contributing factor allowing us to write about the elimination of HAT today.

The activity of inorganic arsenic-based compounds had already been recognized in the mid-19th century and the treatment of "nagana" (animal trypanosomiasis) was described by David Livingstone in 1848 and David Bruce in 1895. This knowledge led to the development of the first organo-arsenic compound Atoxyl® in 1905 by Paul Ehrlich, who used trypanosomes as a model to screen molecules, but was mainly searching for drugs against syphilis. Wolferstan Thomas in Liverpool subsequently showed that Atoxyl® was effective against *T. b. gambiense*. However, Atoxyl®, meaning 'non-toxic', caused severe adverse drug reactions particularly affecting the optic nerve; it was only active against early stage HAT and was followed by tryparsamide in 1919. Tryparsamide was developed in the USA and was the first drug to be active against the late stage, although not very active and also prone to extensive resistance development. Tryparsamide was also very toxic, with a dose dependent risk damaging the optic nerve. This is documented in a horrifying report from 1930 when a lieutenant of the French Army in Cameroon doubled the prescribed dose of tryparsamide to speed up the recovery of 800 patients. Two days later, all these patients were blind. This event prompted the Swiss chemist and physician Dr. Friedheim to investigate alternative drugs. The introduction of a triazine ring lead to the development of melarsen (disodium p-melaminyl-phenyl arsonate) in 1940, which proved to be a very efficient drug against *T. b. gambiense*, but was still very toxic. In 1944, Friedheim first described the trivalent arsenoxide form of melarsan, known as melarsenoxide. He reported its use in treatment of human sleeping sickness in 1948. The main achievement was the reduction of the duration of therapy to six weeks, with two weeks of seven daily injections of 1.5 mg/kg each, spaced by an interval of one month. In a further step, capping the arsenic in melarsen oxide with British anti-Lewisite, an antidote to the arsenical warfare agent Lewisite, reduced the toxicity by a factor of the order of 100, but the trypanocidal activity only by a factor 2.5. The new drug was called melarsoprol (Mel B; Arsobal®) [5]. It remained the mainstay of second stage HAT treatment until the early 2000s despite the long treatment duration of 35 days, the known related adverse drug reactions, particularly the encephalopathic syndrome that occurs in about 10% of the patients treated and leads to their death in about 50% of cases, and the potential for drug resistance.

Another line of research was the molecules with a diamidine structure discovered in the 1930s. These molecules were detected by serendipity in the search for hypoglycaemic compounds, with the idea in mind that this effect might compromise the very prominent and particular glucose metabolism of trypanosomes. Several compounds, however, proved to have a direct trypanocidal effect with the three compounds stilbamidine, pentamidine, and propamidine identified to have the highest activity [6]. Pentamidine does not penetrate the blood brain barrier so its use is limited to first stage HAT; despite this drawback it is still is in use today, for treatment of children below six kilograms. The distinctly better safety profile of the drugs only active against first stage disease (pentamidine and suramin) versus melarsoprol was also the advent of the consistent performance of lumbar puncture to determine the disease stage and make a treatment decision. The need for a lumbar puncture was, for over 50 years, a characteristic of HAT treatment, a source of patient distress, stigma and technical limitation of treatment. Some 70 years after the discovery of pentamidine, the diamidines again became the focus of drug development, although not successful until today.

The development of the organo-arsenicals, diamidines, and also drugs developed much later and still in use like eflornithine and nifurtimox, including their drawbacks related to the potential for drug resistance are described in detail in the contribution of De Koning.

The "scramble for Africa" was an investment with very high political and economic stakes, and sleeping sickness was not just a disease; it had become the colonial disease. Besides drug development, the responses of the Anglophone and Francophone colonial powers to trypanosomiasis differed significantly. Francophone countries chose to concentrate directly on the medical problems presented by the disease in humans. This included the introduction of "mobile teams" actively searching and screening population for HAT cases. This method of systematic case detection and treatment with the aim of elimination of the parasite reservoir was suggested by the French military surgeon Eugène Jamot and such activities started in 1926 in Cameroon ("atoxylisation") [7]. Subsequently, the prevalence of HAT declined from as high as 60% in 1919 to 0.2–4.1% in 1930, leading to an expansion of the methodology to other countries. After the Second World War, Atoxyl® was replaced by pentamidine and a regular application of the drug every six months to the population at risk was introduced ("pentamidinisation"). In the 1950s in the Belgian Congo alone, some two million people were subjected to this preventive mass drug administration [3].

Due to the partial presence of *T. b. rhodesiense* in their territories, the Anglophone countries were confronted with the more widespread problem of disease in domestic livestock, which also presented a reservoir for human disease. Their approach included vector control (traps, spraying), bush clearing, and game destruction [3,7], and later the chemopreventive use of veterinary drugs (diminazene, isometamidium, and homidium).

The control measures were overall very successful and progressively controlled the disease, reaching a very low, generalized transmission by the mid-1960s, with a minimum of 4435 cases declared in Africa in 1964 [8]. However, the measures taken were very costly, but above all very unpopular in the communities. This led to concealment where possible, and made the longterm goal of elimination by chemotherapy difficult, if not impossible [3]. We could observe similar tendencies when conducting clinical trials in the 2000s; potential patients were mostly hiding away or fleeing the villages at the beginning of mobile team campaigns for reasons of fear of stigmatization, lumbar puncture, pain, and the possibility of being treated with the dangerous drug melarsoprol. The in-depth understanding of the communities' beliefs, needs, and approaches is therefore key in a successful elimination attempt; insight on these topics are presented in the papers by and Falisse et al., Lee et al., and Palmer et al.

A factor mentioned by Winslow in 1951, which may still be under-researched today, is the relationship between the disease and poverty, particularly inadequate food supply, as the disease leads to unused land, which creates malnutrition [3]. Such a view would require an even more integrated approach towards disease control and elimination.

When the colonial powers withdrew from Africa between 1960 and 1975, a new era began. The young nations created their own institutions with the goal of continuing research towards the elimination of HAT (e.g., Kenya Trypanosomiasis Research Institute (KETRI), Nigerian Institute for Trypanosomiasis Research (NITR), Uganda Trypanosomiasis Research Organisation (UTRO), and Programme sur la Recherche sur la Trypanosomiase in Côte d'Ivoire (PRCT)). These institutions were reinforced since the 1970s by internationally funded institutes dedicated wholly or partly to trypanosomiasis research (e.g., International Laboratory for Research on Animal Diseases (ILRAD) in Kenya, International Centre of Insect Physiology and Ecology (ICIPE) in Kenya, International Trypanotolerance Centre (ITC) in the Gambia). However, in the course of monetary adjustments in the 1980s, the decreasing funds available, and the emergence or increase of other health priorities, institutions devoted to a single disease were no longer sustainable and they were continuously integrated or transformed into multilateral institutions. Overall, in the years after the independence process, the expenditures for HAT were reduced, and awareness and surveillance of the disease decreased. The number of mobile teams was decreased, and it was attempted to transfer activities to the public health system—without having the respective tools, approaches, and knowledge [9]. This, together with social instability, conflicts, and insecurity constraining disease control interventions led to a significant resurge of Gambiense HAT in the 1980s and 1990s [8], mainly affecting Angola, Congo, Southern Sudan, and the West Nile district of Uganda [1]. At the end of the 1990s, the situation was comparable to the one in the 1920 and 1930; the number of reported cases was almost 30,000 with 300,000 cases suspected [10].

3. The Second Turning Point—The Change for the Better

In 2001, we published a Special Issue in the Journal Tropical Medicine and International Health [11], asking ourselves whether there were new approaches to roll back HAT. Not only was this the time of 300,000 HAT cases suspected in 19 countries of sub-Saharan Africa, it was also the time when the organo-arsenic drug melarsoprol was still the only treatment available for second stage HAT. Treatment with melarsoprol required around 35 days of hospitalization with numerous and very painful injections, very severe adverse drug reactions like an encephalopathic syndrome were common and the mortality rate under treatment was as high as 2–10%.

In those days, an oncologist tried to comfort us, saying that a 95% treatment success rate for a disease with an inevitably fatal course was fantastic. We did not share this view, and rather expressed a dream: to make HAT "an ordinary" disease, which follows the usual pattern "test, treat, track"—without the need of a lumbar puncture to make treatment decisions, without a high mortality rate under treatment, without the pain, without the stigma.

Elimination was a very far-fetched goal at this time, but there were some first positive signals that the dimensions of the problem and its impact on society and development were being recognized. The conclusions adopted by the International Scientific Committee of Trypanosomiasis Research and Control (ISCTRC) in 1999 reflected a new awareness of the disease. The African Union member states were urged to give highest priority ranking to African trypanosomiasis in their development programs, and it was recommended that urgent and particular attention should be given to surveillance and intervention in epidemic areas, to drug availability and resistance, and to the implementation of operational research to respond to the needs of control programs. At their meeting in Lomé in July 2000 the OAU Heads of State and Governments signed a declaration of intent to eradicate tsetse flies on the African continent—something that will likely not happen, but it was the turning point towards manifold activities which make us today work towards elimination of HAT as a public health problem of 2020 and the interruption of transmission by 2030.

At the same time, Médecins sans Frontières' Access to Medicines Campaign were able to make a compelling case that society needed to rethink drug discovery paradigms for neglected diseases. Aventis (now Sanofi) was persuaded to repurpose and develop the failed anti-cancer drug eflornithine for use against HAT and to donate it at no cost to the WHO for distribution in Africa. Millions of dollars were also provided by Aventis/Sanofi to the WHO, who could now develop new screening and intervention programmes [9]. Bayer signed a similar contract with the WHO, a success story and joint effort which has been renewed by both companies until today, and which is one of the strong drivers in control and now elimination. In 2001, the Bill and Melinda Gates Foundation selected HAT to be one of the first diseases they targeted through the Consortium of Parasitic Drug Development (CPDD) and shortly thereafter, the Drugs for Neglected Diseases initiative (DNDi) was founded. The beginning of the century was truly an exciting time for neglected diseases and for HAT in particular. The changes and significant impact on funding were later summarized in the landmark publication "the new landscape of neglected disease drug development" [12].

The changed situation immediately led to the initiation of several large scale activities in drug development and the term "elimination" in the context of HAT was mentioned for the first time by Dr. Jannin, leading the anti-HAT efforts at the WHO in 2004 [13]. Drug development had been virtually dormant for about 50 years. Although the cultivation and test methods for drug screening for anti-trypanosomal drugs had been developed in the 1980s and 1990s [14], the money for pursing lead compounds in preclinical work, translational studies and large-scale trials was too scarce in these days. During the 1990s, some initial limited drug activities were carried out on shoestring budgets: eflornithine, which had initially been developed in the 1970s as a potential anti-cancer drug, was found to be active against second stage Gambiense HAT. This discovery in the 1980s was a scientific breakthrough [15] and eflornithine was shown to be much safer compared to melarsoprol. The drug received orphan drug status by the US Food and Drug Administration in 1990; however, production was stopped after a few years and only resumed after significant public and political pressure. Eflornithine, however, was only introduced for treatment in a limited number of centres by MSF in 2000, but not until 2006 by the National Sleeping Sickness Control programs because of its limited availability, the initial high costs, and particularly the logistical challenge to transport the drug and its associated 56 bottles of sterile water per treatment. The turning point was when WHO launched a kit format and coordinated training of staff from National Sleeping Sickness Control Programs [16]. Furthermore, in the 1990s nifurtimox, developed against Chagas disease was used in experimental settings mainly to treat melarsoprol refractory cases [17].

In the mid-1990s, the pharmacokinetics of melarsoprol was elucidated. The assessment of a subsequently proposed abridged 10 days regimen in a large scale trial with 550 patients in Angola (IMPAMEL I) allowed the replacement of the empirically derived complex schemes lasting from 25–36 days in 2003 [18–20]. Whereas the new regimen had major socio-economic advantages, the disappointment was that the frequency of the worst adverse drug reaction, the encephalopathic syndrome, remained at levels of 5–10% of patients treated, still resulting in death in 10–50% of those in whom encephalopathy developed. The metabolism of melarsoprol was elucidated somewhat later [21]. The finding that the major metabolite melarsenoxide covalently bound to a midsize protein triggered another large-scale clinical trial, which led to the elucidation of the nature of the encephalopathic syndrome. For several reasons, these data by Seixas et al. were so far only published in the form of a thesis, and are now presented in this issue.

The IMPAMEL program (Improved Application of Melarsoprol; financed by the Swiss Agency for Development and Cooperation) may not have been a breakthrough towards a new treatment against second stage HAT, but it comprised the first large scale clinical trial on this disease executed according to Good Clinical Practice, and it demonstrated the feasibility of modern clinical development for neglected diseases under the challenging conditions in countries of Central Africa.

The early 2000s were dominated by the development of the oral prodrug pafuramidine against first stage HAT; the program failed at a late point of development, but it contributed much to the understanding of HAT chemotherapy and the conduct of clinical trials against HAT, which it is described in detail by the paper of Dickie et al.

In parallel, several trials assessing combinations of eflornithine, melarsoprol, and nifurtimox were conducted. In all trials, the efficacy was better in the combination arms compared to the monotherapies. However, combinations containing melarsoprol resulted in very high frequencies of severe adverse drug reactions and were rapidly abandoned [16]. A multiple-centre trial, conducted in the Republic of Congo and the Democratic Republic of the Congo (DRC) compared nifurtimox–eflornithine combination therapy (NECT) with the standard eflornithine therapy. NECT reduces the number of eflornithine infusions from 56 to 14, the total amount of eflornithine by half and the hospitalization time by one-third [22]. Based on the favourable results of the trials conducted, NECT was included for treatment of second stage Gambiense HAT into the WHO's Essential Medicines List in 2009 [23], and for children in 2013 [16]. NECT can be considered a milestone improvement: under optimal conditions, fatality during treatment is 0.5% compared to 5–6% under melarsoprol [24]. The complexity of its application still restricts the use to the second stage disease, meaning that the lumbar puncture for diagnostic staging is still required [24], continuing until today.

To identify better alternatives, the Drugs for Neglected Diseases Initiative initiated a major compound mining effort in 2005 to explore new and old nitroimidazoles as drug leads against human

African trypanosomiasis. One of the 830 compounds screened, fexinidazole, proved to be orally active against *T. b. gambiense* and *T. b. rhodesiense* in animal studies and had an excellent safety profile.

The development of this orally active compound is described in detail in the papers of Neau et al., and Dickie et al., Fexinidazole received a positive scientific opinion from the European Medicines Agency for treatment of Gambiense HAT in late 2018, it was approved by the drug regulatory authority of the DRC and added to the WHO list of essential medicines in 2019, and the first official application in the DRC happened at the end of January 2020 on World NTD day in a public ceremony. This deliberate coincidence of the date depicts the new integrated thinking of HAT control and elimination in the framework of NTDs clearly.

Fexinidazole will be an essential component towards HAT elimination. However, it has some limitations, which will hamper its widespread use in the field: its absorption is dependent on simultaneous food intake, or else only subtherapeutic drug levels are reached; based on the observation of a lowered efficacy in patients with advanced disease, a lumbar puncture for staging still is necessary in such patients; and the drug has not been tested yet for children below six years [25].

Hence, the search for "the magic bullet" [26] continues—with an excellent starting position compared to 20 years ago: for the first time in history, we can speak of a modest pipeline of anti-HAT drugs. One most promising candidate is in late clinical development, several compounds are well advanced in pre-clinical stages, and medicinal chemistry and lead selection work is continued as described in the contributions of Buckner et al., Kariuku et al., Lim et al., and Rao et al.

Currently, the leading novel class of molecules are the boron-containing benzoxaboroles. One candidate, SCYX-7158, acoziborole, entered Phase II/III assessment in 2016 [27]. The compound is described in the publication of Dickie et al. Should the development program be successful, acoziborole would further revolutionize the efforts to eliminate and sustain elimination of HAT. Due to its long half-life of 400 h, it can be potentially used as a single-dose treatment and should it be well tolerated this would provide further options for decentralized use, and maybe even for "ring-treatment" of patient contacts following the example of ring-vaccinations used, e.g., in the control of the Ebola virus. With fexinidazole, and potentially even more with acoziborole, the focus will turn away from the discovery and development of better tools, to the understanding of the implementation, optimal use, including the needs and perception of patients.

The clinical research programs have contributed to the reduction of cases: new strong partnerships were formed as described by Taylor et al. and the conduct of clinical trials in a number of endemic areas per se has had an impact through staff training, attention to disease, and intensified active case search and treatment of a large number of patients as described by Mbo et al.

Besides the improvements of the renewed interest of governments and improved drug treatment, there are several other reasons for the decrease of HAT prevalence: the advances in diagnostics are one of the major factors. The serological card agglutination test for trypanosomes (CATT) first published in 1986 [28] had a paramount impact on how patients could be screened by mobile teams. The test was adapted and improved several times, and despite its disadvantages (insufficient specificity to confirm diagnosis, only available in larger batches, cold chain necessary), it has kept its place in HAT diagnosis. The mini-anion exchange chromatography for trypanosomes (mAECT) which increases the sensitivity to detect the parasite in the blood significantly was already published in 1976 [29,30], however, only the increased funding available allowed its more consistent use and therefore detection of cases with low parasitemia. The introduction of rapid diagnostic tests is a true advancement, but also lacks the specificity needed to make a final treatment decision [31]. Additional tools were recently developed but so far only introduced to a limited extent into routine use (e.g., loop-mediated isothermal amplification (LAMP) [32,33]; immune trypanolysis test [34]), which will both play a role in the "end-game". The question, however, is how such tests will be used in the future, and in what settings. The currently ongoing research program DiTECT-HAT is set up do exactly that: it seeks to validate the performance of diagnostic tools and algorithms for early and rapid diagnosis of Gambiense HAT for passive case detection, post-elimination monitoring, and for assessing the therapeutic response [35].

In addition to the optimization of the technical aspects, however, it is of paramount interest to know about local settings, preferences, and the loss of skills in areas with decreasing patient numbers. The paper by Palmer et al. reports on such investigations carried out in Uganda. Benhamou et al., through a case report on a repeatedly misdiagnosed patient, gives us an insight on future challenges for rapid diagnosis if knowledge and interest in the public health system is not maintained and broadened. Another unresolved caveat of diagnosis is that a number of patients are determined to be seropositive, but thereafter HAT cannot be confirmed. It will be one of the leading discussions when defining future strategies, and what to do in such cases. Nkieri et al. investigated the extent of this phenomenon in the still affected regions of DRC.

On one hand, relapses have always been a major challenge in the treatment of HAT and have made follow-up periods of up 24 months after treatment necessary [23]. On the other hand, until a few years ago, the dogma was "infected, but not treated inevitably leads to the death of the patient". Reports on patients surviving for longer periods despite infection with trypanosomes emerged in the past few years [36]. One of the compartments where trypanosome may survive seems to be the skin [37,38]. This might also explain how HAT can re-emerge in so-called silent foci as illustrated by a nine-year-old child, who was diagnosed with Gambiense-HAT in Ghana in 2013, 10 years after the last detected case [39]. In this light, the findings of Mudji et al. also have importance: over ten years after treatment in the framework of clinical trials, a number of patients revisited presented continued signs and symptoms seen in HAT (lymphadenopathy, severe headaches, sleep disturbances); since no trypanosomes could be identified by any means, the implication of these findings remain open at this point.

In any case, the existence of such long-term cases has a sudden and dramatic impact on the view of HAT epidemiology and HAT elimination [39].

Besides further epidemiological, parasitological, and molecular research, mathematical modelling may help to improve our epidemiological knowledge and inform about elimination strategies [40] and their related costs [41]. This field has significantly developed against all odds in the past years: trypanosomiasis with its extremely focal distribution and the many external factors influencing its transmission has been a true headache over two decades for all modellers and predictive mappers. Studies of existing Gambiense-HAT models in a few foci (i.e., DRC, Guinea, and Chad) suggest that some type of additional infection reservoir is needed to match the observed dynamics of reported HAT cases [42,43]. This could arise from another human reservoir (including undiagnosed and latent infections), an animal reservoir, and/or heterogeneities in human risk exposure and surveillance coverage [39].

The French colonial forces had completely dismissed the value of vector control due the successes of the treatment strategy proposed by Laveran. However, vector control may play a larger role in Gambiense HAT elimination than anticipated. Historical investigations, practical intervention studies, and modelling demonstrate the significant role that vector control can play in the control of Gambiense HAT. Recent models suggest vector control will be essential if we are to reach the set target of elimination of the diseases as a public health problem by 2020 and beyond [44,45]. The fact that neither modelling nor vector control are represented in this edition does not represent a valuation of these topics.

4. Towards Elimination or a Dreadful Comeback?

This Special Issue comes in a very timely moment, because it is now important to secure what has been achieved, to understand missing pieces, and to finish the work. However, several challenges have to be overcome to not to end up, again, in disaster. In 2012, the World Health Organization, which has played an instrumental role in the control, set the goal for the elimination of human African trypanosomiasis (HAT), caused by *Trypanosoma brucei gambiense* (gHAT), as a public health problem for 2020 and for the total interruption of transmission to humans for 2030. The efforts to maximise output and optimize innovation by the WHO has intensified since, and several stakeholders and expert groups have been created and convened [46]. Since 2012, the spectacular decrease of the case number has continued: some 2,164 cases were reported in 2016, far fewer than the targeted 2016 milestone of 4000 cases, and 660 in 2018 [47,48].

First of all, "donor fatigue" must be avoided. The elimination to "no transmission" in the DRC where over 95% of the cases are nowadays occurring is a Herculean task, which will not happen without considerable and continued funding. The conventional measurements of success (e.g., US$ spent per DALY prevented) inevitably fail in an elimination scenario. Naturally, the amount of money spent per patient identified and treated will soar, so the question to the health economists is, rather how much money do we lose in case efforts would not be continued, factoring in the needed future efforts to re-start and control the disease again. Decisions on priorities will be necessary, too: whereas the total number of patients has massively decreased, the area in the DRC they are coming from has not. Therefore, a vast area still has to be kept under surveillance; this area has to be gradually reduced by safely "closing" focus by focus in order to not jeopardize the efforts. The elimination of HAT, malaria, and Guinea worm were all believed at a certain point to only be a matter of time—before new reservoirs became known (Guinea worm), pestidicide, and drug resistance set in (malaria), and interest was decreased in a premature belief in success (malaria and HAT).

Secondly, the human factor will start to play a key role: in theory, fexinidazole could be applied in 1,338 fixed health facilities (2017) an increase up by 52% from 2015 [47], and it will be many more, should acoziborole make it to application in a few years. However, HAT is a massively stigmatized disease, linked to many beliefs and bad spirits. Traditionally, patients after treatment were excluded from working and sexual intercourse for six months [49]. Therefore, the questions are: "will the disease be recognized by the younger physicians and nurses who have never seen a case of HAT?" "Is the medical staff willing to recognize a suspected case, given this will create a massive workload including trouble with the relatives of the patient and village, paperwork, an invasion of specialists for diagnosis and follow up activities?" "Is the medical staff that was told for over 100 years that HAT belongs into the specialized hands of the vertical programs willing to assume this task and challenge?" "Are the patients willing to accept HAT as a diagnosis anymore?" "Can we overcome wrong dogma and information?" and "Will patients falling into the respective category accept a lumbar puncture?" These questions can only be addressed through the thorough understanding of beliefs, perceptions, preferences, and decision-making processes. Therefore, the social and anthropological science, as well as health economics, will start to play a key role in the "end game". The articles presented in this issue by Falisse et al., and Lee et al. are contributing to this area.

Thirdly, peace, stability, and a minimal standard of living for the people in the remote regions most affected are necessary to achieve disease elimination—this condition has not yet been met. There is little the scientific community can directly contribute to this—however, knowing that disease and poverty are inextricably linked [50], our efforts have to continue.

Finally, Rhodesiense HAT (the East African form of the disease) was reduced to as little as 54 cases in 2016 [47], goals have been reached and it may be seen as a quantité négligable. However, the disease with a zoonotic reservoir has the potential for spectacular returns, and this real danger still exists as described in the contribution of Matovu et al. The surveillance and the knowledge of local medical staff has dwindled, innovation was absent for *T. b. rhodesiense* for decades, and serological instead of microscopic tests are used for diagnosis of other diseases making accidental diagnosis impossible. From January to October 2019, a total of 2–8 cases were reported per month from all treatment centres in Malawi; in November 2019 to January 2020, this number surged to 25 and higher. The cases were reported from populations around the two geographically separate wildlife reserve areas, Vwaza and Nkhotakota; the reason for this increase is, so far, unknown (personal communication, World Health Organization, Control of Neglected Tropical Diseases, Geneva). This outbreak causes major concern and should be a serious warning to everyone who is of the opinion that sleeping sickness has been conquered. Similarly, other unexpected priorities, such as the current SARS-CoV-2 epidemic, may at all times derail a fragile health system. As soon as the mental and financial attention and priority is on

Trop. Med. Infect. Dis. **2020**, *5*, 57

another disease, signals of a HAT resurgence may well be overlooked—we should now be well aware about the consequences and impact of late reactions and exponential transmission.

Compared to when I wrote the conclusion of the 2001 HAT Special Issue in [11], we are at a completely different point today. We celebrated several marvellous scientific successes in the meantime, tools were improved, patients numbers down—but to reach the set goals and to get completely rid of this horrible disease, the conclusion is the same again: "The goal must now be to maintain the momentum" and "even the biggest efforts of the research scientists, field workers, development agencies, and companies will fail if they are not paralleled by achievements in the political field bringing peace, stability, and a minimal standard of living to the people in the remote regions most affected".

Conflicts of Interest: The author declares no conflict of interest.

References

1. Steverding, D. The history of African trypanosomiasis. *Parasites Vectors* **2008**, *1*, 3. [CrossRef] [PubMed]
2. de Raadt, P. The history of sleeping sickness. In Proceedings of the Second International Course on African Trypanosomes, Lyon, France, 12–30 November 2001; pp. 249–260.
3. Maudlin, I. African trypanosomiasis—Centennial Review. *Ann. Trop. Med. Parasitol.* **2006**, *100*, 679–701. [CrossRef]
4. Hide, G. The elusive trypanosome. *Parasitol. Today* **1994**, *10*, 85–86. [CrossRef]
5. Burri, C. Pharmacological Aspects of the Trypanocidal Drug Melarsoprol. Ph.D. Thesis, University of Basel, Basel, Switzerland, 1994.
6. Phillips, M.A.; Stanley, S.L.J. Chemotherapy of Protozoal Infections: Amebiasis, Giardiasis, Trichomoniasis, Trypanosomiasis, Leishmania and Other Protozoal Infectious. In *Goodman's & Gilmans—The Pharmacological Basis of Therapeutics*, 12th ed.; Brunton, L.L., Chubner, B.A., Knollmann, B.C., Eds.; McGraw Hill Medical: New York, NY, USA, 2011; pp. 1419–1443.
7. Steverding, D. The development of drugs for treatment of sleeping sickness: A historical review. *Parasites Vectors* **2010**, *3*, 15. [CrossRef] [PubMed]
8. Simarro, P.P.; Franco, J.R.; Diarra, A.; Jannin, J.G. Epidemiology of human African trypanosomiasis. *Clin. Epidemiol.* **2014**, *6*, 257–275. [CrossRef]
9. Jannin, J.; Louis, F.J.; Lucas, P.; Simarro, P.P. Control of human African trypanosomiasis: Back to square one. *Med Trop (Mars).* **2001**, *61*, 437–440.
10. Jannin, J.G. Sleeping sickness—A growing problem? *BMJ* **2005**, *331*, 1242. [CrossRef]
11. Burri, C. Are there new approaches to roll back trypanosomiasis (Editorial). *Trop. Med. Int. Health* **2001**, *6*, 327–329. [CrossRef]
12. Moran, M.; Ropars, A.L.; Guzman, J.; Diaz, J.; Garrison, C. *The New Landscape of Neglected Disease Drug Development*; Wellcome Trust: London, UK, 2005.
13. Jannin, J. Commentary: Sleeping sickness—A growing problem? *BMJ* **2005**, *331*, 1242. [CrossRef]
14. Brun, R.; Balmer, O. New developments in human African trypanosomiasis. *Curr. Opin. Infect. Dis.* **2006**, *19*, 415–420. [CrossRef]
15. Bacchi, C.J.; Nathan, H.C.; Clarkson, A.B., Jr.; Bienen, E.J.; Bitonti, A.J.; McCann, P.P.; Sjoerdsma, A. Effects of the Ornithine Decarboxylase Inhibitors Dl-α-Difluoromethylornithine and α-Monofluoromethyldehydroornithine Methyl Ester Alone and in Combination with Suramin against Trypanosoma brucei brucei Central Nervous System Models. *Am. J. Trop. Med. Hyg.* **1987**, *36*, 46–52. [CrossRef] [PubMed]
16. Eperon, G.; Balasegaram, M.; Potet, J.; Mowbray, C.; Valverde, O.; Chappuis, F. Treatment options for second-stage gambiense human African trypanosomiasis. *Expert Rev. Anti-Infective Ther.* **2014**, *12*, 1407–1417. [CrossRef] [PubMed]
17. Vannieuwenhove, S. Nifurtimox in late-stage arsenical refractory gambiense sleeping sickness. *Bull. Société Pathol. Exot.* **1988**, *81*, 650.

18. Burri, C.; Nkunku, S.; Merolle, A.; Smith, T.; Blum, J.; Brun, R. Efficacy of new, concise schedule for melarsoprol in treatment of sleeping sickness caused by Trypanosoma brucei gambiense: A randomised trial. *Lancet* **2000**, *355*, 1419–1425. [CrossRef]

19. Schmid, C.; Nkunku, S.; Merolle, A.; Vounatsou, P.; Burri, C. Efficacy of 10-day melarsoprol schedule 2 years after treatment for late-stage gambiense sleeping sickness. *Lancet* **2004**, *364*, 789–790. [CrossRef]

20. Schmid, C.; Richer, M.; Bilenge, C.M.M.; Josenando, T.; Chappuis, F.; Manthelot, C.R.; Nangouma, A.; Doua, F.; Asumu, P.N.; Simarro, P.P.; et al. Effectiveness of a 10-Day Melarsoprol Schedule for the Treatment of Late-Stage Human African Trypanosomiasis: Confirmation from a Multinational Study (I mpamel II). *J. Infect. Dis.* **2005**, *191*, 1922–1931. [CrossRef]

21. Keiser, J.; Ericsson, Ö.; Burri, C. Investigations of the metabolites of the trypanocidal drug melarsoprol. *Clin. Pharmacol. Ther.* **2000**, *67*, 478–488. [CrossRef]

22. Priotto, G.; Kasparian, S.; Mutombo, W.; Ngouama, D.; Ghorashian, S.; Arnold, U.; Ghabri, S.; Baudin, E.; Buard, V.; Kazadi-Kyanza, S.; et al. Nifurtimox-eflornithine combination therapy for second-stage African Trypanosoma brucei gambiense trypanosomiasis: A multicentre, randomised, phase III, non-inferiority trial. *Lancet* **2009**, *374*, 56–64. [CrossRef]

23. WHO. *Control and Surveillance of Human African Trypanosomiasis: Report of a WHO Expert Committee*; World Health Organisation: Geneva, Switzerland, 2013.

24. Simarro, P.; Franco, J.; Diarra, A.; Postigo, J.A.R.; Jannin, J. Update on field use of the available drugs for the chemotherapy of human African trypanosomiasis. *Parasitology* **2012**, *139*, 842–846. [CrossRef]

25. Lindner, A.K.; Lejon, V.; Chappuis, F.; Seixas, J.; Kazumba, L.; Barrett, M.P.; Mwamba, E.; Erphas, O.; A Akl, E.; Villanueva, G.; et al. New WHO guidelines for treatment of gambiense human African trypanosomiasis including fexinidazole: Substantial changes for clinical practice. *Lancet Infect. Dis.* **2020**, *20*, e38–e46.

26. Bendiner, E. Louise Pearce: A 'Magic Bullet' for African Sleeping Sickness. *Hosp. Pr.* **1992**, *27*, 207–221. [CrossRef]

27. Acoziborole—DNDi. 2019. Available online: https://www.dndi.org/diseases-projects/portfolio/acoziborole/ (accessed on 30 December 2019).

28. Magnus, E.; Vervoort, T.; Van Meirvenne, N. A card-agglutination test with stained trypanosomes (C.A.T.T.) for the serological diagnosis of T. B. gambiense trypanosomiasis. *Ann. Soc. Belg. Med. Trop.* **1978**, *58*, 169–176.

29. Lejon, V.; Büscher, P.; Nzoumbou-Boko, R.; Bossard, G.; Jamonneau, V.; Bucheton, B.; Truc, P.; Lemesre, J.-L.; Solano, P.; Vincendeau, P. The separation of trypanosomes from blood by anion exchange chromatography: From Sheila Lanham's discovery 50 years ago to a gold standard for sleeping sickness diagnosis. *PLoS Negl. Trop. Dis.* **2019**, *13*, e0007051. [CrossRef]

30. Lumsden, W.G.R.; Kimber, C.D.; Evans, D.A.; Doigs, J. *Trypanosoma brucei*: Miniature anion exchange centrifugation for detection of low parasitemias: Adaptation for field use. *Trans. Roy. Soc. Trop. Med. Hyg.* **1979**, *73*, 313–317. [CrossRef]

31. Büscher, P.; Mertens, P.; Leclipteux, T.; Gilleman, Q.; Jacquet, D.; Mumba-Ngoyi, D.; Pyana, P.P.; Boelaert, M.; Lejon, V. Sensitivity and specificity of HAT Sero-K-SeT, a rapid diagnostic test for serodiagnosis of sleeping sickness caused by Trypanosoma brucei gambiense: A case-control study. *Lancet Glob. Heal.* **2014**, *2*, e359–e363. [CrossRef]

32. Kuboki, N.; Inoue, N.; Sakurai, T.; Di Cello, F.; Grab, D.J.; Suzuki, H.; Sugimoto, C.; Igarashi, I. Loop-Mediated Isothermal Amplification for Detection of African Trypanosomes. *J. Clin. Microbiol.* **2003**, *41*, 5517–5524. [CrossRef] [PubMed]

33. Grab, D.J.; Nikolskaia, O.V.; Courtioux, B.; Thekisoe, O.M.M.; Magez, S.; Bogorad, M.; Dumler, J.S.; Bisser, S. Using detergent-enhanced LAMP for African trypanosome detection in human cerebrospinal fluid and implications for disease staging. *PLoS Negl. Trop. Dis.* **2019**, *13*, e0007631. [CrossRef] [PubMed]

34. Dama, E.; Camara, O.; Kaba, D.; Koffi, M.; Camara, M.; Compaoré, C.; Ilboudo, H.; Courtin, F.; Kaboré, J.; N'Gouan, E.K.; et al. Immune trypanolysis test as a promising bioassay to monitor the elimination of gambiense human African trypanosomiasis. *Parasite* **2019**, *26*, 68. [CrossRef] [PubMed]

35. DiTECT-HAT Consortium. Diagnostic Tools for Human African Trypanosomiasis Elimination and Clinical Trials (DiTECT-HAT). 2020. Available online: https://www.ditect-hat.eu/g (accessed on 16 February 2020).

36. Jamonneau, V.; Ilboudo, H.; Kabore, J.; Kaba, D.; Koffi, M.; Solano, P.; Garcia, A.; Courtin, D.; Laveissière, C.; Lingue, K.; et al. Untreated Human Infections by Trypanosoma brucei gambiense Are Not 100% Fatal. *PLoS Negl. Trop. Dis.* **2012**, *6*, e1691. [CrossRef]

37. Capewell, P.; Cren-Travaillé, C.; Marchesi, F.; Johnston, P.; Clucas, C.; Benson, R.; Gorman, T.-A.; Calvo-Alvarez, E.; Crouzols, A.; Jouvion, G.; et al. The skin is a significant but overlooked anatomical reservoir for vector-borne African trypanosomes. *eLife* **2016**, *5*, 157. [CrossRef]
38. Caljon, G.; Van Reet, N.; De Trez, C.; Vermeersch, M.; Pérez-Morga, D.; Abbeele, J.V.D. The Dermis as a Delivery Site of Trypanosoma brucei for Tsetse Flies. *PLoS Pathog.* **2016**, *12*, e1005744. [CrossRef] [PubMed]
39. Buscher, P.; Bart, J.M.; Boelaert, M.; Bucheton, B.; Cecchi, G.; Chitnis, N.; Courtin, D.; Figueiredo, L.M.; Franco, J.; Grébaut, P.; et al. Do cryptic reservoirs threaten gambienses-leeping sickness elimination? *Trends Parasitol.* **2018**, *34*, 197–207. [CrossRef] [PubMed]
40. Rock, K.; Stone, C.M.; Hastings, I.; Keeling, M.J.; Torr, S.; Chitnis, N.; Stone, C.M. Mathematical Models of Human African Trypanosomiasis Epidemiology. *Adv. Parasitol.* **2015**, *87*, 53–133. [PubMed]
41. Sutherland, C.S.; Stone, C.M.; Steinmann, P.; Tanner, M.; Tediosi, F. Seeing beyond 2020: An economic evaluation of contemporary and emerging strategies for elimination of Trypanosoma brucei gambiense. *Lancet Glob. Heal.* **2017**, *5*, e69–e79. [CrossRef]
42. Rock, K.; Torr, S.; Lumbala, C.; Keeling, M.J. Quantitative evaluation of the strategy to eliminate human African trypanosomiasis in the Democratic Republic of Congo. *Parasites Vectors* **2015**, *8*, 532. [CrossRef]
43. Pandey, A.; Atkins, K.E.; Bucheton, B.; Camara, M.; Aksoy, S.; Galvani, A.P.; Ndeffo-Mbah, M.L. Evaluating long-term effectiveness of sleeping sickness control measures in Guinea. *Parasites Vectors* **2015**, *8*, 550. [CrossRef]
44. Ndeffo-Mbah, M.L.; Pandey, A.; Atkins, K.E.; Aksoy, S.; Galvani, A.P. The impact of vector migration on the effectiveness of strategies to control gambiense human African trypanosomiasis. *PLoS Negl. Trop. Dis.* **2019**, *13*, e0007903. [CrossRef]
45. Aksoy, S.; Büscher, P.; Lehane, M.; Solano, P.; Abbeele, J.V.D. Human African trypanosomiasis control: Achievements and challenges. *PLoS Negl. Trop. Dis.* **2017**, *11*, e0005454. [CrossRef]
46. All Past Events/Information Related to Human African Trypanosomiasis. 2020. Available online: https://www.who.int/trypanosomiasis_african/archives/en/ (accessed on 16 February 2020).
47. Franco, J.R.; Cecchi, G.; Priotto, G.; Paone, M.; Diarra, A.; Grout, L.; Simarro, P.P.; Zhao, W.; Argaw, D. Monitoring the elimination of human African trypanosomiasis: Update to 2016. *PLoS Negl. Trop. Dis.* **2018**, *12*, e0006890. [CrossRef]
48. Mudji, J.; Benhamou, J.; Mwamba, E.; Burri, C.; Blum, J. The Flipside of Eradicating a Disease; Human African Trypanosomiasis in a Woman in Rural Democratic Republic of Congo: A Case Report. *Trop. Med. Infect. Dis.* **2019**, *4*, 142. [CrossRef]
49. Falisse, J.-B.; Mwamba, E.; Mpanya, A. Whose Elimination? Frontline Workers' Perspectives on the Elimination of the Human African Trypanosomiasis and Its Anticipated Consequences. *Trop. Med. Infect. Dis.* **2020**, *5*, 6. [CrossRef] [PubMed]
50. Poverty and Health. 2020. Available online: https://www.who.int/hdp/poverty/en/ (accessed on 16 February 2020).

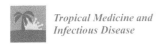

Tropical Medicine and Infectious Disease

MDPI

Article

Product Development Partnerships: Delivering Innovation for the Elimination of African Trypanosomiasis?

Emma Michelle Taylor [1,]* and James Smith [2]

1   Department of Social Anthropology, University of Edinburgh, Edinburgh, EH8 9LD, UK
2   Centre of African Studies, University of Edinburgh, Edinburgh, EH8 9LD, UK; James.Smith@ed.ac.uk
*   Correspondence: E.M.Taylor@ed.ac.uk

Received: 2 December 2019; Accepted: 30 December 2019; Published: 15 January 2020

Abstract: African trypanosomiasis has been labelled as a 'tool-deficient' disease. This article reflects on the role that Product Development Partnerships (PDPs) have played in delivering new tools and innovations for the control and elimination of the African trypanosomiases. We analysed three product development partnerships—DNDi, FIND and GALVmed—that focus on delivering new drugs, diagnostic tests, and animal health innovations, respectively. We interviewed key informants within each of the organisations to understand how they delivered new innovations. While it is too early (and beyond the scope of this article) to assess the role of these three organisations in accelerating the elimination of the African trypanosomiases, all three organisations have been responsible for delivering new innovations for diagnosis and treatment through brokering and incentivising innovation and private sector involvement. It is doubtful that these innovations would have been delivered without them. To varying degrees, all three organisations are evolving towards a greater brokering role, away from only product development, prompted by donors. On balance, PDPs have an important role to play in delivering health innovations, and donors need to reflect on how best to incentivise them to focus and continue to deliver new products.

Keywords: product development partnerships; research and development; medical innovation; donor policy; African trypanosomiasis

1. Introduction

"Markets work well for society when there is price competition, comprehensive and accurate information, an adequate supply of drugs, where consumers are able to make informed unpressured choices between competing products, and when there are few barriers for entry to market. However, substantial evidence shows that markets have failed to work". [1] (p. 1590)

For the better part of half a century, innovation for the African Trypanosomiases stalled. Following the introduction of drug melarsoprol in 1949, it took 41 years for eflornithine to be registered for the treatment of stage 2 *T. b. gambiense*, and a further 19 years for that drug to be put to full use in a combination therapy (Nifurtimox-Eflornithine Combination Therapy). The Card Agglutination Test for Trypanosomiasis (CATT), launched in 1978, remained the sole screening test for *T. b. gambiense* for over thirty years. And yet, none of these products constituted 'perfect' tools, fit for purpose (melarsoprol is dangerous and subject to treatment failure, Nifurtimox-Eflornithine Combination Therapy is expensive and logistically challenging to deliver, and the CATT test lacks sensitivity and cannot provide a confirmatory diagnosis). Rather, a failure of the market and public policy in the years following African independence meant that there was little incentive for the private sector to invest in product innovation for a disease that only affected poor and marginalised communities living along the tsetse belt of Sub-Saharan Africa.

African Trypanosomiasis is often depicted as the quintessential colonial disease [2]. Caused by unicellular protozoan parasites from the genus Trypanosoma, the disease commonly affects humans (*T. b. gambiense* and *T. b. rhodesiense*) and valuable domestic livestock (*T. vivax, T. congolense* and *T. brucei* subspecies) [3]. A major epidemic at the start of the twentieth century threatened to obstruct imperial pursuits on the African continent, making trypanosomiases a pan-African priority to unite colonial interests. Neill has documented how the imperative to control Human African Trypanosomiasis (HAT) during this period gave rise to a new medical specialty—tropical medicine—and stimulated the creation of international networks of experts to propose solutions [4]. This networked approach proved successful. By the 1960s, HAT was almost eliminated using a toolkit of interventions devised during the colonial period [5].

Following African independence, basic research into the trypansomiases continued, attracting vast investment from development agencies and their colonial pre-cursors. However, it was the failure to translate this research into new tools and approaches that disappointed [5,6].

Around the turn of the millennium, a HAT epidemic, coupled with a threat to the manufacture and supply of all HAT drugs [7], provided a case example of what Médecins Sans Frontières (MSF) later termed the "fatal imbalance" of research and development for HAT and other diseases of poverty [8]. According to MSF, HAT was not just a neglected disease but, by virtue the market and public policy failings that had rendered it "tool deficient" [8] (p. 13), it was a "most neglected disease" [8] (p. 11). A number of surveys examining the state of the product development pipelines for Neglected Tropical Diseases (NTDs) confirmed this distinction [6,9]. In response, MSF launched the Access to Essential Medicines campaign. Access to Essential Medicines identified three gaps in the drug development process for neglected disease, emphasising the first gap—between basic research and pre-clinical research—as most significant [8]. Access to Essential Medicines argued that in the current profit-driven system, "It is a matter of simple economics: potential return on investment, not global health needs, determines how companies decide to allocate R&D funds" [8] (p. 18). The campaign set out that traditional profit-driven models of innovation could no longer be relied upon to deliver for the world's poorest and most vulnerable populations. Instead, new models of partnership, driven by patient needs, were urgently required. This position has since gained widespread support in light of the augmented demands posed by disease elimination goals [10].

International development, and global health in particular, has recognised the role of partnerships to deliver impact. The Millennium Development Goals recognised the role of partnerships in ensuring development activity was harmonised, locally relevant and mutually accountable. The current Sustainable Development Goals emphasis partnerships even more strongly [11]. But partnerships can and do have many meanings. There is a broad literature exploring the realities of partnerships in international development and global health, mainly around the extent to which they are truly reciprocal or equal, but this is beyond the scope of this paper [12,13]. For our purposes, we define a partnership as 'a collaborative relationship among organisations in which risks and benefits are shared in pursuit of a common goal that would not otherwise be attainable'.

A partnership model prioritising a need-based approach to research and development (R&D) is now operational, delivering for a host of neglected tropical and zoonotic infections previously underserved by the market. It is known as a Product Development Partnership (PDP). While different permutations exist, certain key features define PDPs: they are "not-for-profit organisations that drive product development for neglected diseases in conjunction with external partners;" they "are formal organisations rather than one-off collaborations between public and private groups and share a number of characteristics in the way they work. They focus on one or more neglected diseases and develop products suitable for use in developing countries" and "they generally use private sector management practices" in their R&D activities [14] (p. 116). For the African trypanosomiases, PDPs are proving to be a game changer, with some examples delivering not just single products but product pipelines for the first time in history.

Today, *T. b. gambiense* stands on the cusp of elimination (in 2017 just 1447 new cases were reported [15]). Yet, product development for this disease continues unabated. PDPs have already contributed to the global campaign to see HAT eliminated as a public health problem by 2020 —delivering new diagnostics and treatments—but their larger contribution is yet to be realised: delivering at scale the products that could see the transmission of HAT eliminated by 2030. Reaching and sustaining this goal requires HAT services, which have traditionally been run vertically, to be integrated into national healthcare structures. This paradigm shift is only made possible by the development of new, safe, easy to use products that can deployed at point of need (in addition to the active participation of public bodies in disease endemic countries). PDPs have been instrumental in prioritising these types of products for the African Trypanosomiases, through the setting of minimal performance and operational characteristics that place product users at their core, aka Target Product Profiles.

This paper explores the models and contribution of three PDPs set up to deliver product innovation for the African Trypanosomiases (as part of larger disease portfolios): the Drugs for Neglected Disease Initiative (DNDi), the Foundation for Innovative New Diagnostics (FIND) and the Global Alliance for Livestock Veterinary Medicines (GALVmed). Drawing on empirical research and documentary data, we describe their working models, explore their product portfolios, and set out the stories behind some of their most high profile projects.

Our analysis reveals that PDPs are not static entities fulfilling singular product development functions. Rather, they are heterogeneous and evolving organisational forms. Having served up much of the 'low hanging fruit' from the product pipelines in their early years, they are being driven to transform by a number of factors, including donor pressures for greater impact and value for money, and the changing nature of R&D partnerships.

The Emergence of Product Development Partnerships

While minimal collaboration between the public and private sectors had been the norm up until the mid-1970s, in the late 1970s and early 1980s, disillusionment with the state and the rise of a neoliberal agenda carved out a bigger space for the private sector. The latter half of the 1990s witnessed a burgeoning of Public-Private Partnerships (PPPs) for health. Conceived with the aim of overcoming market and policy failures, such collaborations leveraged new financial resources and proposed innovative solutions to intractable global health problems. A continued appetite for these "networked approaches" [16] (p. 2) into the first and second decades of the twenty-first century can be explained by three factors: the global burden of disease [17]; unprecedented levels of funding for health favouring the PPP approach (including from philanthropic and private sources) [18]; and new developments in the science and technology sectors [19].

Under the umbrella of PPPs for health, sub-categorisations have emerged, including: product-based or access PPPs, which seek to extend access to existing products for which there exists limited demand/ability to pay); issues or systems-based PPPs, which might, for instance, include PPPs seeking to improve health system capacity; and product development-based or PDPs [17]. The focus of this paper is largely on the third category, although the PDPs included in this review also provide some functions of access PPPs.

While Moran et al. sought to define PDPs using the criteria cited above, they also underlined that their summary definition—while expressing many of the shared characteristics of the PDP model—failed to convey the many differences that can still exist between different PDP entities [14]. For instance, while some have in-house laboratory and manufacturing capacity, others depend entirely on collaboration with others for these functions; and while some PDPs limit their operations to product development, others pursue additional objectives, including capacity building and technology transfer. Subsequently, identifying the key differences between PDPs is an important first step in understanding their scope and contribution.

Over the past ten years, a sea change has occurred in how PDPs for health are viewed. Once perceived as an unknown quantity [20], today, they occupy a central position in the global health infrastructure, and are credited as the main driving force behind an "unrecognised revolution in global health" [21]. To expand, Policy Cures noted that over a period of 15 years 485 neglected disease product candidates had entered the product pipeline, 58% of which came from PDPs and other PPPs [21] (p. 1). In addition, "Because these groups are driven by public health goals, their products are designed to be affordable and appropriate for developing countries" (ibid.). A review by Berdud, Towse and Kettler seconded this position [22]. Their work suggests that for malaria, at least, PDPs are one of the only incentivising mechanisms with a proven track record at this time.

In the new millennium, the case was made that a number of tropical infections, including HAT, should be taken forward as a group by virtue of their 'neglected' status and shared geographic overlap, and because cost savings and synergies could be levied if the different disease programmes acted together [23]. The resulting categorisation—Neglected Tropical Disease (NTD)—has subsequently become a successful "brand identity," leveraging attention and resources for the named diseases [24,25].

The International AIDS Vaccine Initiative and the Medicines for Malaria Venture were the first PDPs to be established in the mid-1990s. In the new millennium, the Access to Essential Medicines and NTD movements helped catalyse the establishment of PDPs for NTDs. Prior to this, the World Health Organisation's Special Programme for Research and Training in Tropical Diseases (WHO/TDR) had been "essentially the 'only game in town'" for tropical disease for several decades [26] (p. 3).

In 2017, 14% (US$506m) of all R&D funding for neglected diseases was channeled through PDPs [27] (p. 99).

2. Materials and Methods

This paper reports on a mixed methods research project which employed a multiple case study design influenced by Yin and Blaikie [28,29]. We focused our research on the three PDPs that have an explicit focus on product development for the African Trypanosomiases. The objective of this study was to track the emergence and evolution of our PDPs over a prolonged period, noting the need to place empirical studies in a series of broader contexts if they are to be generalisable [30].

Between 2013 and 2019, a number of semi-structured interviews were undertaken with staff—past and present—from the three case study PDPs ($n = 11$); and with representatives from partner organisations, such as the Institute of Tropical Medicine, Antwerp; the Swiss Tropical and Public Health Institute; Dundee University's Drug Discovery Unit; and the International Livestock Research Institute ($n = 14$). In addition, our research project joined the HAT Platform during the study period [31], providing opportunities to gain more informal insights into the work of DNDi and FIND.

Extensive notes were taken at conferences where the work of the foci PDPs was presented and discussed, for instance, DNDi's tenth anniversary conference (Nairobi 2013), ISNTD D$_3$ (London 2016), and the NTD Summit (Geneva 2017).

Finally, a discourse analysis of primary and secondary documentation was undertaken. This included strategy papers and annual reports produced by the PDPs themselves, and the academic and grey literature around PDPs more generally, for instance, the G-FINDER public search tool and reports, which collect funding data on R&D for neglected diseases [32]. We also drew on evaluation reports commissioned by some of the main donors currently supporting the PDP model.

Qualitative data (interview transcripts, primary and secondary documentation) were managed and analysed using NVivo—a software package for qualitative research. Quantitative data were managed in Microsoft Excel.

Ethics approval was attained from the University of Edinburgh's formal ethics approval process in the School of Social and Political Science and the broader project was granted ethics approval by the European Research Council.

Work in relation to this output was conducted over an extended period. While our research project closed in February 2018, change in our case study organisations continued unabated. Therefore, in order to bring this paper up to date, we conducted follow up interviews where feasible (at GALVmed), and drew on other sources where not (e.g., conference notes, strategy papers and annual reporting). It is a limitation of our study that we were not able to conduct follow-up interviews at all three organisations.

3. Results: Product Development Partnerships for the African Trypanosomiases

3.1. Drugs for Neglected Disease Initiative (DNDi)

DNDi was launched in 2003 on the back of recommendations made by the Drugs for Neglected Diseases Working Group, a thinktank set up by MSF to investigate the crisis in R&D for neglected diseases. DNDi's primary objective is to deliver new treatments for patients suffering from the most neglected diseases, through the development of new drugs or the reformulation of existing ones. Its original strategy was based on a "two-pronged approach to R&D," which sought to address urgent need in the short term while attempting to deliver entirely new treatments in the long term [33] (p. 6). DNDi now operates a three-prong approach: managing short- (1–3 years), medium- (3–5 years) and long-term projects (6–15 years) [34].

DNDi is registered as a not-for-profit legal entity in Switzerland. It was founded by seven public and private institutions: MSF; the Oswaldo Cruz Foundation; the Indian Council for Medical Research; the Kenya Medical Research Institute; the Ministry of Health, Malaysia; Institut Pasteur, France; and WHO/TDR. It has headquarters in Geneva, and eight regional offices in New York, Kenya, India, Brazil, Malaysia, Japan, South Africa and the Democratic Republic of Congo.

DNDi's early portfolio focused primarily on the kinetoplastid diseases, although its portfolio always remained open to other R&D projects where "glaring gaps" were apparent [33] (p. 3). In 2015, DNDi formally broadened its mission from neglected diseases to neglected patients, thus adopting "a more dynamic approach to the evolution" of its portfolio that has seen it take on paediatric HIV, Hepatitis C and antimicrobial resistance [34] (p. 10). DNDi's 2019 portfolio tackles seven diseases and includes over 47 R&D projects. From this position, DNDi now aims to deliver 16 to 18 new treatments by 2023, and to ensure equitable access to these treatments. It has already delivered eight [34].

DNDi's original not-for-profit R&D model was said to be characterised by four tenets: "a concretely patient-centred, needs-driven approach; a commitment to both equitable access to treatment for patients and open access to knowledge; financial and scientific independence; and the leveraging of existing knowledge and expertise by building solid alliances with public and private partners" [33] (p. 3). In 2019, its model is more clearly rearticulated as having six tenets: needs-driven; independent; collaborative, transparent and open; globally networked and access-orientated [34].

To expand on a few of these, DNDi has always prioritised a needs-driven approach to R&D by "beginning with the end in mind" [33] (p. 3). It has done this through the setting of Target Product Profiles (TPPs), in conjunction with other partners and, where possible, patient representatives. TPPs are a description of the ideal specifications needed for a given product, considering the needs of the patient and the main characteristics of the health system that serves them. Today, DNDi promotes the setting of "Public-Interest Target Product Profiles" in support of its needs-based agenda [34].

The main way DNDi maintains financial and scientific independence is through its funding policy, which seeks to prevent any single funder imposing undue influence or creating financial dependency. Accordingly, DNDi seeks to maintain a balance of public and private support, to minimise restricted funding, and to ensure that no one donor contributes more than 25% of the overall budget. DNDi has been much more successful at securing unrestricted funding than other PDPs, receiving 47% of its income as unrestricted contributions [34]. DNDi's funding model does not require it to recoup R&D investments or finance future research through the sale of products or revenues generated by Intellectual Property. Instead, donor contributions pay upfront for R&D, delinking the financing of R&D from the price of the final product. In 2018, DNDi received Euros 66.4 million in multi-year funds (for DNDi and the Global Antibiotic Research and Development Partnership), as well as Euros 20.2 million in the form of in kind contributions from partners [35] (p. 3).

DNDi operates through a virtual R&D model, meaning it does not have any in-house laboratory or manufacturing capacity. This is why the building of successful alliances is so fundamental to its work. DNDi depicts its role as the "conductor of a virtual orchestra" [33] (p. 5), through which it draws on the capabilities and expertise of a host of partners straddling academia, public-sector research institutions, pharmaceutical and biotechnology companies, non-governmental organisations, other PDPs, and national governments. The PDP currently has 180 partnerships in over 40 countries [34] (p. 13). As of 2018, 34% of its partners were in low- and middle-income countries (LMICs) [34] (p. 21).

DNDi is committed to open and collaborative science, on which its operations depend. From 2012 to 2018, 57% of the compounds screened to evaluate their potential as drug candidates were made available to DNDi free of cost [35] (p. 7). It is through such arrangements that the PDP has begun to challenge the much-cited di Masi et al. (1991) figure, which puts the price of bringing a new drug to market at US\$ 500 million. DNDi estimates it can develop and register a new treatment based on existing drugs for Euros 4–32 million and a novel chemical entity for Euros 60–190 million (attrition in the pipeline included) [34] (p. 18).

DNDi's mission has always set out to utilise and strengthen R&D capacities in the countries where its portfolio diseases are endemic. Now, however, its ambition has grown, and it aspires "to contribute to new innovation eco-systems," driven by scientific leaders in LMICs [34] (p. 22). This, it hopes, will change how research priorities are defined and where health R&D in the public interest is conducted. As part of this vision, the PDP has helped establish five disease-specific clinical research platforms. This includes the HAT Platform, established in the DRC in 2005, to build and strengthen treatment methodologies and clinical trial capacity. It is a common feature of the evolution of the PDPs under study that they seek to deepen and support LMIC leadership of disease control and elimination, primarily in recognition of the need to learn from and engage with the sites in which new technologies will be deployed.

In the past, drugs candidates for neglected diseases were progressed one at a time through a chain model. This was the model DNDi began with, but it quickly moved on (Simon Croft addressing ISNTD D3 conference 25 May 2016). Taking its cue from big pharma and other PDPs like the Medicines for Malaria Venture, DNDi switched to a portfolio model, whereby a pipeline is created with back-ups in place to replace, succeed or even synergise with other drug candidates already further along the development pathway. Table 1 depicts DNDi's HAT portfolio.

Table 1. DNDi's HAT portfolio.

Research >	Translation >	Development >	Implementation
Oxaborole SCYX-1330682		Acoziborole	Fexinidazole for T. b. gambiense
Oxaborole SCYX-1608210		Fexinidazole for *T. b. rhodesiense*	Nifurtimox-Eflornithine Combination Therapy (NECT)

Product Backstory: NECT, Fexinidazole and Acoziborole

DNDi's three-pronged approach to R&D is well exemplified through its HAT portfolio. Initially targeting an urgent unmet need, the newly registered DNDi built on earlier work conducted by MSF Epicentre and WHO/TDR to move the HAT drug eflornithine into a combination therapy (to protect it from resistance and improve its efficacy). The chagas drug nifurtimox provided a new lead when, in 2006, it was registered for the compassionate treatment of melarsoprol-refractory HAT cases in combination with other trypanocidal drugs. Several trials were conducted, testing three different combinations. While all three combinations proved more efficacious than their monotherapy counterparts, the nifurtimox-eflornithine combination emerged as the safest option [36,37]. A multi-centre trial was initiated, with the results supporting the adoption of Nifurtimox-Eflornithine Combination Therapy (NECT) as the preferred treatment option for late-stage *T. b. gambiense* [38]. In 2009, NECT was added to the WHO's Essential Medicines List, scoring an early success for DNDi.

Trop. Med. Infect. Dis. **2020**, 5, 11

Hoping to develop a wholly new treatment for HAT, DNDi carried out a major survey of previously discarded compounds known as nitroheterocycles for trypanocidal activity. A systematic review and profiling of more than 700 nitroheterocyclic compounds was undertaken in 2005. From this search, the nitroimidazeole compound fexinidazole was identified as a promising drug candidate [39]. In this manner, fexinidazole is said to have been 'rediscovered' by DNDi, as the drug (once known as Hoe 239) had previously been in preclinical development as a broad spectrum anti-protozoal drug by Hoechst AG, Frankfurt, Germany (now Sanofi, Paris, France) during the 1970s and 1980s. DNDi went on to develop fexinidazole in conjunction with Sanofi. The drug entered clinical development in September 2009. In November 2018, fexinidazole was approved by the European Medicines Agency as the first all-oral treatment for both stages of T. b. gambiense. In 2019, it was added to the WHO's list of Essential Medicines.

Fexinidazole eliminates the need for systemic hospitalisation for late-stage patients and will reduce the number of lumbar punctures required for diagnosis and follow up. In short, fexinidazole proposes to change the paradigm of HAT care by making treatment simpler and safer. Nevertheless, within DNDi and the broader HAT community, there remains further momentum to improve HAT treatment. To explain, while a *good enough* drug might suffice for disease control, given the goal of reaching and sustaining HAT elimination, something more closely resembling a *perfect* drug is desirable. Fexinidazole is not considered a perfect drug, given concerns around dosage (once a day for ten days), and the fact that it has to be metabolised to work (Interview 30 March 2013). This again, is where DNDi's portfolio model comes into play, driving the PDP to explore several back-up compounds, even as fexinidazole progressed through clinical trials.

Between 2007 and 2008, DNDi worked to establish the HAT Lead Optimization Consortium (in conjunction with SYNEXIS, and Pace University), which seeks to optimise new classes of compounds identified from screening activities. In 2008, DNDi was approached by the biotech company Anacor Pharmaceuticals Inc., Palo Alto, CA, United States, with a promising new chemical series known as oxaboroles. In 2009, it opted to advance the compound SCYX-7158—now known as acoziborole—into preclinical development [33].

Acoziborole is an entirely novel chemical entity with the potential of becoming the first oral, single-dose treatment for T. b. gambiense. The drug is currently in a Phase II/III study in the Democratic Republic of Congo, with results expected by the end of 2020 [35].

3.2. Foundation for Innovative New Diagnostics (FIND)

FIND was launched at the World Health Assembly in May 2003. Its purpose is to develop and deliver innovative, field-adapted diagnostics for use in low-resource settings. FIND is an independent Swiss Foundation, established as a not-for-profit legal entity. It has its headquarters in Geneva and four regional hubs in India, Kenya, South Africa and Vietnam.

Initially focused on tuberculosis, HAT was the first NTD to be included in FIND's portfolio (in 2006). FIND's 'NTD portfolio' was subsequently expanded to include leishmaniasis (in 2010) and chagas disease (in 2012). It has since been augmented further to include buruli ulcer and schistosomiasis. Inclusive of NTDs, FIND's portfolio incorporates four main programme areas (tuberculosis and acute febrile respiratory infections; malaria and acute febrile syndrome; Hepatitis C) and several mini portfolios. Under its current strategy (2015–2020), FIND is attempting to catalyse the development of 15 new diagnostic technologies [40]; ten of which have already completed all phases of development [41] (p. 9).

In 2010, FIND underwent something of a crisis, having accumulated a significant financial deficit that served to raise serious concerns around the organisation's governance and management structure ("Original accounting policies had led to an inappropriate recognition of income and the reinstatement of income revealed an accumulated deficit of USD 6.03 mill in 2010, which was mostly due to overhead spending without related funding base" [42] (p23)). The situation was so grave that questions were raised around whether FIND should continue to operate at all, or whether it should be merged with another PDP. This did not happen. Instead, between 2011 and 2013, FIND restructured (becoming a "lean, expert organization" that outsources work to consultants) [40] (p. 35), overhauled its financial systems, and rearticulated its role in product development. Today, FIND is again deemed "a viable PDP" [42] (p. 18).

In its new incarnation, FIND is guided by a five-year strategy that has placed greater emphasis on its roles as 'mobilizer', 'bridge builder', and 'enabler' [40]. It has moved away from a primary focus on developing individual diagnostic technologies in conjunction with private companies to supporting complete diagnostic solutions, termed *packages*. This revision recognises that a diagnostic test requires a suite of ingredients to support its roll out and use, in what are often weak health systems (see Figure 1).

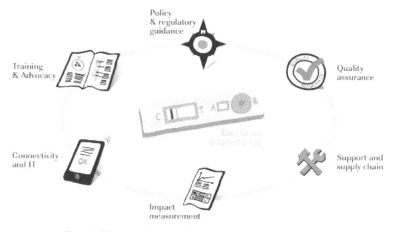

Figure 1. Elements of a complete diagnostic solution [40] (p. 23).

Given this premise, FIND now works around four strategic goals: (1) **catalyse development** by identifying needed diagnostic solutions and removing barriers to their development; (2) **guide policy and use** by leading products through the clinical trials pathway to global policy on use and market entry; (3) **accelerate access** by supporting uptake and appropriate use of diagnostics to achieve health impact (4) **shape agenda** by improving understanding of the value of diagnostics and strengthen the commitment to their funding and use [40].

Like DNDi, FIND operates through a virtual model, relying on partners to realise its goals. Where once the PDP operated through bilateral partnerships, under its current strategy it aspires to adopt coalition- and initiative-based approaches, in order "to achieve broader reach and stronger outcomes" [40] (p. 36). FIND also hopes to establish more output-orientated partnerships, for example, with other PDPs "where alignment of disease-level strategies is pursued and development of complementary, rather than duplicative or conflicting initiatives is encouraged" (ibid). It is thought that such collaborations would facilitate joint funding and implementation opportunities.

FIND's donors include the Global Fund to Fight AIDS, tuberculosis and malaria, the UK's Department for International Development (DFID), the Bill and Melinda Gates Foundation (BMGF), and the Australian Department of Foreign Affairs and Trade. In 2017, FIND's funding from donors was nearly US $56 million, with a further US $3.9 million given as in-kind donations [41] (annex p. 8). Unlike DNDi, FIND does not have an explicit policy to prevent one donor emerging as dominant, and in its early years found itself heavily dependent on funding from the BMGF. That said, it was able to achieve significant funding diversification in the period of 2009–2013, and is now in a less precarious position [42]. FIND has had some success in reducing the proportion of restricted funding it receives (bringing the total down from 100% in 2010) but it has not been as successful as DNDi [41,42].

FIND's portfolio (see Table 2) for HAT is based on two objectives: (i) increase detection of HAT through improved case finding; and (ii) facilitate faster, less burdensome confirmation of HAT through improved tools [40].

Table 2. FIND's HAT portfolio.

Catalyse Development >	Guide Use and Policy >	Delivered
HAT/Malaria combo RDT	2nd generation rapid diagnostic test (RDT), using recombinant antigens	1st generation RDT, using native antigens
		Primo Star iLED fluorescence microscope (iLED FM)
		Loop-mediated isothermal amplification (LAMP) of DNA

Product Backstory: Competing Rapid Diagnostic Tests for HAT

The Institute of Tropical Medicine, Antwerp (ITM) enjoyed a de facto monopoly over HAT diagnostics for several decades years prior to the establishment of FIND in 2003. The CATT was developed at ITM, and launched in 1978. Yet, it was not adopted at scale until the mid-1990s. Our fieldwork revealed that the right people had to be persuaded of the scientific merit of the CATT in order to abandon tried and tested techniques. That this took nearly 20 years points to missing elements in the innovation puzzle for HAT prior to the establishment of PDPs: product promotion and access (Interview 24 June 2015). FIND, in its current incarnation, recognises this fact through its endorsement of complete diagnostic solutions.

In the new millennium, FIND and ITM initially set out to work together to develop a rapid diagnostic test (RDT) for HAT, but when disagreements arose between the two parties, ITM determined to develop a competing test in parallel (Interview 19 November 2013). This period of competition proved fruitful, and in 2012 and 2013, two new RDTs for HAT were launched: the SD BIOLINE HAT, co-developed by FIND and manufactured by Standard Diagnostics, Suwon, S. Korea; and ITM's HAT Sero K-SeT, manufactured by the Coris BioConcept, Gembloux, Belgium.

In theory, ITM boasted certain advantages that should have seen its test dominate: ITM manufactures the native antigens used in both tests (meaning in theory it can set a ceiling on how many tests FIND can produce); it is also the WHO collaborating centre for HAT diagnostics. However, FIND has proved an astute political player. At its product launch in December 2012, FIND formally credited ITM with helping develop the test, glossing over their rivalry to paint the relationship as collaborative (Interview 19th November 2013). It has also carved out a role for its RDT in low areas of low endemicity (knowing the ITM test would be used in areas of high endemicity), framing its usefulness in support of elimination efforts [43]. Finally, FIND secured a lower unit price for its tests (less than US $1 per test as opposed to ~ US $2.50) (Interview 19 November 2013) [44], thus contributing to a narrative—that its research arm helps to perpetuate—that the SD RDT is notably cost-effective [45]. Implementation research conducted by the Diagnostic Tools for HAT Elimination and Clinical Trials project (DiTECT-HAT) has since suggested that the ITM and FIND RDTs do not even necessarily need to compete; that potentially, they can both be incorporated into algorithms for passive case detection and post-elimination monitoring [46]. This is because while both tests use the same native antigens, their separate development pathways have produced RDTs with slightly different performance characteristics in field settings that enable them to identify overlapping but nevertheless immunologically different patient populations.

In recent years, both FIND and ITM have continued to innovate, setting out—again, in parallel—to develop second generation RDTs for HAT based on recombinant antigens. And while our research suggests that the relationship between ITM and FIND has at times been privately strained, the external view of the ensuing rivalry has been largely positive, suggesting competition is both a fertile catalyst of innovation and a means of securing production:

"A healthy competition exists between several groups to develop HAT rapid diagnostic tests, which should improve quality and provide options in case one test fails to improve diagnostic accuracy. As a neglected tropical disease and with decreasing disease prevalence, progressive commercial disinterest is a possibility for HAT. Thus, reliance on a single rapid diagnostic test for which production could be stopped for economic reasons is dangerous, and could harm the elimination strategy" [47] (e306–e307).

Indeed, the heightened activity in this field has since attracted other players to explore HAT diagnostics [48]. In short, the establishment of FIND has done much to energise a field that had for several decades, lain dormant.

3.3. Global Alliance for Livestock Veterinary Medicines (GALVmed)

GALVmed, formerly the Global Alliance for Livestock Vaccines (GALV), was launched in 2004. GALVmed is set up to make livestock medicines, vaccines and diagnostics accessible and affordable to farmers in developing countries. GALVmed's goal is to develop and advocate for the benefits of animal health products to meet the needs of small-scale livestock producers, passing them onto others to manufacture and distribute. Trypanosomiasis has been an important strand of GALVmed's work since the beginning. Besides the impacts of livestock health, mortality and productivity, an important element of this work would be to reduce the role of livestock as a reservoir of the zoonotic *T. b. rhodesiense* form of sleeping sickness [49].

Since its inception, the majority of GALVmed's funding and all of its core funding has come from DFID and the BMGF. GALVmed (then GALV) had been established to explicitly focus on vaccines but this rapidly expanded to include other veterinary products. Between 2005 and 2017 DFID and the BMGF provided almost US $60 million of support (DFID project record [50]). Initially DFID has been the majority funder but this balance of funding responsibility has gradually reversed. In 2011, DFID awarded an additional grant of just over US $10 million to support the development of an integrated package of tools and policies for the cost-effective control of animal African trypanosomosis (AAT). This package aspires to deliver a new field diagnostic tool and new trypanocidal drugs, and to establish the basis for the development of a vaccine for AAT (DFID project record). The BMGF has since complemented this grant twice in support of project Phase 1 and Phase 2 (the BMGF awarded US $1.4 million in January 2014). The stated purpose of the BMGF grant was to develop safe and effective drugs against drug-resistant AAT, to develop a diagnostic test for field diagnosis in cattle, and to improve quality control of existing trypanocidal drugs used by smallholder livestock keepers in sub-Saharan Africa [51].

GALVmed's early work included the development of an anti-trypanosomiasis vaccine candidate, but this failed to progress beyond exploratory stages due to numerous technical difficulties (Interview 27 March 2013). Over the past ten years, GALVmed's work has evolved. Generally, there has been a significant shift away from R&D, through testing of pilot field projects to assess commercial development, towards the current establishment of large-scale, market-based initiatives. In a similar vein to the other PDPs, GALVmed now sees its work as having two strands. One remains new product development, with perhaps a greater focus on improving products to meet the specific needs of smallholder farmers. The second is commercial development—utilising the commercial value of products to ensure their sustainable availability to smallholder farmers.

The 'product development' strand has also broadened (See Table 3 [52]). Product improvement requires working with different stakeholders, including more directly with smallholders. Product development is increasingly delivered through complex consortia, as can be seen with GALVmed's AAT programme.

Table 3. GALVmed's programme objectives for Animal African Trypanosomaisis.

Objective	Activities
The development of a new class of trypanocides for therapeutic and prophylactic field use.	Drug discovery work is taking place through a substantial network of partners and is the major focus of the Tryps 2 programme. The specific objectives of this work are one therapeutic candidate and one late-stage prophylactic compound to be transferred to a commercial company for full development. Additionally, a comprehensive backup pipeline of compounds to be made available.
The development of a pen-side diagnostic for field use.	One new pen-side diagnostic test will be licensed to a commercial company for subsequent production and marketing.
The development of improved integrated control methods at the farm/village level resulting in more effective use of the full range of vector and disease control measures.	Under the Tryps 2 programme, continuing support for improved trypanocide regulation and quality control is being provided through capacity building activities in two African laboratories.
Improved quality and regulatory control of trypanocides in Africa to counter the growing problem of counterfeit and substandard drugs.	Developing a better understanding of the integrated use of diagnostics, trypanocides, trypanotolerant breeds and vector control methods at the farm/community level in different farming and eco-systems.

In response to technical difficulties in the creation of an effective vaccine against AAT, GALVmed diversified its AAT portfolio. Its multi-pronged approach, which placed an emphasis on improving the systems through which animal health technologies would be delivered, required a different approach to partnerships. GALVmed now facilitates more than 20 often-complex research partnerships that include global pharmaceutical companies, universities, public research groups and organisations representing farmers. This has led to the current state of affairs with the marketing of a pen-side diagnostic test by a commercial animal health company and the trypanocide moving into development with a commercial partner.

Over the last decade we can see a tangible shift in GALVmed's approach [53]. It is now less concerned with picking 'low hanging' technological fruits—many of which have been picked—and more concerned with understanding the needs of smallholders, delivering sustainable services and advocating for better policy to ensure appropriate products are developed and delivered. This means understanding the complex interplay between retailers, veterinary services and smallholders in multiple contexts, engaging much more in policy circles, and giving more thought to market needs and commercial concerns.

This broader approach to the delivery of animal health products is mirrored to an extent by GALVmed's two main donors, the BMGF and DFID. The BMGF and DFID recently (2018) funded a new US $50 million programme with GALVmed called VITAL (Veterinary Innovations Transforming Animal Health and Livelihoods) which aims for sectoral transformational change—focusing on the development of six new vaccines and partnering with the animal health industry to develop five large-scale product development networks in Asia and Africa.

In one key respect, animal health product delivery is markedly different from human health: there is more potential for commercial profit in delivering new products. This is often much less clear, especially for NTDs like HAT, given their close relationship to poverty. GALVmed is therefore much more interested in understanding the commercial context in which new health products will exist than either FIND or DNDi. Indeed, GALVmed sees itself as having a catalytic role to "educate industry that LMICs are interesting" (Interview 8 August 2019). GALVmed's trypanosomiasis programme in particular is focused on consortium building given its immediate focus on a pen-side test and new drugs. GALVmed's consortium building and commercial engagement, ostensibly to ensure the immediate commercial viability of its products, can play an important role in future-proofing its activities. Many of the most pressing future concerns in the livestock sector in developing countries—population growth/demand for high quality protein due to an emerging middle class, the rise of antimicrobial resistance, and the impacts of climate change—have strong commercial drivers that GALVmed could be well-placed to engage with to lever the delivery of new technologies.

Product Backstory: Pen-Side Diagnostic Test

Drugs to treat AAT do exist, but most were introduced over 40 years ago. One strand of GALVmed activity is focused on incentivising pharmaceutical companies to search for new classes of trypanocides [3]. Another important strand of work is the development of more effective diagnostic approaches. There are no specific clinical signs of infection by *T. vivax*, *T. congolense* or *T. b. rhodesiense*, so differential diagnosis is difficult. Currently, the only way to confirm a diagnosis in infected animals is to demonstrate and identify the parasites in blood and other bodily fluids (which is in itself difficult as parasite numbers are generally low). Most treatment of AAT is therefore presumptive, which has costs for farmers and their perception of the efficacy of treatment [54,55]. The lack of a simple diagnostic test similarly makes it difficult to identity and deal with parasitic reservoirs within livestock populations. Developing a simple pen-side diagnostic test, focused on *T. b. rhodensiense*, may therefore have implications for both animal and human health [56].

GALVmed funded a number of laboratories with different approaches to antigen discovery in a competitive manner. This portfolio approach preserved the diversity of promising antigen candidates that were discovered and could then be tested. One of the partners included the University of Dundee where promising *T. vivax* proteins were identified and developed into prototype lateral flow and ELISA tests [54]. A further collaboration with BBI Solutions, who specialise in immunoassay development, led to the development of a simple lateral flow test that could be used in situ as the favoured approach (hence 'pen-side'). This required no electricity, additional equipment or diagnostic expertise. Not coincidentally, the BBI Solutions-Dundee partnership was built on earlier work in relation to the development of a lateral flow diagnostic test for HAT, supported by FIND. GALVmed also worked with the pharmaceutical company CEVA, the University of Bordeaux, the French research agency CIRAD and teams of researchers from across Africa to develop the first commercially available rapid field diagnostic test against AAT, a lateral flow test, which can detect infection with both the *T. congolense* and *T. vivax* strains. This is now being used in several regions in Cameroon.

These new generation tests are not perfect. In particular, they remain expensive (currently more expensive than simply treating a cow so there are issues as to whom they are of utility to). The cost of the test means that it may currently be of more interest to academics. And the targeting of the tests on *T. congolense* and *T. vivax* means they are not a tool of utility to reduce *T. b. rhodesiense* parasite burdens within cattle as a means of reducing the risk of human infection. GALVmed has, however, demonstrated its ability to build a new diagnostic pipeline from lab to livestock.

4. Discussion: Innovation, Evolution and Sustainability

To date the majority of studies on PDPs have examined them only as relatively static entities [14,57], noting their differences from one another with less emphasis on their progression over time. In this article, we attempted to sketch the emergence, evolution and contributions of three PDPs closely associated with the African trypanosomiases. All three have delivered for the archetypal neglected tropical disease and been changed in the process.

DNDi changed tack early on to mirror the portfolio approach of big pharma, building a product pipeline for HAT for the first time in history. At the same time, it broke with the profit-driven model of industry—delinking R&D from the price of products—to assert that product development in the public interest is possible. FIND's entry into HAT diagnostics shook up a field that had lain dormant for decades. Its early work contributed to the development of competing, yet complementary screening tests that will help secure the supply chain for elimination, and hopefully drive further advancements that could help simplify HAT's complex diagnostic tree [58]. GALVmed cast off its (inherited) vaccine pursuit to prioritise a more user-focused product portfolio. In doing so, it produced a successful pen-side test even if it was not able to stick to the 'cost' component of its target product profile. This achievement has provided a proof of concept for its approach, which should help drive further projects, and hopefully donor confidence.

All three PDPs have also evolved in the sense that they have expanded their portfolios and extended their missions, moving away from a narrow focus on product development to encompass a broader suite of complementary functions to ensure products are accessible and impactful. Our research suggests all three case study PDPs are being driven to evolve by three interlinked factors: funding, an impetus to show impact and the changing nature of R&D partnerships.

The most important factor is funding—primarily to ensure sufficient investment in research and that incentives exist to encourage private sector actors to engage in product development. The years 2000–2010 are now viewed as a 'golden era' for global health funding. During that decade, development assistance for health grew at an annual rate of 11.2%. By contrast, from 2010–2017, the total growth was just 1% annually [59]. And where once PDPs were channeling around a quarter of all R&D funding for neglected diseases, in 2017, that proportion had dropped to 14% [27] (p. 99). While there are many external reasons to explain the constrained funding environment (the aftermath of the financial crisis, rising nationalism), it must be frustrating for PDPs, given that in many ways, they represent a 'best buy' in global health. From a donor perspective, not only are our case study PDPs productive, they reduce financial risk, incur lower R&D costs (through portfolio approaches), and present donors with lower management responsibilities than if they were to give to multiple product developers. Moreover, from the perspective of public sector investment, PDPs provide an avenue for public-funded basic research to feed into public goods and much-needed products.

However, where PDPs are less successful is in demonstrating impact, at least in the short term. During their formative years, all three organisations were incentivised by their major donors to deliver new technological innovations. There were set product delivery targets and focused on delivering new innovations above all else. This resulted in multiple new products that would not have been taken forward by industry. However, a move towards what we term a 'post-low hanging fruit phase' characterises DNDi, FIND and GALVmed. In short, the easy wins have been achieved. Increasingly, PDPs are being asked to show not just outputs but outcomes as donors have become more concerned with measuring the impacts of their investments. Yet, the type of health products that our case study PDPs produce—drugs, diagnostics and vaccines—tend to incur long lead times to impact (there is a long development times for drugs and vaccines, and uncertain patient pathways from diagnostics to treatment). Moreover success in these fields is an anomaly rather than a given, hence why DNDi has to factor 'attrition' into its drug development calculations. Donors clearly have a concern with value for money and impact, as is demonstrated by the growing number of donor evaluations into the PDPs they support [42,60].

Each of our case study PDPs exists in an ever more complex institutional context. Traditional institutions jostle for funding and prioritisation—and the NTD sector is a good example of this [25]. Meanwhile, new actors emerge as bilateral funders like DFID increasingly look to experiment with private sector approaches and work through other organisations, given concerns around the ability of traditional aid to drive efficiency, value and scalability [61]. Funders like the BMGF are now providing more funding directly to manufacturers [40,42]. FIND has flagged this up, pointing to the "increased but fragmented" participation in product development [40] (p. 19). There are potentially advantages to this—more opportunities for collaboration, information sharing and building a portfolio-driven approach, but also disadvantages—increased transaction and opportunity costs, imperfect access to information hampering decision-making, and collaboration turning into competition if budgets are tight. There needs to be an important role for donors in this complex, evolving environment. Giving incentives and impetus to working across PDPs can create new opportunities—witness the GALVmed lateral flow diagnostic test genesis described above—but the "absence of an overarching and sustainable framework to govern and drive public interest R&D" threatens to hamper progress [34] (p. 38).

PDPs find themselves in a bind. The three PDPs described here have all developed innovations (although it is too early to assess their impacts). It can be argued that each has already picked its 'low-hanging fruit' and future innovations will be more expensive and harder work to deliver. They all operate in a funding environment which is contingent on a very small number of donors, who are increasingly focused on results, impacts and managing risk [42]. There is a tension here between ability to deliver and expectation of impact, and the response of the PDPs has been to diversify the breadth of their disease portfolios and the nature of their partnerships. Allied to this, donors are exploring other private sector delivery mechanisms, forcing PDPs to re-position themselves as 'brokers', 'enablers' and 'interpreters' within this new, ever more complex global health innovation arena; the end goal being to diversify their funding base by demonstrating their value to the private sector and venture capitalists.

5. Conclusions

It is too soon to judge the contributions of DNDi, FIND and GALVmed to the elimination of African Trypanosomiasis. Most of the products described here are too new or still under trial and in any case, it would be an enormously complex question to answer given technological innovations can only ever be a contingent component of any successful health intervention or system. Instead, this paper has attempted to describe the broader role of PDPs as deliverers of new tools to combat the archetypal "tool-deficient" NTD. New tools have and are being delivered. It is unclear that these new tools would have been delivered so quickly without the role of PDPs to broker, connect and fund research and innovation.

PDPs have also helped (in conjunction with WHO and other partners) rebuild and reinvigorate the epistemic community around tropical medicine. This is perhaps the biggest shake up of that network since it first emerged during the colonial period [4]. PDPs have helped attract big pharma back into this network, but even more importantly, they have helped formalise the central role played by public bodies in disease endemic countries. The HAT platform established with the help of DNDi, is a case in point [31].

PDPs have already contributed to the global campaign to see HAT eliminated as a public health problem by 2020—in delivering new diagnostics and treatments—but their larger contribution is yet to be realised: delivering at scale the products that could see the transmission of HAT eliminated by 2030. Reaching and sustaining this goal requires HAT services be integrated into national healthcare structures. This paradigm shift is complex to engineer—but from a technical perspective, it is only made possible by the development of new, safe, easy to use products that can be deployed at point of care. PDPs have been instrumental in prioritising these types of products for the trypanosomiases, through the setting of performance and operational attributes that place patients and product users at their core. It is telling that PDPs like DNDi, FIND and GALVmed are broadening their partnership networks and integrating their activities into nascent health and pastoral systems. This can facilitate innovations more closely tailored to the needs of countries, clinics and farms. It can also facilitate spillovers between PDPs and other actors. There is a danger, however, that PDPs—in trying to do too much to stay relevant to donors—could lose their important singular focus. This is a lesson for donor, PDP and policymakers alike if the elimination of African trypanosomiasis is to not only be attained, but sustained.

Author Contributions: Conceptualization, E.M.T. and J.S.; methodology, E.M.T. and J.S.; formal analysis, E.M.T. and J.S.; investigation, E.M.T. and J.S.; data curation, E.M.T. and J.S.; writing—original draft preparation, E.M.T. and J.S.; writing—review and editing, E.M.T. and J.S. All authors have read and agreed to the published version of the manuscript.

Funding: This research was funded by European Research Council, grant number 295845.

Acknowledgments: We would like to thank our research participants who generously shared their perspectives and time. We would like to thank Jennifer Palmer (London School Hygiene and Tropical Medicine), who commented on an earlier proof of the diagnostic case study. Finally, we would like to thank our reviewers whose suggestions greatly improved the final paper.

Trop. Med. Infect. Dis. **2020**, *5*, 11

Conflicts of Interest: The authors declare no conflict of interest. The funders had no role in the design of the study; in the collection, analyses, or interpretation of data; in the writing of the manuscript, or in the decision to publish the results.

Abbreviations

AAT	Animal African Trypanosomiasis
BMGF	Bill and Melinda Gates Foundation
CATT	Card Agglutination Test for Trypanosomiasis
CIRAD	French Agricultural Research Centre for International Development
DFID	UK's Department for International Development
DNDi	Drugs for Neglected Diseases Initiative
FIND	Foundation for Innovative New Diagnostics
GALV	Global Alliance for Livestock Vaccines
GALVmed	Global Alliance for Livestock Veterinary Medicines
HAT	Human African Trypanosomiasis
ITM	Institute of Tropical Medicine, Antwerp
LMICs	Low- and Middle-Income Countries
MSF	Médecins Sans Frontières
NECT	Nifurtimox-Eflornithine Combination Therapy
NTD	Neglected Tropical Disease
PDP	Product Development Partnership
PPP	Public-Private Partnership
R&D	Research and Development
RDT	Rapid Diagnostic Test
SD	Standard Diagnostics
TPP	Target Product Profile
WHO/TDR	World Health Organisation's Special Programme for Research and Training in Tropical Diseases

References

1. Henry, D.; Lexchin, J. The pharmaceutical industry as a medicines provider. *Lancet* **2002**, *360*, 1590–1595. [CrossRef]
2. Lyons, M. *The Colonial Disease*; Cambridge University Press: Cambridge, UK, 1992.
3. Giordani, F.; Morrison, L.J.; Rowan, T.G.; De Koning, H.P.; Barrett, M.P. The animal trypanosomiases and their chemotherapy: A review. *Parasitology* **2016**, *143*, 1862–1889. [CrossRef]
4. Neill, D.J. *Networks in Tropical Medicine: Internationalism, Colonialism, and the Rise of a Medical Specialty, 1890–1930*; Stanford University Press: Stanford, CA, USA, 2012; ISBN 9780804781053.
5. Molyneux, D.; Ndung'u, J.; Maudlin, I. Controlling sleeping sickness—"when will they ever learn?". *PLoS Negl. Trop. Dis.* **2010**, *4*, e609. [CrossRef]
6. Trouiller, P.; Olliaro, P.; Torreele, E.; Orbinski, J.; Laing, R.; Ford, N. Drug development for neglected diseases: A deficient market and a public-health policy failure. *Lancet* **2002**, *359*, 2188–2194. [CrossRef]
7. Barrett, M.P. Problems for the chemotherapy of human African trypanosomiasis. *Curr. Opin. Infect. Dis.* **2000**, *13*, 647–651. [CrossRef]
8. Drugs for Neglected Diseases Working Group, Médecins Sans Frontières. *Fatal Imbalance The Crisis in Research and Development for Drugs for Neglected Diseases*; Médecins Sans Frontières: Geneva, Switzerland, 2001; Available online: www.accessmed-msf.org (accessed on 2 December 2019).
9. Pedrique, B.; Strub-Wourgaft, N.; Some, C.; Olliaro, P.; Trouiller, P.; Ford, N.; Pécoul, B.; Bradol, J.H. The drug and vaccine landscape for neglected diseases (2000–11): A systematic assessment. *Lancet Glob. Heal.* **2013**, *1*, e371–e379. [CrossRef]
10. WHO. *Accelerating Work to Overcome the Global Impact of Neglected Tropical Diseases: A Roadmap for Implementation*; WHO: Geneva, Switzerland, 2012; Available online: https://www.who.int/neglected_diseases/NTD_RoadMap_2012_Fullversion.pdf (accessed on 26 August 2019).

11. Smith, J.; Taylor, E.M. What is Next for NTDs in the Era of the Sustainable Development Goals? *PLoS Negl. Trop. Dis.* **2016**, *10*, e0004719. [CrossRef]

12. Crewe, E.; Harrison, E. *Whose Development?: An Ethnography of Aid*; Zed Books: London, UK, 1998; ISBN 1856496066.

13. Crawford, G. Partnership or Power? Deconstructing the "Partnership for Governance Reform" in Indonesia. *Third World Q.* **2003**, *24*, 139–159. [CrossRef]

14. Moran, M.; Guzman, J.; Ropars, A.L.; Illmer, A. The role of Product Development Partnerships in research and development for neglected diseases. *Int. Health* **2010**, *2*, 114–122. [CrossRef]

15. WHO. Outlines Criteria to Assess Elimination of Sleeping Sickness. World Health Organization: Geneva, Switzerland. Available online: https://www.who.int/neglected_diseases/news/criteria-eliminate-sleeping-sickness/en/ (accessed on 10 January 2020).

16. Buse, K.; Tanaka, S. Global public-private health partnerships: Lessons learned from ten years of experience and evaluation. *Int. Dent. J.* **2011**, *61*, 2–10. [CrossRef]

17. Widdus, R. Public-private partnerships for health: Their main targets, their diversity, and their future directions. *Bull. World Health Organ.* **2001**, *79*, 713–720.

18. Moran, M.; Guzman, J.; Henderson, K.; Liyanage, R.; Wu, L.; Chin, E.; Chapman, N.; Abela, O.; Gouglas, D.; Kwong, D. *G-FINDER 2012: Neglected Disease Research and Development: A Five Year Review*; Policy Cures: Sydney, Australia, 2012.

19. Buse, K.; Walt, G. Global public-private partnerships: Part I—A new development in health? *Bull. World Health Organ.* **2000**, *78*, 549–561. [PubMed]

20. Moran, M.; Ropars, A.-L.; Guzman, J.; Diaz, J.; Garrison, C. *The New Landscape of Neglected Disease Drug Development*; Wellcome Trust: London, UK, 2005; Available online: http://www.policycures.org/downloads/The_new_landscape_of_neglected_disease_drug_development.pdf (accessed on 9 August 2017).

21. Policy Cures. *The Unrecognised Revolution in Global Health*; Policy Cures: Sydney, Australia, 2015. Available online: http://projectreporter.nih.gov/project_info_description (accessed on 2 December 2019).

22. Berdud, M.; Towse, A.; Kettler, H. Fostering incentives for research, development, and delivery of interventions for neglected tropical diseases: Lessons from malaria. *Oxf. Rev. Econ. Policy* **2016**, *32*, 64–87. [CrossRef]

23. Molyneux, D.H.; Hotez, P.J.; Fenwick, A. "Rapid-Impact Interventions": How a Policy of Integrated Control for Africa's Neglected Tropical Diseases Could Benefit the Poor. *PLoS Med.* **2005**, *2*, e336. [CrossRef]

24. Molyneux, D.H. The "Neglected Tropical Diseases": Now a brand identity; Responsibilities, context and promise. *Parasites Vectors* **2012**, *5*, 23. [CrossRef]

25. Smith, J.; Taylor, E.M. MDGs and NTDs: Reshaping the global health agenda. *PLoS Negl. Trop. Dis.* **2013**, *7*, e2529. [CrossRef]

26. Olliaro, P.L.; Kuesel, A.C.; Reeder, J.C. A Changing Model for Developing Health Products for Poverty-Related Infectious Diseases. *PLoS Negl. Trop. Dis.* **2015**, *9*, e3379. [CrossRef]

27. Chapman, N.; Doubell, A.; Oversteegen, L.; Barnsley, P.; Chowdhary, V.; Rugarabamu, G.; Ong, M.; Borri, J. G-FINDER 2018: Neglected Disease Research and Development: Reaching New Heights. 2019. Available online: www.policycuresresearch.org (accessed on 26 August 2019).

28. Yin, R.K. *Case Study Research Design and Methods*, 5th ed.; Sage Publications, Inc.: London, UK, 2014; ISBN 978-1-4522-4256-9.

29. Blaikie, N.W.H. *Designing Social Research: The Logic of Anticipation*; Polity Press: Cambridge, UK, 2000; ISBN 9780745643380.

30. Burawoy, M. *The Extended Case Method: Four Countries, Four Decades, Four Great Transformations, and One Theoretical Tradition*; University of California Press: Berkeley, CA, USA, 2009; ISBN 9780520943384.

31. HAT Platform—DNDi. Available online: https://www.dndi.org/strengthening-capacity/hat-platform/ (accessed on 10 January 2020).

32. G-FINDER—Public Search Tool. Available online: https://gfinder.policycuresresearch.org/PublicSearchTool/ (accessed on 10 January 2020).

33. DNDi. *An Innovative Approach to R&D for Neglected Patients: Ten Years of Experience & Lessons Learned by DNDi*; DNDi: Geneva, Switzerland, 2014; Available online: https://www.dndi.org/wp-content/uploads/2009/03/DNDi_Modelpaper_2013.pdf (accessed on 2 December 2019).

34.   DNDi. *15 Years of Needs-Driven Innovation for Access: Key Lessons, Challenges, and oppoRtunities for the Future*; DNDi: Geneva, Switzerland, 2019; Available online: https://www.dndi.org/wp-content/uploads/2019/10/DNDi_ModelPaper_2019.pdf (accessed on 2 December 2019).

35.   DNDi. *Annual Report 2018: Making Medical History to Meet the Needs of Neglected Patients*; DNDi: Geneva, Switzerland, 2019; Available online: https://www.dndi.org/wp-content/uploads/2019/07/DNDi_2018_AnnualReport.pdf (accessed on 2 December 2019).

36.   Priotto, G.; Fogg, C.; Balasegaram, M.; Erphas, O.; Louga, A.; Checchi, F.; Ghabri, S.; Piola, P. Three Drug Combinations for Late-Stage Trypanosoma brucei gambiense Sleeping Sickness: A Randomized Clinical Trial in Uganda. *PLoS Clin. Trials* **2006**, *1*, e39. [CrossRef]

37.   Bisser, S.; N'Siesi, F.; Lejon, V.; Preux, P.; Van Nieuwenhove, S.; Miaka Mia Bilenge, C.; Büscher, P. Equivalence Trial of Melarsoprol and Nifurtimox Monotherapy and Combination Therapy for the Treatment of Second-Stage Trypanosoma brucei gambiense Sleeping Sickness. *J. Infect. Dis.* **2007**, *195*, 322–329. [CrossRef]

38.   Priotto, G.; Kasparian, S.; Mutombo, W.; Ngouama, D.; Ghorashian, S.; Arnold, U.; Ghabri, S.; Baudin, E.; Buard, V.; Kazadi-Kyanza, S.; et al. Nifurtimox-eflornithine combination therapy for second-stage African Trypanosoma brucei gambiense trypanosomiasis: A multicentre, randomised, phase III, non-inferiority trial. *Lancet* **2009**, *374*, 56–64. [CrossRef]

39.   Torreele, E.; Trunz, B.B.; Tweats, D.; Kaiser, M.; Brun, R.; Mazué, G.; Bray, M.A.; Pécoul, B. Fexinidazole—A new oral nitroimidazole drug candidate entering clinical development for the treatment of sleeping sickness. *PLoS Negl. Trop. Dis.* **2010**, *4*, e923. [CrossRef] [PubMed]

40.   FIND. *FIND Strategy 2015–2020: Turning Complex Diagnostic Challenges into Simple Solutions*; FIND: Geneva, Switzerland, 2014; Available online: https://www.finddx.org/wp-content/uploads/2016/01/FIND_Strategy.pdf (accessed on 2 December 2019).

41.   FIND. *FIND Annual Report 2017: Partnering for Diagnostic Excellence*; FIND: Geneva, Switzerland, 2018; Available online: https://www.finddx.org/wp-content/uploads/2019/03/Annual-Report-2017_21-11_web-cpr.pdf (accessed on 2 December 2019).

42.   Boulton, I.; Meredith, S.; Mertenskoetter, T.; Glaue, F. Evaluation of the Product Development Partnerships (PDP) Funding Activities-The UK Department for International Development (DFID)-The German Ministry for Education and Research (BMBF). 2015. Available online: https://assets.publishing.service.gov.uk/media/57a0897140f0b649740000b0/Evaluation_of_the_Product_Development_Partnerships_funding_activities.pdf (accessed on 3 June 2019).

43.   Palmer, J.J.; Robert, O.; Kansiime, F. Including refugees in disease elimination: Challenges observed from a sleeping sickness programme in Uganda. *Confl. Health* **2017**, *11*, 22. [CrossRef] [PubMed]

44.   Büscher, P.; Gilleman, Q.; Lejon, V. Rapid Diagnostic Test for Sleeping Sickness. *N. Engl. J. Med.* **2013**, *368*, 1069–1070. [CrossRef]

45.   Bessell, P.R.; Lumbala, C.; Lutumba, P.; Baloji, S.; Bieler, S.; Ndung'u, J.M. Cost-effectiveness of using a rapid diagnostic test to screen for human African trypanosomiasis in the Democratic Republic of the Congo. *PLoS ONE* **2018**, *13*, e0204335. [CrossRef] [PubMed]

46.   Study Overview|DiTECT HAT. Available online: https://www.ditect-hat.eu/about-us/study-overview/ (accessed on 10 January 2020).

47.   Jamonneau, V.; Bucheton, B. The challenge of serodiagnosis of sleeping sickness in the context of elimination. *Lancet Glob. Heal.* **2014**, *2*, e306–e307. [CrossRef]

48.   Sternberg, J.M.; Gierliński, M.; Biéler, S.; Ferguson, M.A.J.; Ndung'u, J.M. Evaluation of the Diagnostic Accuracy of Prototype Rapid Tests for Human African Trypanosomiasis. *PLoS Negl. Trop. Dis.* **2014**, *9*, e0003613. [CrossRef]

49.   Welburn, S.C.; Picozzi, K.; Fèvre, E.M.; Coleman, P.G.; Odiit, M.; Carrington, M.; Maudlin, I. Identification of human-infective trypanosomes in animal reservoir of sleeping sickness in Uganda by means of serum-resistance-associated (SRA) gene. *Lancet* **2001**, *358*, 2017–2019. [CrossRef]

50.   Research for Development Outputs—GOV.UK. Available online: https://www.gov.uk/dfid-research-outputs (accessed on 10 January 2020).

51.   Global Alliance for Livestock Veterinary Medicines—Bill & Melinda Gates Foundation. Available online: https://www.gatesfoundation.org/How-We-Work/Quick-Links/Grants-Database/Grants/2014/01/OPP1100291 (accessed on 10 January 2020).

52. Animal African Trypanosomosis (AAT) Overview and Objectives—GALVmed. Available online: https://www.galvmed.org/work/product-development/large-ruminant-programmes-east-coast-fever-contagious-bovine-pleuropneumonia-animal-african-trypanosomosis-rift-valley-fever-and-brucellosis/ (accessed on 10 January 2020).

53. GALVmed. *GALVmed at 10: A Decade of Protecting Livestock, Improving Human Lives*; GALVmed: Edinburgh, UK, 2018; Available online: https://www.galvmed.org/galvmedat10/GALVmed_at_10.pdf (accessed on 2 December 2019).

54. Fleming, J.R.; Sastry, L.; Wall, S.J.; Sullivan, L.; Ferguson, M.A.J. Proteomic Identification of Immunodiagnostic Antigens for Trypanosoma vivax Infections in Cattle and Generation of a Proof-of-Concept Lateral Flow Test Diagnostic Device. *PLoS Negl. Trop. Dis.* **2016**, *10*, e0004977. [CrossRef]

55. Pinto Torres, J.E.; Goossens, J.; Ding, J.; Li, Z.; Lu, S.; Vertommen, D.; Naniima, P.; Chen, R.; Muyldermans, S.; Sterckx, Y.G.J.; et al. Development of a Nanobody-based lateral flow assay to detect active Trypanosoma congolense infections. *Sci. Rep.* **2018**, *8*, 9019. [CrossRef]

56. Sones, K. Protecting livestock, improving human lives. *Vet. Rec.* **2012**, *170*, 611–613. [CrossRef]

57. De Pinho Campos, K.; Norman, C.D.; Jadad, A.R. Product development public-private partnerships for public health: A systematic review using qualitative data. *Soc. Sci. Med.* **2011**, *73*, 986–994. [CrossRef] [PubMed]

58. Bonnet, J.; Boudot, C.; Courtioux, B. Overview of the Diagnostic Methods Used in the Field for Human African Trypanosomiasis: What Could Change in the Next Years? *Biomed Res. Int.* **2015**, *2015*, 583262. [CrossRef] [PubMed]

59. Institute for Health Metrics and Evaluation. *Financing Global Health 2017: Funding Universal Health Coverage and the Unfinished HIV/AIDS Agenda*; Institute for Health Metrics and Evaluation: Seattle, WA, USA, 2018; Available online: http://www.healthdata.org/policy-report/financing-global-health-2017 (accessed on 2 December 2019).

60. Mostert, B.; de Jongh, T.; Nooijen, A.; Ploeg, M. Review of the Product Development Partnerships Fund 2011–2014: Final Report to the Dutch Ministry of Foreign Affairs. 2014. Available online: https://www.technopolis-group.com/wp-content/uploads/2014/11/141118_PDP_Review_Technopolis_Group4.pdf (accessed on 3 June 2019).

61. Dodsworth, S.; Cheeseman, N. Risk, politics, and development: Lessons from the UK's democracy aid. *Public Adm. Dev.* **2018**, *38*, 53–64. [CrossRef]

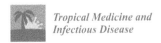

*Tropical Medicine and
Infectious Disease*

Review

Innovative Partnerships for the Elimination of Human African Trypanosomiasis and the Development of Fexinidazole

Philippe Neau [1,*], Heinz Hänel [2], Valérie Lameyre [1], Nathalie Strub-Wourgaft [3] and Luc Kuykens [4]

[1]   Sanofi France, 82 avenue Raspail, 94250 Gentilly, France; valerie.lameyre@sanofi.com
[2]   Sanofi Deutschland, Industriepark Höchst, Bldg. H831, 65926 Frankfurt am Main, Germany; Heinz.Haenel@sanofi.com
[3]   Drugs for Neglected Diseases initiative (DNDi), 15 Chemin Louis-Dunant, 1202 Geneva, Switzerland; nstrub@dndi.org
[4]   Sanofi US, 55 Corporate Drive, Bridgewater, NJ 08807, USA; Luc.Kuykens@sanofi.com
*   Correspondence: Philippe.neau@sanofi.com

Received: 3 December 2019; Accepted: 10 January 2020; Published: 27 January 2020

Abstract: Human African Trypanosomiasis (HAT or sleeping sickness) is a life-threatening neglected tropical disease that is endemic in 36 sub-Saharan African countries. Until recently, treatment options were limited and hampered by unsatisfactory efficacy, toxicity, and long and cumbersome administration regimens, compounded by infrastructure inadequacies in the remote rural regions worst affected by the disease. Increased funding and awareness of HAT over the past two decades has led to a steady decline in reported cases (<1000 in 2018). Recent drug development strategies have resulted in development of the first all-oral treatment for HAT, fexinidazole. Fexinidazole received European Medicines Agency positive scientific opinion in 2018 and is now incorporated into the WHO interim guidelines as one of the first-line treatments for HAT, allowing lumbar puncture to become non-systematic. Here, we highlight the role of global collaborations in the effort to control HAT and develop new treatments. The long-standing collaboration between the WHO, Sanofi and the Drugs for Neglected Diseases *initiative* (Geneva, Switzerland) was instrumental for achieving the control and treatment development goals in HAT, whilst at the same time ensuring that efforts were led by national authorities and control programs to leave a legacy of highly trained healthcare workers and improved research and health infrastructure.

Keywords: sleeping sickness; human African trypanosomiasis; *T. b. gambiense*; g-HAT; *T. b. rhodesiense*; r-HAT; elimination; neglected tropical diseases; fexinidazole

1. Introduction

Human African Trypanosomiasis (HAT), or sleeping sickness, is a life-threatening, neglected tropical disease (NTD). It is considered endemic in 36 sub-Saharan African countries, where around 60 million people are estimated to be at some level of risk of HAT, primarily those living in 'foci' in poor and remote rural areas where health infrastructure is poor or non-existent [1–3]. HAT is transmitted to humans by the bite of tsetse flies and the etiological agent of HAT is the kinetoplastid protozoan parasite *Trypanosoma brucei (T. b.)*. Two subspecies of this parasite are pathogenic for humans: *T. b. gambiense* (g-HAT) responsible for the chronic form of the disease occurring in western and central Africa, and *T. b. rhodesiense* (r-HAT) responsible for a more acute form occurring in eastern and southern Africa [4]. *T. b. gambiense* is currently responsible for 98% of HAT cases [5], with the highest disease burden in the Democratic Republic of Congo (DRC) where 37.5 million people were estimated to be at some level of risk of g-HAT between 2012 and 2016 [1,2]. Humans are the principal reservoir for g-HAT and the progressive disease course occurs in two stages: a hemolymphatic phase (stage 1 with a mean duration of around 18 months) with common signs and symptoms including fever, headache, pruritus, weakness, asthenia, anemia, and lymphadenopathy; and a meningo-encephalic stage (stage 2 with a mean duration of around 8 months) occurring when the parasites have crossed the blood–brain barrier with resulting sleep disturbances and neuropsychiatric symptoms that may lead to coma and death if left untreated [4–6].

In this review, we highlight the role of global collaborations in the effort to control HAT and develop new treatments. In particular, we emphasize the role played by the public–private partnership between Sanofi (formerly Aventis) and the Drugs for Neglected Diseases *initiative* (DND*i*, Geneva, Switzerland), together with a range of governmental national sleeping sickness control programs (NSSCPs; such as the Le Programme National de Lutte contre la Trypanosomiase Humaine Africaine of the DRC [PNLTHA]) and non-governmental organizations (NGOs), in development of the first oral-only treatment for HAT, Fexinidazole Winthrop (fexinidazole).

2. A Strategy to Eliminate HAT

2.1. Global Alliances and Innovative Partnerships

Devastating epidemics of HAT have occurred throughout the 20th century. Following the neglect of control efforts implemented up to the 1960s, a dramatic resurgence of the disease was observed in the 1990s, with the World Health Organization (WHO, Geneva, Switzerland) estimating that 300,000 new cases were occurring each year in endemic areas, although only 30,000 cases were being diagnosed and treated [7]. In response to this relapse, the WHO passed a resolution in 1997 to raise awareness of the disease, promote access to diagnosis and treatment, and strengthen control and surveillance [8]. Around 20 years ago, the WHO launched an intensified coordination initiative [9] to achieve these goals by forming global alliances with United Nations Agencies (under the Program Against African Trypanosomiasis, PAAT), national governments (under NSSCPs), and the Organization of African Unity who established the Pan African Tsetse and Trypanosomiasis Eradication Campaign (PATTEC) in June 2000. Another key alliance with the WHO was the formation of what would become a longstanding public–private partnership with Sanofi in 2001, which made it possible to distribute vital drugs for the treatment of HAT and other NTDs in endemic areas free of charge. This partnership between the WHO and Sanofi also provided funds to support screening and surveillance efforts, improving treatment centers and training of local health workers, and, to contribute to research and development programs for new treatments. Under this agreement, renewed in 2006, 2011, and again 2016, Sanofi provided on average 5 million dollars per year for combating HAT (25% donated through drug donation and 75% as financial support for capacity building, patient screening, and other projects), totaling more than 85 million dollars [10]. In 2012, Sanofi cemented its commitment to the goal of eliminating HAT by signing the 'London Declaration on Neglected Tropical Diseases' [11]. This declaration focused on the commitment of a range of actors from public and private sectors to control or eliminate 10 infections, including HAT, affecting the world's poorest populations. In this context, Sanofi was contributing to the elimination of HAT as a public health issue by aligning its objectives with the elimination goals of the WHO, by continuing to freely supply drugs to ensure that all patients had access to appropriate treatment, and by developing new therapeutic options, through an innovative partnership with the DND*i* for the development of fexinidazole, improving the management of the disease.

In addition to the pivotal partnership between the WHO and Sanofi, similar private collaborations were formed with Bristol-Myers-Squibb and Bayer Healthcare for the supply of raw materials and other treatments. The WHO also coordinated partnerships between NGOs and research institutions, leading to collaborations with the Bill and Melinda Gates Foundation, Doctors Without Borders (Médecins Sans Frontières [MSF], Geneva, Switzerland) and the DND*i*.

2.2. The Success of Collaborative Strategies for HAT Elimination

As a result of the substantial collaborative efforts of the global alliance initiative, with the key role in strengthening control and surveillance activities being played by the NSSCPs of endemic countries, there has been a steady decline in HAT cases over the past two decades (Figure 1) [2,12,13]. Since 2001, more than 40 million HAT screening tests have been performed, and over 210,000 cases detected and treated [14]. A 96% decline in reported HAT cases was observed between 2000 and 2018, with 26,550 cases reported in 2000 and a historic low of 977 cases reported in 2018 [2,15]. In 2012, HAT was included in the WHO's roadmap for the control, elimination or eradication of NTDs and a target date was set for global elimination of g-HAT as a public health problem (<1 case/10,000 inhabitants in at least 90% of endemic foci) by 2020, with complete interruption of transmission in Africa targeted for 2030 [16]. Representatives of partners in the HAT global alliance attending the third WHO meeting of stakeholders on the elimination of g-HAT in Geneva in April 2018 concluded that global targets for reducing the number of cases had been met and that the goal of eliminating HAT was in sight [17].

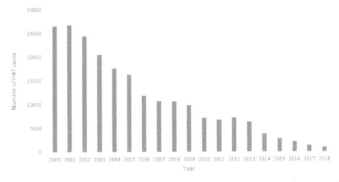

Figure 1. Total number of Human African Trypanosomiasis (HAT) cases reported per year (2000–2018) using data provided by national sleeping sickness control programs, non-governmental organizations, and research institutions, and assembled in the Atlas of HAT published in [2,15].

2.3. The Need for New Treatment Options

Despite the overwhelming success of HAT initiatives in reducing the number of cases, new diagnostic tools and treatments were deemed essential to facilitate the integration of the specialized HAT control, surveillance and management programs into national health systems and to maintain the goal of g-HAT elimination [17,18]. Historically, the diagnostic tools and algorithms—and the treatments available to manage HAT—have been complex and cumbersome, particularly given that the most at-risk populations are primarily located in the most remote, resource-poor, and politically unstable regions of endemic countries [19]. Indeed, even in 2016 around 28% of the population at highest risk of g-HAT (more than 200,000 people) were >5 h travel from a competent fixed diagnostic and treatment facility [2].

One of the major drawbacks of the treatments available before the development of fexinidazole (summarized in Table 1) was that a complicated sequence of events was required before hospital treatment could be accessed: serological screening, generally performed via active surveillance, followed by laboratory-based microscopy analyses to confirm the presence of the parasite in the lymph and blood, and, finally, disease staging involving patients undergoing lumbar puncture to determine the presence of trypanosomes and the levels of white blood cells (WBCs) in the cerebrospinal fluid (CSF) [16]. In a first effort to improve treatment, which at the time consisted of melarsoprol (a highly efficient but toxic arsenic-based treatment), a short-term research and development strategy evaluating the effectiveness of combining available treatments was implemented. This initiative—instigated by MSF and Epicentre and then the DNDi, with Sanofi and Bayer and other alliance partners—led to the nifurtimox–eflornithine combination therapy (NECT) becoming available to treat stage 2 g-HAT in 2009 [20]. Clinical trials demonstrated that NECT was a safe and effective treatment [21] and led to this combined therapy being used as a first-line therapy for stage 2 HAT in all endemic African countries. NECT helped to drastically reduce the number of HAT cases, with a steep decline in cases from around 7000 cases in 2010 to under 1000 cases in 2018 (Figure 1). However, NECT posed logistical concerns in remote locations (weight per treatment: 9 kg; volume per treatment 37.5 dm^3; Figure 2a,b), and required hospitalization and trained nursing staff to administer [22,23].

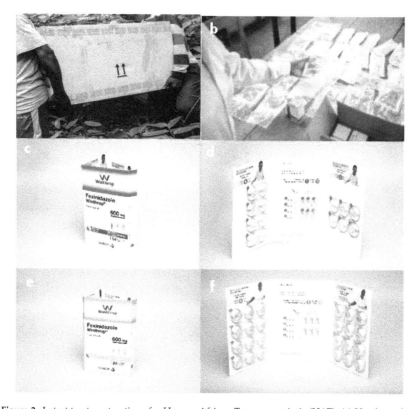

Figure 2. Latest treatment options for Human African Trypanosomiasis (HAT). (**a**) Heath workers transporting a Nifurtimox–Eflornithine Combination Therapy (NECT) kit in a remote region of the Democratic Republic of the Congo. The package contains four treatments and weighs approximately 36 kg [23]. (**b**) NECT required for the treatment of one patient. Nifurtimox is supplied in glass bottles, each containing 100 tablets of 120 mg and is given orally at a dose of 15 mg/kg/day, every 8 h for 10 days. Eflornithine is supplied in glass bottles (200 mg/mL in 100 mL bottles), is given by intravenous infusion 400 mg/kg/day every 12 h for 7 days, and once opened must be stored in the fridge (for up to 24 h) [23]. (**c**) and (**d**) Fexinidazole treatment for children (aged ≥ 6 years and weighing ≥ 20 and <35 kg): each wallet contains 14 tablets (1 aluminum foil blister of 6 tablets and 1 aluminum foil blister of 8 tablets) to be taken once daily with food as 2 tablets (1200 mg) once a day for the first 4 days of treatment, and 1 tablet (600 mg) once a day for the remaining 6 days. (**e**) and (**f**) Fexinidazole treatment for adults (weighing ≥ 35 kg): each wallet contains 24 tablets (2 aluminum foil blisters of 12 tablets) to be taken once daily with food with 3 tablets (1800 mg) once a day for the first 4 days of treatment, and 2 tablets (1200 mg) once a day for the remaining 6 days [24].

Table 1. Summary of former treatments available for HAT before development of fexinidazole.

HAT Stage	Drug Name (Marketing Date)	Route, Dose	Comments
Stage 1	Pentamidine (1940)	Single IM dose of 4 mg/kg/day for 7 days (preferred) or IV injections	Skilled health workers, adverse events (metabolic disorders, pancreatitis, local abscesses), heavy treatment burden (for patients and families), parasite resistance. Effective in stage-1 g-HAT only
	Suramin (1920s)	Test dose then weekly IV injections for 5 weeks	Primarily for stage-1 r-HAT rarely used for g-HAT, adverse events (anaphylactic reactions, renal toxicity), heavy treatment burden (for patients and families)
Stage 2	NECT (2009)	Nifurtimox: 5 mg/kg PO every 8 h (15 mg/kg/day) for 10 days. Eflornithine: 200 mg/kg/day IV infusion every 12 h (400 mg/kg/day) for 7 days	Systematic hospitalization, skilled health workers, logistical concerns. First-line treatment for stage 2 g-HAT
	Eflornithine or DFMO (1990)	100 mg/kg/day IV infusion every 6 h (400 mg/kg/day) for 14 days	Systematic hospitalization, skilled health workers, long therapy, heavy treatment burden (for patients and families). Mainly used as a second-line treatment for stage-2 g-HAT
	Melarsoprol (1949)	2.2 mg/kg/day slow IV injection for 10 days	Highly toxic, painful, parasite resistance, skilled health workers. Restricted to cases refractory to NECT for stage-2 g-HAT. Remains the only drug effective in stage-2 r-HAT

Abbreviations: g-HAT, Human African Trypanosomiasis due to *T. b. gambiense*; IM, Intramuscular; IV, Intravenous; NECT, Nifurtimox-Eflornithine Combination Therapy; PO, Per Oral; r-HAT, Human African Trypanosomiasis due to *T. b. rhodesiense*.

Thus, the HAT Platform, supported by DND*i*, defined new target product profile characteristics for HAT treatments, namely for a safe treatment that was effective in both stages of HAT with the same dosing regimen and could avoid the need for systematic lumbar puncture for staging [25].

3. The Development of a New Oral Treatment for HAT: The Story of Fexinidazole

Fexinidazole is the first drug to be developed to fulfil this target product profile. This 5-nitroimidazole derivative DNA synthesis inhibitor [26] is the only, all-oral treatment for HAT and is indicated for use by adults and children (aged ≥ 6 years and weighing ≥ 20 kg) for both g-HAT stages [24,27]. The weight-based dose of fexinidazole (adults > 35 kg:1800 mg/d loading dose for 4 days and 1200 mg/d maintenance dose for 6 days; children aged ≥ 6 years and weighing ≥ 20 kg and <35 kg:1200 mg/d loading dose for 4 days and 600 mg/d maintenance dose for 6 days) is administered in the form of tablets to be taken once daily with food, with the treatment course being provided in the form of a simple wallet (Figure 2c–f) [24]. This revolutionary new treatment for HAT has the potential to transform disease management for both patients and healthcare workers [18,27,28]. As fexinidazole is effective for both disease stages, depending on the severity of the clinical signs, systematic lumbar puncture is no longer required for determination of the treatment strategy. Adherent patients, with adequate food intake, no psychiatric disorders or history of psychiatric disorders, or signs of advanced disease, can benefit from outpatient treatment administration under daily supervision by trained staff, reducing the risk of the disease having a major impact on their livelihood and daily activities, as well as those of their families. This simplified treatment regimen also has major benefits for healthcare infrastructure: fexinidazole is easy to store (<30 °C) and transport, and outpatient treatment will free-up vital resources for other health concerns [24,28].

3.1. The Rediscovery of Fexinidazole

Fexinidazole was developed over 15 years (illustrated in Figure 3), through partnership between Sanofi and the DND*i*, with clinical studies being conducted by investigators from endemic African nations coordinated by the NSSCP in the DRC, via support from the HAT Platform [29] and partners of the WHO global alliance initiative [9]. Shortly after its creation in 2003, the DND*i* began the search for a new oral treatment for HAT. The DND*i*'s expert group first identified nitroimidazoles, a group of compounds with known antiprotozoal activity, as a class to target in the search for a new HAT treatment. Among the reports identified was a review published by Raether and Hänel [30] on nitroheterocyclic compounds. One of the authors of the review (Prof. H. Hänel, Sanofi, Paris, France), working together with a representative of the DND*i* (Dr B. Bourdin Trunz), selected fexinidazole (designated HOE239) as a potential candidate for further development [31,32]. Prof. Hänel had conducted research on fexinidazole in the 1970s as a student working for Hoechst AG Frankfurt/Main in Germany (now part of Sanofi). It was one of several hundred compounds produced by Hoechst chemists between 1950 and 1980 as part of a project to identify antiprotozoal agents [32]. The project was abandoned in the 1980s due to changes in company strategy, but not before pre-clinical tests of fexinidazole showed that this agent displayed promising efficacy against *T. brucei* infections in mice, accompanied by good oral availability and toxicity profiles [33,34]. After an extensive search of the Hoechst archives, Prof. Hänel was able to provide detailed chemical synthesis, preclinical safety, efficacy and pharmacokinetic data for Fexinidazole, together with a few milligrams of the compound [32].

Fexinidazole was just one of over 700 nitroheterocyclic compounds evaluated and profiled as part of the mining exercise conducted in collaboration with the Swiss Tropical and Public Health institute (Swiss TPH, Basel, Switzerland). The positive pre-clinical profile obtained for fexinidazole [35] led, in 2009, to a new agreement between Sanofi and the DND*i* for the development of fexinidazole. Under the terms of this agreement, the DND*i* was responsible for preclinical, clinical and pharmaceutical development and Sanofi was responsible for the industrialization, production, registration and distribution of the drug [27,36].

3.2. Clinical Trials

The first in-human clinical trials involving fexinidazole began in 2009 [37]. These phase I studies were conducted in France in healthy males of African origin to assess the safety, tolerance and pharmacokinetic properties of fexinidazole, as well as bioavailability under different food intake conditions [27,37]. After consultation on the design of the clinical development plan with both the European Medicines Agency (EMA, Amsterdam, Netherlands)–under the article 58 procedure–and U.S. Food and Drug Administration (FDA, Silver Spring, Maryland,MD, USA), in the presence of WHO observers [38], the phase II/III clinical trials of fexinidazole began in 2012 (summarized in Table 2). The efficacy of fexinidazole in the treatment of g-HAT was demonstrated by a pivotal multicenter, randomized, open-label, phase II/III trial comparing fexinidazole and NECT in adult patients (aged ≥ 15 years) with late stage 2 g-HAT (DNDiFEX004; [18,39]). As its primary efficacy outcome, based on a predetermined acceptability margin for the difference in success rates between the two treatments of −13%, this trial showed that fexinidazole met the non-inferiority objective concerning treatment success rates at 18 months. After the end of treatment, success rates of >90% were observed for both agents (91.2% for fexinidazole and 97.6% for NECT). Two non-comparative, prospective, "plug-in" trials then reported treatment success rates of 98.7% 12 months after the end of treatment in a further cohort of stage 1 or early stage 2 adult (≥15 years) g-HAT patients (DNDiFEX005; [24,28]), and rates of 97.6% in children (aged 6–14 years) with any stage of g-HAT (DNDiFEX006; [24,28]). However, among stage 2 patients with baseline WBCs in the CSF of >100 /μL, the treatment success rate at 18 months was found to be lower with fexinidazole than with NECT (86.9% versus 98.7%, respectively) [24,28]. A further clinical trial (DNDiFEX09HAT) is currently ongoing to assess the efficacy and safety of fexinidazole in population groups not included in the previous trials (including pregnant or breastfeeding women, and patients with poor nutritional status or with chronic diseases) and include both patients treated in health centers and those treated in an outpatient setting [18,27,37].

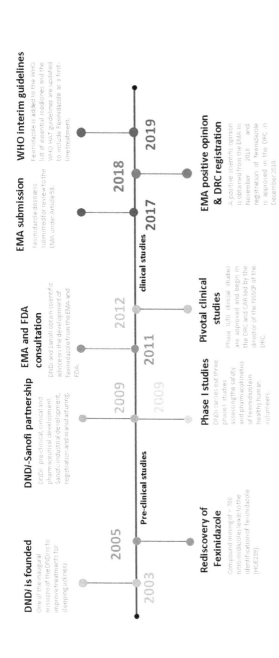

Figure 3. Timeline of the fexinidazole development project. DND*i*, Drugs for Neglected Diseases *initiative*; EMA, European Medicines Agency; FDA, Food and Drug Administration; DRC, Democratic Republic of Congo; CAR, Central African Republic; NSSCP, National Sleeping Sickness Control Program; WHO, World Health Organization; HAT, Human African Trypanosomiasis.

Table 2. Summary of phase II/III clinical trials evaluating the efficacy of fexinidazole in Human African Trypanosomiasis caused by *Trypanosoma brucei gambiense*.

Study Name, Designation, Phase and Duration	Study Description	Patients	Key Results
DNDiFEX004 NCT01685827 (II/III: 2012–2015)	Efficacy and safety of fexinidazole compared to NECT in patients (aged ≥ 15) with late stage 2 g-HAT: a pivotal, non-inferiority, multicenter, randomized, open-label study	394 (264 fexinidazole; 130 NECT)	Study confirms the efficacy of fexinidazole in late stage 2 g-HAT patients: success rate at 18 months post-treatment of 91.2% for fexinidazole, versus 97.6% for NECT within the margin of acceptable difference (97.06% CI −11.2 to −1.6; p = 0.0029). [18,39]
DNDiFEX005 NCT02169557 (II/III: 2014–2017)	Efficacy and safety of fexinidazole in patients (aged ≥ 15) with stage 1 or early stage 2 g-HAT: a prospective, multicenter, open-label and single arm cohort study, plug-in to the pivotal study	230	Studies confirm the efficacy of fexinidazole in stage-1 and early-stage-2 g-HAT patients: success rates in adults of 98.7% (95% CI [96.2%–99.7%]) and in children of 97.6% (95% CI [93.1%–99.5%]) at 12 months post-treatment. [24]
DNDiFEX006 NCT02184689 (II/III: 2014–2017)	Efficacy and safety of fexinidazole in children (≥6 years and <15; ≥20 kg) with g-HAT of any stage: a prospective, multicenter, open-label and single arm cohort study, plug-in to the pivotal study	125	
DNDiFEX09HAT NCT03025789 \(IIIb:2016–ongoing)	An open-label study assessing effectiveness, safety and compliance with fexinidazole in patients with g-HAT at any stage	174	Follow up ongoing [37]

Abbreviations: g-HAT, Human African Trypanosomiasis caused by *Trypanosoma brucei gambiense*; NECT, Nifurtimox–Eflornithine Combination Therapy; CI, Confidence Interval.

Fexinidazole treatment was well tolerated, particularly by patients with stage 1 disease, and pooled analysis of the safety data from the three clinical studies indicated that fexinidazole had an acceptable safety profile: the most common adverse events (AEs) considered as being related to fexinidazole were mild or moderate (vomiting, nausea, asthenia, decreased appetite, headache, insomnia, tremor, and dizziness) and only four serious AEs considered as possibly related to fexinidazole were reported (two reports of personality change, one of acute psychosis and one of hyponatremia) [24,27,28]. The pivotal clinical trial showed that there were no differences in the frequency of patients experiencing at least one AE between patients that received fexinidazole and those that received NECT (94% versus 93%, respectively) [39]. However, several of the most frequently observed treatment-emergent AEs occurred more commonly in the fexinidazole group than in the NECT group, including headache, insomnia, nausea, asthenia, tremor, and dizziness. Conversely, a lower proportion of patients taking fexinidazole than NECT experienced hyperkalemia, pyrexia, convulsions, and chills. Vomiting was reported in a similar percentage of patients in the fexinidazole (28.4%) and NECT groups (28.5%) [39]. With the exception of vomiting shortly after fexinidazole administration (20% of pediatric patients versus 6% of adult patients vomited within 30 min of drug intake), the safety profile of fexinidazole in the pediatric study population was similar that in adults [24].

The pivotal clinical trial was conducted at 10 sites in the DRC and Central African Republic (CAR) by African investigators under the guidance of the principal investigator and director of the NSSCP in the DRC, Dr V Kande ([39]; Figure 4). Extensive collaboration with partners of the HAT Platform, with support from the Swiss TPH and the Société Française et Francophone d'Éthique Médicale (SFFEM) were required to enable these clinical trials to be conducted in accordance with Good Clinical

Practice guidelines and international ethics standards [38]. This was achieved by strengthening the capacity and improving the infrastructure of local facilities in the often remote geographical regions of the DRC and CAR (Figure 4), resulting in the renovation and refurbishment of nine referral treatment units, training of over 200 researchers, monitors and practitioners (Table 3), and provision of support and training to active surveillance teams for the screening of over 2 million people in the DRC [40].

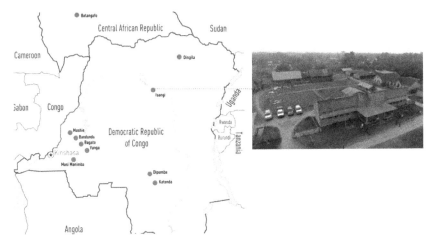

Figure 4. Locations of the 10 sites involved in the phase II/III clinical trials of fexinidazole led by the director of Le Programme National de Lutte contre la Trypanosomiase Humaine Africaine (PNLTHA). Inset: the Isangi clinical site along the Congo river in Democratic Republic of Congo.

Table 3. Strengthening the local capacity of clinical sites in remote regions of the Democratic Republic of Congo and the Central African Republic.

Infrastructure	• Renovation and refurbishment of 9 referral units in rural district hospitals • Provision of solar energy equipment and generators • Installation of Internet and satellite connections to transmit care report forms • Improvement of waste management
Supply of Equipment	• Medical equipment: oxygen concentrators, defibrillators, ECG devices etc. • Diagnostic equipment: microscopes, Piccolo analyzers etc. • Incinerators for waste management
Training of Staff	• Good Clinical Practice guidelines • Universal standard precautions • Laboratory diagnosis • Patient examination techniques and treatment procedures • Pharmacovigilance • Waste management

3.3. A Positive Opinion from the European Medicines Agency

The dossier was submitted to the EMA on the 14 December 2017, under Article 58 of (EC) No. Regulation 726/2004 which allows medicines intended for markets outside the European Union to be evaluated by the EMA in the context of collaboration with the WHO and other non-EU authorities, such as regulators from the endemic African nations [38,41]. On the 15 November 2018, fexinidazole gained a positive scientific opinion from the EMA as an oral monotherapy for the treatment of both stages of g-HAT at the same dosing regimen [27,38,41]. This positive opinion paves the way for applications for marketing authorization and registration of fexinidazole in endemic countries, and for its free distribution by the WHO under the global alliance agreement made with Sanofi covering all anti-HAT medicines [9,27,42].

The involvement of the WHO and regulators from the DRC and Uganda in the EMA submission process under article 58 has facilitated the registration process in these countries: fexinidazole was approved for use in the DRC in December 2019, an unprecedented time-scale [42]. The registration process in Uganda is also underway.

The positive scientific opinion from the EMA was followed by the inclusion of fexinidazole in the WHO List of Prequalified Medicinal Products by March 2019 and then in the WHO Model List of Essential Medicines that same year [43]. The WHO has also updated its guidelines for the treatment of g-HAT [5], recommending that the 10-day oral treatment with fexinidazole is used as the first-line treatment for g-HAT patients aged ≥ 6 years (weighing ≥ 20 kg) with the exception of patients with a WBC > 100/µL in the CSF after lumbar puncture performed due to clinical suspicion of severe stage 2 disease. These updated guidelines specified the need for medically supervised administration and monitoring to ensure adequate food intake. It was also noted that convenience for the patient and their family, development of side effects, existing comorbidities and the capacity of the healthcare system needed to be considered in the decision to administer fexinidazole on an outpatient basis. Hospitalization was deemed mandatory for patients with psychiatric disorders or a history of psychiatric disorders, those at risk of poor compliance to treatment, children under 35 kg, and patients with a WBC > 100/µL in the CSF exceptionally treated with fexinidazole [5].

Animal toxicity data from the regulatory preclinical studies indicated that fexinidazole did not have any direct or indirect harmful effects on reproductive function or teratogenicity at therapeutic doses [24]. As a precautionary measure, the use of fexinidazole should be avoided during the first trimester of pregnancy, and fexinidazole should be used during the second and third trimesters only if the potential benefits outweigh the potential risks to both the mother and the fetus [24]. As pharmacokinetic studies indicate that fexinidazole and its metabolites are excreted in breast milk, the benefits of therapy for the mother and the benefits of breastfeeding for the child need to be considered before initiating fexinidazole treatment [24]. A clinical trial is currently ongoing to further assess the efficacy and safety of fexinidazole in patients with g-HAT, including pregnant and breastfeeding women.

3.4. The Cost of Developing a New Chemical Entity

The DND*i* estimates the cost involved in the development of fexinidazole, from data mining activities in 2005 through to submission of the EMA dossier in 2018–2019, at 55 million Euros (Figure 5a) [40]. Donations from a range of partners also played a key role in funding this project, with around 31 million Euros being donated by the Bill & Melinda Gates Foundation, and around 25 million Euros being donated by the UK Department for International Development, other public donors, MSF and other private donors (Figure 5b). In addition, Sanofi estimates a further 13 million Euros has been spent on regulatory, human resource and industrial activities during the course of fexinidazole development. However, the value of many of the contributions involved in the development of this new treatment cannot be included in these figures, such as free access to Sanofi's assets and active pharmaceutical agents for trials, or the expertise and materials for research and development studies and product registration. The scale of the costs involved in the development of fexinidazole underscores the commitment undertaken by all the public and private partners that have supported the HAT elimination initiative, either through core funding or resources specifically earmarked for fexinidazole (Figure 5b), and highlights the true value of global collaboration to achieve this common goal.

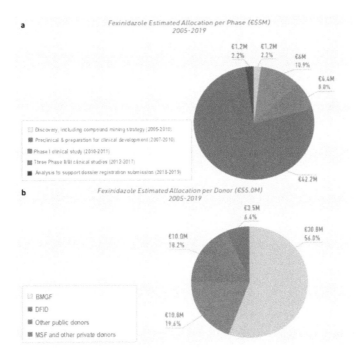

Figure 5. Estimated cost and funding of the fexinidazole development project. (**a**) Estimated allocation of funds per phase of development: 55 million Euros from 2005–2019. (**b**) Estimated allocation per donor. Donors: the Bill & Melinda Gates Foundation (BMGF, Seattle, WA, USA), the UK Department for International Development (DFID, London, UK), the Dutch Ministry of Foreign Affairs, the German Federal Ministry of Education and Research, the German Development Agency, the French Development Agency, the French Ministry of Foreign and European Affairs, the Norwegian Agency for Development Cooperation, the Spanish Agency for International Development Cooperation, the Republic and Canton of Geneva, Switzerland, the Swiss Agency for Development and Cooperation, Médecins Sans Frontières (MSF)/Doctors without Borders, Brian Mercer Charitable Trust, and other donors from the HAT campaign.

4. Conclusions

The resounding successes of the HAT elimination initiative and the fexinidazole development project are undoubtedly due to the strategy of global alliance and collaboration with highly dedicated and motivated individuals and organizations, and public and private collaborators. In forming an alliance to combat 21st century HAT epidemics, the HAT program and fexinidazole development project have demonstrated the effectiveness of public–private partnership in tackling global health issues. Furthermore, NSSCPs played a major role in both the control and surveillance program, and during the clinical phase of fexinidazole development, leaving behind a legacy of improved health and research infrastructure. Following on from the success of the fexinidazole program, similarly collaborative frameworks–involving private–public partnerships—are ongoing to further improve therapeutic options for g-HAT (for example, acoziborole [44]).

Main Partners: Amatsi Aquitaine (formerly Bertin Pharma), France; Aptuit, Italy; Biotral, France; Cardiabase, France; CBCO, DRC; Eurofins-Optimed, France; Institute of Tropical Medicine Antwerp, Belgium; Institut de Recherche pour le Développement, France; Institut National de Recherche Biomédicale (INRB), DRC; HAT Platform; National Control Programs of the Democratic Republic of Congo, the Central African Republic, and Guinea, Médecins Sans Frontières (Doctors without Borders); Phinc, France; Sanofi, France; SGS, Belgium; SGS, France; Swiss Tropical and Public Health Institute, Switzerland, and the World Health Organization NTD department.

Donors: The Bill & Melinda Gates Foundation (BMGF); the UK Department for International Development (DFID); the Dutch Ministry of Foreign Affairs (DGIS); the German Federal Ministry of Education and Research (BMBF) through KfW; the German international cooperation (GIZ); the French Development Agency (AFD); the French Ministry of Foreign and European Affairs (MEAE); the Norwegian Agency for Development Cooperation (Norad); the Spanish Agency for International Development Cooperation (AECID); the Republic and Canton of Geneva, Internal Solidarity Office, Switzerland; the Swiss Agency for Development and Cooperation (SDC), Médecins Sans Frontières (Doctors without Borders), Brian Mercer Charitable Trust, UK aid, UBS Optimus Foundation, Switzerland; Stavros Niarchos Foundation, USA and other private foundations and individual donors from the HAT campaign.

Author Contributions: All authors contributed to the preparation of this review. All authors have read and agreed to the published version of the manuscript.

Funding: Medical writing services were funded by Sanofi and provided by Emma Pilling and Marielle Romet (Santé Active Edition).

Conflicts of Interest: H.H., V.L., P.N., and L.K. are all employees of Sanofi. N.S. is an employee of DND*i*.

References

1. Drugs for Neglected Diseases Initiative. About Sleeping Sickness. Available online: https://www.dndi.org/diseases-projects/hat/ (accessed on 11 November 2019).
2. Franco, J.R.; Cecchi, G.; Priotto, G.; Paone, M.; Diarra, A.; Grout, L.; Simarro, P.P.; Zhao, W.; Argaw, D. Monitoring the elimination of human African trypanosomiasis: Update to 2016. *PLoS Negl. Trop. Dis.* **2018**, *12*, e0006890. [CrossRef]
3. Cecchi, G.; Paone, M.; Franco, J.R.; Fevre, E.M.; Diarra, A.; Ruiz, J.A.; Mattioli, R.C.; Simarro, P.P. Towards the Atlas of human African trypanosomiasis. *Int. J. Health Geogr.* **2009**, *8*, 15. [CrossRef]
4. Brun, R.; Blum, J.; Chappuis, F.; Burri, C. Human African trypanosomiasis. *Lancet* **2010**, *375*, 148–159. [CrossRef]
5. World Health Organization. WHO Interim Guidelines for the Treatment of Gambiense Human African Trypanosomiasis. 2019. Available online: https://www.who.int/trypanosomiasis_african/resources/9789241550567/en/ (accessed on 17 December 2019).
6. Checchi, F.; Funk, S.; Chandramohan, D.; Haydon, D.T.; Chappuis, F. Updated estimate of the duration of the meningo-encephalitic stage in gambiense human African trypanosomiasis. *BMC Res. Notes* **2015**, *8*, 292. [CrossRef] [PubMed]
7. WHO. Expert Committee on the Control and Surveillance of African Trypanosomiasis & World Health Organization. In *Control and Surveillance of African Trypanosomiasis: Report of A WHO Expert Committee*; WHO technical report series; World Health Organization: Geneva, Switzerland, 1998; p. 881.
8. World Health Organization. Resolutions and decisions, annexes. In Proceedings of the Fiftieth World Health Assembly, Geneva, Switzerland, 5–14 May 1997. Available online: https://apps.who.int/iris/handle/10665/179638 (accessed on 17 December 2019).
9. World Health Organization. WHO Programme to Eliminate Sleeping Sickness: Building A Global Alliance 2002. Available online: https://www.who.int/trypanosomiasis_african/resources/who_cds_csr_eph_2002.13/en/ (accessed on 17 December 2019).
10. World Health Organisation. WHO HAT Elimination Partners: Donors. Available online: https://www.who.int/trypanosomiasis_african/partners/partners_donors/en/ (accessed on 11 November 2019).
11. World Health Organisation. London Declaration on Neglected Tropical Diseases. Available online: https://www.who.int/neglected_diseases/London_Declaration_NTDs.pdf (accessed on 11 November 2019).
12. Franco, J.R.; Cecchi, G.; Priotto, G.; Paone, M.; Diarra, A.; Grout, L.; Mattioli, R.C.; Argaw, D. Monitoring the elimination of human African trypanosomiasis: Update to 2014. *PLoS Negl. Trop. Dis.* **2017**, *11*, e0005585. [CrossRef] [PubMed]
13. Simarro, P.P.; Cecchi, G.; Franco, J.R.; Paone, M.; Diarra, A.; Ruiz-Postigo, J.A.; Fevre, E.M.; Mattioli, R.C.; Jannin, J.G. Estimating and mapping the population at risk of sleeping sickness. *PLoS Negl. Trop. Dis.* **2012**, *6*, e1859. [CrossRef] [PubMed]
14. SANOFI. Fighting Negleted Tropical Diseases Factsheet. Available online: https://www.sanofi.com/.../Fighting_Neglected_Tropical_Diseases_2018.pdf (accessed on 11 November 2019).

15. World Health Organisation. Global Health Observatory Data Repository, Human African Trypanosomiasis. Available online: http://apps.who.int/gho/data/node.main.A1635 (accessed on 25 November 2019).

16. World Health Organization. *Control and Surveillance of Human African Trypanosomiasis: Report of A WHO Expert Committee*; WHO Technical Report Series; World Health Organization: Geneva, Switzerland, 2013; pp. 1–237.

17. Barrett, M.P. The elimination of human African trypanosomiasis is in sight: Report from the third WHO stakeholders meeting on elimination of gambiense human African trypanosomiasis. *PLoS Negl. Trop. Dis.* **2018**, *12*, e0006925. [CrossRef] [PubMed]

18. Chappuis, F. Oral fexinidazole for human African trypanosomiasis. *Lancet* **2018**, *391*, 100–102. [CrossRef]

19. Tong, J.; Valverde, O.; Mahoudeau, C.; Yun, O.; Chappuis, F. Challenges of controlling sleeping sickness in areas of violent conflict: Experience in the Democratic Republic of Congo. *Confl. Health* **2011**, *5*, 7. [CrossRef]

20. Yun, O.; Priotto, G.; Tong, J.; Flevaud, L.; Chappuis, F. NECT is next: Implementing the new drug combination therapy for Trypanosoma brucei gambiense sleeping sickness. *PLoS Negl. Trop. Dis.* **2010**, *4*, e720. [CrossRef]

21. Priotto, G.; Kasparian, S.; Mutombo, W.; Ngouama, D.; Gharashian, S.; Arnold, U.; Ghabri, S.; Baudin, E.; Buard, V.; Kazadi-Kyanza, S.; et al. Nifurtimox-eflornithine combination therapy for second-stage African Trypanosoma brucei gambiense trypanosomiasis: A multicentre, randomised, phase III, non-inferiority trial. *Lancet* **2009**, *374*. [CrossRef]

22. Babokhov, P.; Sanyaolu, A.O.; Oyibo, W.A.; Fagbenro-Beyioku, A.F.; Iriemenam, N.C. A current analysis of chemotherapy strategies for the treatment of human African trypanosomiasis. *Pathog. Glob. Health* **2013**, *107*, 242–252. [CrossRef] [PubMed]

23. Drugs for Neglected Diseases Initiative. NECT Dossier. Available online: https://www.dndi.org/achievements/nect/ (accessed on 11 November 2019).

24. Sanofi. *Summary of Product Characteristics: Fexinidazole Winthrop 600 mg Tablets*; Sanofi-Aventis Groupe: Paris, France, 2019.

25. Drugs for Neglected Diseases Initiative. Target Product Profile—Sleeping Sickness. Available online: https://www.dndi.org/diseases-projects/hat/hat-target-product-profile/ (accessed on 11 November 2019).

26. Patterson, S.; Wyllie, S. Nitro drugs for the treatment of trypanosomatid diseases: Past, present, and future prospects. *Trends Parasitol.* **2014**, *30*, 289–298. [CrossRef] [PubMed]

27. Deeks, E.D. Fexinidazole: First Global Approval. *Drugs* **2019**, *79*, 215–220. [CrossRef]

28. Deeks, E.D.; Lyseng-Williamson, K.A. Fexinidazole in human African trypanosomiasis: A profile of its use. *Drugs Ther. Perspect.* **2019**, *35*, 529–535. [CrossRef]

29. Drugs for Neglected Diseases Initiative. Human African Trypanosomiasis (HAT) Platform. Available online: https://www.dndi.org/strengthening-capacity/hat-platform/ (accessed on 11 November 2019).

30. Raether, W.; Hanel, H. Nitroheterocyclic drugs with broad spectrum activity. *Parasitol. Res.* **2003**, *90* (Suppl. S1), S19–S39. [CrossRef]

31. Sanofi. Sleeping Sickness: Providing Hope for the Forgotten. *Connectome* **2011**, *2*, 5.

32. Hänel, H.; (Sanofi-Aventis Deutschland, Frankfurt am Main, Germany). Personal Communication, 2019.

33. Jennings, F.W.; Urquhart, G.M. The use of the 2 substituted 5-nitroimidazole, fexinidazole (Hoe 239) in the treatment of chronic *T. brucei* infections in mice. *Zeitschrift für Parasitenkunde* **1983**, *69*, 577–581. [CrossRef]

34. Raether, W.; Seidenath, H. The activity of fexinidazole (HOE 239) against experimental infections with *Trypanosoma cruzi*, trichomonads and *Entamoeba histolytica*. *Ann. Trop. Med. Parasitol.* **1983**, *77*, 13–26. [CrossRef]

35. Torreele, E.; Bourdin Trunz, B.; Tweats, D.; Kaiser, M.; Brun, R.; Mazue, G.; Bray, M.A.; Pecoul, B. Fexinidazole—A new oral nitroimidazole drug candidate entering clinical development for the treatment of sleeping sickness. *PLoS Negl. Trop. Dis.* **2010**, *4*, e923. [CrossRef]

36. Drugs for Neglected Diseases Initiative. *European Medicines Agency Recommends Fexinidazole, the First All-Oral Treatment for Sleeping Sickness*; [press release]; Drugs for Neglected Diseases Initiative: Geneva, Switzerland, 2018.

37. Drugs for Neglected Diseases Initiative. Clinical Trials. Available online: https://www.dndi.org/category/clinical-trials/ (accessed on 11 November 2019).

38. *European Medicines Agency Assessment Report: Fexinidazole Winthrop 2018*; European Medicines Agency: London, UK, 2018.

39. Mesu, V.; Kalonji, W.M.; Bardonneau, C.; Mordt, O.V.; Blesson, S.; Simon, F.; Delhomme, S.; Bernhard, S.; Kuziena, W.; Lubaki, J.F.; et al. Oral fexinidazole for late-stage African *Trypanosoma brucei gambiense* trypanosomiasis: A pivotal multicentre, randomised, non-inferiority trial. *Lancet* **2018**, *391*, 144–154. [CrossRef]

40. Drugs for Neglected Diseases Initiative. Achievements: Fexinidazole. Available online: https://www.dndi.org/achievements/fexinidazole/ (accessed on 11 November 2019).

41. Pelfrene, E.; Harvey Allchurch, M.; Ntamabyaliro, N.; Nambasa, V.; Ventura, F.V.; Nagercoil, N.; Cavaleri, M. The European Medicines Agency's scientific opinion on oral fexinidazole for human African trypanosomiasis. *PLoS Negl. Trop. Dis.* **2019**, *13*, e0007381. [CrossRef] [PubMed]

42. Drugs for Neglected Diseases Initiative. *Fexinidazole, the First All-Oral Treatment for Sleeping Sickness, Approved in Democratic Republic of Congo*; [press release]; Drugs for Neglected Diseases Initiative: Geneva, Switzerland, 2019.

43. World Health Organization. WHO Model Lists of Essential Medicines, 21st List 2019. Available online: https://www.who.int/medicines/publications/essentialmedicines/en/ (accessed on 17 December 2019).

44. Drugs for Neglected Diseases Initiative. Acoziborole. Available online: https://www.dndi.org/diseases-projects/portfolio/acoziborole/ (accessed on 18 December 2019).

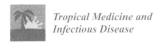
Tropical Medicine and
Infectious Disease

MDPI

Article

How Clinical Research Can Contribute to Strengthening Health Systems in Low Resource Countries

Florent Mbo [1,2,*], Wilfried Mutombo [3], Digas Ngolo [2], Patrice Kabangu [2], Olaf Valverde Mordt [4], Nathalie Strub Wourgaft [4] and Erick Mwamba [2]

[1] HAT Platform, Drugs for Neglected Diseases initiative, Avenue Milambo, N 4, Quartier Socimat, Gombe, Kinshasa 7948, Democratic Republic of Congo
[2] Le Programme Nationale de Lutte contre la Trypanosomiase Humaine Africaine (PNLTHA), croisement du Boulevard Triomphal avec l'avenue de la Libération, Commune de Kasa-Vubu, Kinshasa 7948, Democratic Republic of Congo; dngolo@dndi.org (D.N.); pkabangu@dndi.org (P.K.); erickmwamb2002@yahoo.fr (E.M.)
[3] Drugs for Neglected Diseases initiative (DNDi), Avenue Milambo, N 4, Quartier Socimat, Gombe, Kinshasa 7948, Democratic Republic of Congo; wmutombo@dndi.org
[4] Drugs for Neglected Diseases initiative, 15 Chemin Louis-Dunant, 1202 Geneva, Switzerland; ovalverde@dndi.org (O.V.M.); nstrub@dndi.org (N.S.W.)
* Correspondence: fmbo@dndi.org; Tel.: +243814313838

Received: 31 January 2020; Accepted: 20 March 2020; Published: 29 March 2020

Abstract: Clinical research on neglected tropical diseases is a challenge in low-resource countries, and the contribution of clinical and operational research to health system strengthening is poorly documented. Developing new, simple, safe, and effective treatments may improve the effectiveness of health systems, and conducting research directly in health structures may have an additional impact. This study describes the process of conducting clinical trials in the Democratic Republic of Congo (DRC) in compliance with international standards, and the role of the trials in strengthening health system functions, including governance, human resources, health information, provision of care, and the equipping of health services with the necessary supplies and infrastructure. We conclude that conducting clinical trials in endemic areas has not only reinforced and supported the aim of conducting high-level clinical research in endemic countries, but has also brought lasting benefits to researchers, staff, and hospitals, as well as to broader health systems, which have positive knock-on effect on patients outside of the clinical trials and their communities. Sustainability, however, remains a challenge in an underfunded health system, especially with respect to specialized equipment. Clinical research in most of sub-Saharan Africa is highly dependent on international input and external technical support; there are areas of weaknesses in trial design and documentation, as well as in data management and analysis. Financing remains a critical issue, as African investigators have difficulties in directly accessing sources of international research funding.

Keywords: human African trypanosomiasis; clinical research; health system strengthening

---

1. Introduction

The scientific and social value of research can be difficult to quantify, but it is generally based on three factors:

- the quality of the information produced;
- its relevance to significant health problems;
- its contribution to the creation or evaluation of interventions, policies, or practices that promote individual or public health.

Research needs to show that it is responding to needs or priorities by demonstrating that new knowledge will be generated about the best ways to address a pathology present in the target community. It is possible to measure the impact of health system improvements brought to patients and their communities when clinical trials are conducted in low-resource settings [1].

The Council for International Organizations of Medical Sciences/World Health Organization International Ethical Guidelines for Health-related Research Involving Humans states that for health-related research involving humans to be ethically justified, there must be the prospect of generating knowledge and the means necessary to protect and promote people's health. After successful completion of clinical research, the introduction of a new treatment into general practice may significantly increase the effectiveness of the health system itself. This is particularly true in the field of neglected tropical diseases, which is classified as "tool-deficient" and in need of well-adapted simpler, safer, and/or more effective treatments [2].

Human African trypanosomiasis (HAT) is a neglected tropical disease, predominating in remote areas of Africa where health services are sometimes deficient or poorly equipped. When communities or policymakers identify research on new treatment tools as a public health priority, plans for clinical trials to address this particular need should aim to bring social value to the affected population, and thus respond to broader health needs [1]. The degree to which this will be possible will depend on the relevance of the information that the study is intended to produce for the community in addition to the introduction of specialized training, equipment, and supplies. This approach adds value to the direct justification for the conduct of clinical trials for treatments for HAT. Managers of the national sleeping sickness control program and their research partners in endemic countries determined the target product profile for a new drug for HAT treatment in response to information gathered through interviews with physicians, technicians on the ground, and mobile teams who had experienced serious adverse reactions associated with the use of Melasoprol, such as encephalopathy. The review process, starting from a draft proposed by Drugs for Neglected Diseases initiative (DND*i*), involved two rounds of discussion in a general scientific meeting, followed by a restricted meeting in which each proposed product quality was debated and agreed on by the participants.

Benefits other than those directly associated with participation in the study may be devolved to communities or populations, particularly in low-resource settings. These benefits include improved health infrastructure, trained laboratory personnel, and education of the public about the nature of the research and the benefits of a study. Clinical trials on treatments for HAT also contribute to improvements in management by virtue of staff training and equipping the hospitals involved. [1]

Sleeping sickness was historically managed separately within a strong vertical system, which was separated from the often-underfunded and ill-equipped general health service. The focus of the clinical trials is to address the primary need for developing simplified tools. Integrating NTD care into the general health system is a long process that risks a loss of quality unless the structures and staff are reinforced and supported. As clinical trials are limited in time, this process needs to concentrate on improving the capacity of health staff and providing adequate means for them to perform their roles.

The objective of this work is to examine the contribution made by clinical trials to strengthen the health services involved and the various components of the health system in general, namely, governance, human resources, health information, equipment, and the provision of care. By examining clinical trial site activities, skill levels, and procedures after the end of the trials, we determined the impact on routine health care of the extensive support given outside of specific trial activities and were able to observe any improvements.

2. Materials and Methods

We analyzed the contribution of HAT clinical trials in terms of the six health system pillars, focusing on activities conducted during studies in the DRC. The World Health Organization (WHO) conceptual framework approaches the health system as a six-pillar package [3] in Figure 1:

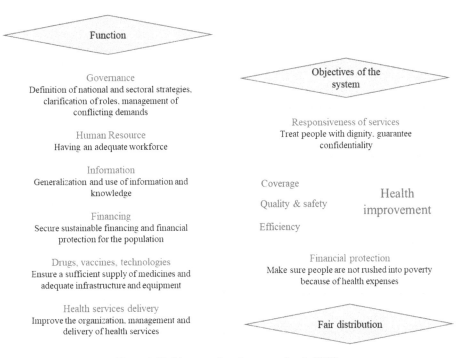

Figure 1. Health system functions according to WHO.

Within this framework, the health system is strengthened by acting on its six pillars in order to improve health services and the health of the population in a sustainable and equitable way. A global vision is needed, and action must be taken in a balanced way to avoid compromising any successes [3].

3. Results

3.1. Leadership and Governance

A consultation organized by WHO in 2007 found that leadership and management capacities are currently inadequate in both the private and public sectors and that few low-income countries are concerned with systematic management issues [4]. For these clinical trials, capacity was built in terms of training and further coaching all members of the research team. The study's national coordinating team solicited the commitment of provincial and local health authorities not to move staff who were involved in the clinical trials.

3.2. Human Resources

To be effective, a health system must have a critical mass of human and material resources. This resource gap is particularly keenly felt when it comes to human capital—the cornerstone of a successful health system [3]. Staff (doctors, nurses, and laboratory technicians) from 10 hospitals participated in the fexinidazole study (Bandundu, Mushie, Bagata, Vanga, Masimanimba, Dipumba, Katanda, Isangi, Dingila, and Batangafo in Central African Republic(CAR). The staff involved in the clinical trials were trained on good clinical and laboratory practice as well as on hospital waste management and universal standard precautions, in accordance with the international standards required for clinical trials. In collaboration with the HAT Platform (a clinical research and access-supporting network that brings together key regional actors involved in the control of HAT in endemic countries, notably ministries of health, national control programs, regulatory agencies, academia, clinicians,

WHO, and NGOs), clinical or operational trials have also contributed to capacity building in endemic countries through the training of researchers, monitors, and practitioners on good clinical practice, laboratory diagnosis, pharmacovigilance, and patient examination techniques, including specific testing techniques. Since the creation of the HAT platform in 2005, more than 400 people have been trained in Africa in 22 training sessions with the support of universities and other African and foreign research institutions [5]. Table 1 shows the different training sessions organized in order to support clinical trials within the health service, both for the fexinidazole trials, with which this paper is primarily interested, and also for previous trials dating from 2006.

Table 1. The number of training sessions and people trained as part of HAT clinical trials since 2006 [5].

Trainings Conducted (Number of People Trained)	Venue and Year
Training in ethical review of research (142)	Kinshasa 2007 Khartoum 2007 Kampala 2007 Luanda 2008 Juba 2009 Bangui 2010
Training of physicians in good clinical practice (GCP) (96)	Nairobi 2006, Kinshasa 2011 and 2012, Juba 2012
Training of physicians on clinical examination of the patient (25)	Kinshasa 2007
Training of clinical monitors (13)	Kampala 2008
Participation at ICAT6 and -7 (26)	Kinshasa 2014, Kampala 2017
HAT training in Dinamadji health district (30)	Dinamadji 2015
HAT clinical training in South Sudan (41)	Juba 2015
Training of Guinean physician in DRC (1)	Kinshasa 2014
Training of laboratory technicians from South Sudan in DRC (3)	Kinshasa 2016
Training of mobile team technicians on HAT diagnosis in DRC (36)	Kinshasa 2016
Waste management training at clinical trial sites in DRC (182)	Mushie, Vanga, Bagata, Masi 2016

Regular supervision was carried out in the test sites, which resulted in an improvement in the quality of care. During these supervisions, each provider was assessed using an evaluation grid. If the nurse under assessment failed 20 percent or more of the tasks in question, they then received additional training and practical support.

3.3. Organization of Services

Even when the necessary input and enough financial support are provided, failures in service provision occur, which are often due to the dysfunctional organization of the health system [6]. Both the overall configuration of health systems and the structure of service delivery need to be addressed. For the HAT trials, the research team established a work structure with tasks for each professional category from the local investigator, nurses, and laboratory technicians to the on-duty cleaner. Training, supervision, and monitoring visits to the field research teams made it possible to improve the organization of the health service not only within the research teams but also in other departments of the hospitals involved. External monitoring and supervision were performed by a team from the Swiss Tropical and Public Health Institute.

3.4. Organization of Health Information

Health information is vital for decision-making and the monitoring and evaluation of the performance of the health system. In the HAT trials, research teams were reminded of the importance of documentation at all levels (investigators, nurses, and laboratory technicians) with the key maxim:

"If it isn't written down, it doesn't exist". The archiving of study subjects' case report files was improved by means of the visits conducted by the clinical monitors and the information, education, and communication systems facilitated by the trial clinical coordination team based in Kinshasa.

3.5. Material Resources

To be efficient, a health system must have a critical mass of material resources [3]. The trials were planned at existing treatment centers in the most endemic areas. Given the limitations of the health system in DRC, each center was assessed to determine its specific material needs so that adequate conditions for conducting a clinical trial could be guaranteed. Material needs were met by providing food, guaranteeing accommodation, and facilitating personal hygiene for staff and patients. Adequate office space for the research team and trial documentation was provided, as was waste management, energy, and communication equipment. Laboratories were refurbished (Table 2). The overall cost of preparing a single hospital for the clinical trial varied between USD 20,000 and 100,000, depending on the different needs of the sites; some had recently been rehabilitated, and others were located in cities with electricity and water supplies.

Table 2. List of material needs for the improvement of clinical trial sites and how these needs were addressed.

Material Need.	Provision
Food	Provided for all HAT patients, irrespective of trial participation
Accommodation	Beds repaired or purchased; new mattresses and mosquito nets; dedicated wards repainted; floors, windows repaired
Personal hygiene	Latrines and shower blocks built; water supply arranged, including rainwater reservoirs, for the benefit of staff and patients
Office space	A nursing room, investigator's office, lockable cupboards, and furniture were provided for the research team and trial documentation
Waste management	A closed waste disposal area with three separated pits was provided or improved; incinerators were built or rehabilitated
Laboratory space	Refurbishment through rebuilding of interiors, including working surfaces and necessary equipment
Energy	Generators and solar systems for lightning, electric equipment, and a cold chain were provided.
Communication equipment	Computers, printers, internet access, and telephone cards were provided

Medical equipment such as defibrillators, tools such as the PiccoloXpress analyzer (an easy-to-use fully automated system for biochemistry blood testing), and sophisticated laboratories was supplied. Internet access allowed for the transmission of case report forms, which are essential for monitoring safety parameters, including distance reading of ECG. This has helped to improve the overall care environment in the health structures involved [7]. These improvements in infrastructure supported or sustained other activities after the end of the studies. The introduction of a microscope with a video-camera in all study structures has enabled the storing of information about HAT cases, given that the best way to identify the mobile parasites is usually in fresh samples that cannot be physically stored. This microscope, together with the archiving computer program that allows for quick transmission of the images taken, plays a very important role in quality assessment and for the training of new staff. After the end of the HAT trials, this equipment may be used for the detection of other endemic diseases, such as malaria.

3.6. Funding

Countries in the African region are facing enormous difficulties in terms of health financing. Financial resources are inadequate, poorly managed, not strategically allocated, and not well-coordinated with what is provided by external sources [8]. The investigators were trained and supported in the efficient management of the funds placed at their disposal. Most of the HAT trial sites used the training to improve financial management and staffing of their respective hospitals. Funding was important for these trials, not only for improving the general clinical trial site environment, but also in terms of supervision visits and monitoring of field research teams who require significant logistical resources (boat, motorcycle, vehicles), and for the referral of patients who often live far from the trial sites. When providing new equipment, caution was taken to provide goods with low maintenance costs. However, it was not feasible to use the biochemistry analyzer after the trial, due to the high individual cost of the reagent discs. Instead, it was recovered after the end of the trials for use where there was external support, including in other clinical trials (Table 3).

Table 3. Cost of the main material resources provided to a model hospital.

Items	Unit Cost in USD (Euro Converted at USD 1.1)
Rehabilitation Works	
Preparation and construction of waste areas	USD 10,150
Latrine and shower construction	USD 8730
Rainwater collection system	USD 5000
Preparation of investigators' offices	USD 750
Lab preparation for routine exams	USD 17,500
5kva solar panels	USD 21,000
Medical Equipment	
Pavilion equipment with 12 beds	USD 1800
Foldable examination table	USD 164
Mechanical weight and height scale	USD 227
Life support equipment	USD 2443
Emergency bag kit	USD 811
Laboratory Equipment	
Microscopes with Camera	USD 3470
8-tube electric centrifuges	USD 1122
Electric Hematocrit Centrifuges	USD 1467
HemoCue Hb 301	USD 548
Eppendorf'' automatic pipette	USD 242
Cold Chain	
Vestfrost refrigerator	USD 895
Cold chain (Freezer + specific solar panels + batteries)	USD 24,074
Transport and Office Equipment	
Motorbike Yamaha AG100	USD 4600
Laptop	USD 1000
Internet connection kit	USD 2760
Printer, scanner, photocopier	USD 300

4. Discussion

Most African countries face challenges related to material and human resources, health information, health financing, and the organization of service delivery. A sector-wide approach (SWAp), reported in six countries (Ghana, Malawi, Mozambique, Tanzania, Uganda, and Zambia), has been taken as an example of how to face the challenge of strengthening health systems and health system reform [3].

For the future, there are political opportunities, both in countries and regional bodies, as well as opportunities for international and technical partnerships [3]. There are opportunities for clinical and operational research within health services of low- and middle-income countries, enabling them to capitalize as much as possible on decisive progress in strengthening health systems [3].

We here describe a case study on the impact of clinical trials on the strengthening of health services, using the WHO pillar framework. These trials on fexinidazole for HAT were conducted by the Drugs for Neglected Diseases initiative (DND*i*) between 2012 and 2017 in collaboration with the Ministry of Health of DRC and Central African Republic, through their Sleeping Sickness National Control Programs. These clinical trials took place in 10 hospitals in 5 provinces of the DRC (Kwilu, Maï-Ndombe, Kasaï Oriental, Tshopo, and Bas-Uélé) and one site in Batangafo, Central African Republic. The results of the main study have been published in The Lancet [9].

In addition to the stated aim of developing trypanocidal drugs, several pillars of the health system were strengthened before and during clinical trials, improving the provision of services to populations living in rural areas or HAT endemic villages where the health system is deficient. The training enabled the investigating physicians, laboratory technicians, and nurses to systematically examine the health problems of the target population, to take better care of the patients included in the study, including those with problems other than sleeping sickness. Provision of additional technical equipment helped with the care of other patients not included in clinical trials, and the use of new diagnostic tools improved levels of trust for medical staff amongst patients.

Watson Tawaba, a nurse in a clinical trial site in the DRC said: "With the clinical trial on fexinidazole, everything has changed. Not only does our hospital no longer look like a farm, but the community benefits from a modern facility, and our work is easier" [10].

In the former Bandundu province in DRC, hospital staff involved in HAT clinical trials have increased the capacity of staff at other rural hospitals not involved in clinical trials in terms of patient record-keeping and the execution of nursing techniques such as venous catheterization, as reported by the North Bandundu Trypanosomiasis Coordination (2009–2012, unpublished report). Prior to the HAT trials, trypanosomiasis unit nurses in one of the clinical trial sites would request support from pediatric nurses for the venous catheterization of patients. After training in the introduction of venous catheters, the research team nurses began to assist their pediatric colleagues in the placement of venous catheters in children and in the handling of resuscitation devices or oxygen concentrators.

The research teams have become an example within their hospitals because they have been well-trained. For remaining staff who were not involved in the study, there is still a long way to go before the improved diagnostic tools, standard precautions, and evidence-based medical care, including careful attention to the patient's clinical evolution, are strictly implemented in the hospitals.

The goal of the training was for clinical trial teams to be able to include, treat, and follow patients in accordance with protocol (goal achievement). The investigators had to adapt to the rules and principles that clinical trials impose (adaptation to the research environment) and maintain the functionality of the health facilities (organizational culture).

Using the impact analysis framework in Figure 2, we found that the HAT clinical study was successful because it considered the dynamic balance of all functions [11].

In these clinical trials, patients with HAT were recruited according to inclusion and exclusion criteria after obtaining informed consent. These patients were diagnosed either by hospitals involved in clinical trials or by mobile teams who actively screen at-risk populations in endemic villages to identify patients who were subsequently referred to clinical trial sites. In 2016–2017, DRC's Programme National de Lutte contre la Trypanosomiase Humaine Africaine (PNLTHA) mobile screening teams, supported by DND*i*, which were active around trypanocidal drug trial sites, examined one-third of the 2 million people examined annually nationwide. A strengthening of the current network of passive screening set up by the PNLTHA around clinical trials research centers is underway. This measure should not only makes it possible to identify additional patients for clinical trials but also to create a passive surveillance system for the sustainable elimination of trypanosomiasis [7].

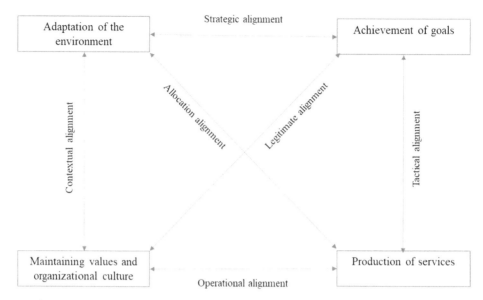

Figure 2. Four functional systems of health care organizations and their six interchange subsystems [11].

5. Conclusions

DND*i*'s experience of conducting clinical trials in collaboration with the national sleeping sickness program in the DRC through the support of the HAT platform has shown that it is possible to create an enabling environment in an endemic country for the conduct of quality clinical trials. Conducting clinical trials in endemic areas has not only reinforced and supported the aim of strengthening high-level clinical research, but has also brought lasting benefits to researchers, staff, and hospitals, as well as to broader health systems. This has a positive knock-on effect on patients outside of the clinical trials and their communities because clinical trial physicians and nurses or lab technicians have shared their new knowledge and experience in governance, GCP, and waste management with staff in their own and other hospitals [7].

When planning to set up this clinical trial, the epidemiology of the target disease was assessed, and this information was used to direct the process of site selection. The trial was conducted in existing health structures that were already treating patients, which facilitated trial execution. Adequate material resources and technologies were needed to ensure that the trial could be conducted up to international research standards and fulfill the requirements of good clinical practice. The sustainability of the improvements after the end of the trial depends mainly on infrastructure improvements, added knowledge, and improved staff practices. The sustainability of equipment depends on the ability of local health services to fund maintenance and consumables; it was not feasible to maintain the biochemistry machine PiccoloXpress®, but other simple laboratory techniques that were introduced will certainly remain. Standard hygiene precautions and waste management require continuous supervisory input, and sustainability will depend on the motivation of the staff and the leadership at each structure.

Clinical research in most of sub-Saharan Africa remains very dependent on international input and external technical support, especially in the HAT-endemic countries of central Africa. Although efforts are being made to build capacity and infrastructure, weak points remain in terms of trial design and documentation, as well as data management and analysis. Financing is a critical issue, as African investigators find it difficult to directly access international research funding sources and rely on international partnerships.

Author Contributions: Conceptualization, F.M. and N.S.W.; Methodology, F.M.; Validation, O.V.M. and N.S.W.; Formal Analysis, F.M.; Investigation, F.M., W.M., D.N., and P.K.; Resources, E.M.; Writing—Original Draft Preparation, F.M.; Writing—Review and Editing, all; Supervision, E.M.; Project Administration, F.M.; Funding Acquisition, N.S.W. All authors have read and agreed to the published version of the manuscript.

Funding: The Drugs for Neglected Diseases initiative (DND*i*) is grateful to its donors, public and private, who have provided funding to DND*i* since its inception in 2003. A full list of DND*i*'s donors can be found at http://www.dndi.org/donors/donors/.

Acknowledgments: We extend our thanks to the team at the DND*i* offices in DRC and Switzerland and thank the DRC PNLTHA team for their contributions. We also thank Louise Burrows (DND*i*) for help with editing the manuscript.

Conflicts of Interest: The authors declare no conflict of interest.

References

1. CIOMS/WHO. *International Ethical Guidelines for Health-Related Research Involving Humans*; World Health Organization: Geneva, Switzerland, 2016.
2. Hotez, P.J.; Pecoul, B. "Manifesto" for Advancing the Control and Elimination of Neglected Tropical Diseases. *PLoS Negl. Trop. Dis.* **2010**, *4*, e718. [CrossRef]
3. Amidou, B.; Saidou Pathé, B.; Kandjoura, D. Renforcement des systèmes de santé dans les pays de la région africaine de l'OMS: Répondre au défi. *Afr. Health Monit.* **2012**, *14*, 4–13. Available online: http://afrolib.afro.who.int/index.php?lvl=notice_display&id=29235 (accessed on 4 March 2020).
4. WHO. *Renforcer la Gestion Dans Les Pays à Faible Revenu, Document de Travail No. 1*; WHO/EIP: Geneva, Switzerland, 2005.
5. Mbo, F.; Valverde, O. The human African trypanosomiasis (HAT) platform. In *Trop Med International Health, Proceedings of the 10th ECTMIH, Antwerp, Belgium, 11–19 October 2017*; John Wiley & Sons Ltd.: Hoboken, NJ, USA, 2017; Volume 22, (Suppl. S1), pp. 115–345.
6. WHO. *Rapport Mondial sur la Santé Dans le Monde 2000: Pour un Système de Santé Performant*; World Health Organization: Geneva, Switzerland, 2000.
7. Valverde, O. Impact des études cliniques visant à développer des médicaments trypanocides sur les efforts d'élimination de la maladie. In Proceedings of the 4th Joint HAT Platform-EANETT Scientific Meeting, Conakry, Guinea, 16 September 2016. Available online: https://tinyurl.com/syc5637 (accessed on 17 March 2020).
8. WHO. *La Santé Des Populations—Rapport Sur la Santé Dans la Région Africaine*; OMS, Bureau régional de l'Afrique: Brazzaville, Congo, 2006.
9. Mesu, V.K.B.K.; Kalonji, W.M.; Bardonneau, C.; Mordt, O.V.; Blesson, S.; Sc, F.S.; Delhomme, S.; Bernhard, S.; Kuziena, W.; Med, J.-P.F.L.M.; et al. Oral fexinidazole for late-stage African *Trypanosoma brucei gambiense* trypanosomiasis: A pivotal multicentre, randomised, non-inferiority trial. *Lancet* **2018**, *391*, 144–154. [CrossRef]
10. Drugs for Neglected Diseases Initiative. Available online: https://www.dndi.org/strengthening-capacity/hat-platform/ (accessed on 16 January 2020).
11. Sicotte, C.; Champagne, F.; Contandriopoulos, A.P.; Barnsley, J.; Béland, F.; Leggat, S.G.; Denis, J.L.; Bilodeau, H.; Langley, A.; Brémond, M.; et al. A conceptual framework for the analysis of health care organizations' performance. *Health Serv. Manag. Res.* **1998**, *11*, 24–41. [CrossRef] [PubMed]

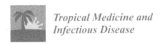

Tropical Medicine and Infectious Disease

Article

Centering Patient Expectations of a Novel Home-Based Oral Drug Treatment among *T. b. rhodesiense* Human African Trypanosomiasis Patients in Uganda

Shona J Lee [1,*], Renah J Apio [2] and Jennifer J Palmer [1,3]

1   Department of Global Health & Development, London School of Hygiene and Tropical Medicine, Keppel Street, London WC1H 9SH, UK; jennifer.palmer@lshtm.ac.uk
2   Dokolo Health Centre, Dokolo, Uganda; apiojanetrenah9@gmail.com
3   Centre of African Studies, University of Edinburgh, 15a George Square, Edinburgh EH8 9LD, UK
*   Correspondence: shona.lee@lshtm.ac.uk; Tel.: +44-77060-46495

Received: 2 December 2019; Accepted: 13 January 2020; Published: 21 January 2020

Abstract: The recent approval of fexinidazole for human African trypanosomiasis (HAT) caused by *T. b. gambiense* enables improved patient management that is pivotal to elimination. Effective in both the early and late stages of the disease, it obviates the need for invasive lumbar punctures which guide therapy, in some patients. Unlike existing injectable treatments requiring systematic hospitalisation, fexinidazole's oral administration will allow many patients to be treated in an outpatient or home-based setting. Drawing on interviews with 25 *T. b. rhodesiense* HAT patients managed under existing protocols in Uganda where trials of fexinidazole will begin shortly, this article explores patient expectations of the new protocol to help HAT programmes anticipate patient concerns. Alongside frightening symptoms of this life-threatening illness, the pain and anxiety associated with lumbar punctures and intravenous injections of melarsoprol contributed to a perception of HAT as a serious illness requiring expert medical care. While preferring a new protocol that would avoid these uncomfortable procedures, patients' trust in the care they received meant that nearly half were hesitant towards shifting care out of the hospital setting. Clinical observation is an important aspect of existing HAT care for patients. Programmes may need to offer extensive counselling and monitoring support before patients are comfortable accepting care outside of hospitals.

Keywords: human Africa trypanosomiasis; fexinidazole; home-based treatment; patient-centred care; Uganda; elimination

1. Introduction

The recent regulatory approval of fexinidazole for the treatment of human African Trypanosomiasis (HAT, also known as sleeping sickness) caused by the most common, *T. b. gambiense* form, has been hailed as a "big step toward the gradual elimination of this disease from sub-Saharan Africa" [1]. The World Health Organisation (WHO) added fexinidazole to the Essential Medicines List for treatment of *gambiense* HAT, following successful clinical trials in the Democratic Republic of Congo (DRC) and Central African Republic [2]. Apart from the adoption of a shorter and safer dosing schedule for melarsoprol in 2010 [3,4], patients suffering from *T. b. rhodesiense* HAT have benefitted little from wider efforts to reform HAT treatment since the early 1980s [5–11]. Trials to test fexinidazole's efficacy against *rhodesiense* HAT, however, are also currently underway in Malawi and about to begin in Uganda [12]. Fexinidazole, a nitroimidazole treatment that can be taken orally once a day for 10 days [11–13], in many ways simplifies HAT treatment regimens, enabling new forms of patient management.

One simplification relates to the use of invasive lumbar punctures. Until recently, HAT programmes have had to balance the risks of administering drugs that were either ineffective or too toxic. Melarsoprol, for example, the only drug effective against the second meningo-encephalitic stage of *rhodesiense* HAT, is notoriously painful to administer and can cause post-treatment reactive encephalopathy, contributing to a treatment-associated fatality rate of about 6% [13,14]. Suramin, a safer drug, can only be used for the first haemo-lymphatic stage because it cannot penetrate the blood–brain barrier. Likewise, in *gambiense* HAT, the safer but less effective drug, pentamidine, is used in the first stage while nifurtimox-eflornithine combination therapy (NECT) is reserved for the second stage. Lumbar punctures are routinely used to determine whether parasites are present in the cerebrospinal fluid to guide HAT treatment decisions.

Capable of penetrating the blood–brain barrier, however, fexinidazole is safe and effective in both the first and second stages of *gambiense* disease [15]. NECT is still recommended as a first-line treatment for patients in "severe second stage" [16] (p.7), defined immunologically as corresponding to a white blood cell count of ≥100/µL of cerebrospinal fluid. Recent ('interim') changes to the WHO HAT treatment guidance, however, empower clinicians to use their clinical judgement in categorizing disease severity by evaluating patients' presenting symptoms. This guidance advises them to perform lumbar punctures only when severe disease is suspected. The use of fexinidazole as a first-line treatment for the first and early second stage of the disease therefore obviates the need for invasive lumbar punctures in many patients.

Another simplification relates to hospitalisation. Unlike existing treatments, which involve labour-intensive intravenous infusions and carry a risk of catheter or needle-related infection [16], fexinidazole's oral administration route is also believed to be safe enough not to require systematic hospitalisation. A subset of patients who are deemed sufficiently healthy and have a supportive caregiving network could be cared for in an outpatient or home-based setting. While the WHO's interim guidelines currently recommend home-based treatment using fexinidazole only if its administration is supervised directly by a healthcare worker [16], home-based treatment administered by caregivers is currently being trialled in a Phase 3b implementation study in the DRC [17].

Toxic medicines, lumbar punctures, and long-term hospitalisation have been hallmark, negative experiences of HAT patient care since the early 20th century [18–20], and collective memories of past control campaigns influence present day HAT awareness and perceptions of risk [21–23]. In the colonial period, lumbar punctures were sometimes administered with violence and patients were forced to stay in treatment camps for years [19]. In the contemporary context, fear of lumbar punctures has been implicated in patients' reasons not to attend mass screening campaigns for HAT or complete diagnostic referrals from peripheral facilities [24,25], and the financial costs of hospitalisation are thought to dissuade patients from completing treatment because of the need to pay for transportation, medical supplies, and food while also dealing with interrupted employment [26].

While a new patient management protocol that circumvents lumbar punctures, more toxic alternatives, and systematic hospitalisation would presumably be welcomed by patients and healthcare workers in endemic settings, these peoples' receptivity towards such technological changes remains unexplored. Introducing novel technologies and strategies into an established ecosystem of care can have unintended effects on the socio-technical relationships that have been formed around HAT case management [25]. Compliance with a new treatment protocol, particularly in a home-based setting, is likely to be contingent not only on patients' trust in the new drug, but also on the institutions and people introducing them [25,27]. Moreover, studies on the extension of hospital care into the home have demonstrated how experiences with older interventions can 'resurface' in contemporary programmes through the "historical longevity of similar groupings of practices and ideas" [28] (p.156), highlighting the importance of examining patient receptivity towards home-based treatments in relation to past and present associations with hospital-based care.

Drawing on interviews with *T. b. rhodesiense* HAT patients managed under existing protocols at two regional treatment centres in Uganda where trials of fexinidazole will begin shortly, this article explores patient receptivity towards key elements of the new fexinidazole patient management protocol. Reflecting on their experiences of hospital treatment and the prospect of an alternative future of HAT care, it describes, from a patient perspective, the existing context of care into which fexinidazole will be introduced. In so doing, we hope to help HAT elimination programmes anticipate key patient concerns and find ways that they can introduce fexinidazole that are culturally appropriate and relevant [29].

2. Materials and Methods

2.1. Context

In Uganda, cases of *T. b. rhodesiense* HAT have declined from 1417 reported in 1990 to only 4 in 2018 [14,30–32]. This study took place between January and March 2016 in Lwala and Dokolo treatment centres in northern Uganda, which manage HAT cases from the historically endemic districts of Dokolo, Kaberamaido, Apac, and Lira. These are now the sites of a clinical trial that will compare the efficacy and safety of fexinidazole to melarsoprol in *T. b. rhodesiense* patients led by the national HAT control programme in partnership with a global product development partnership organisation, the Drugs for Neglected Diseases Initiative (DNDi) under the HAT-r-ACC consortium [32,33].

At the time of fieldwork, suramin and melarsoprol were the treatments used for first and second stage HAT, respectively, and were given according to the WHO's guidelines [34]. Lumbar punctures were systematically done to guide treatment decisions. Suramin was administered intravenously in five weekly doses and melarsoprol in 10 daily doses alongside a 12-day course of prednisolone. Most patients were therefore hospitalized for between 2 and 6 weeks.

2.2. Study Design

T. b. rhodesiense HAT patients were interviewed to document their experiences of HAT and the HAT control programme, including their experiences of treatment-seeking, diagnosis, disease staging, treatment, and post-treatment follow-up. At the time, fexinidazole was undergoing phase 3 trials in the DRC. With such a transformative treatment on the horizon, patients and healthcare workers were invited to reflect on their experiences of the diagnostic staging process and treatment to explore their hopes and concerns about an alternative oral treatment that could be given on the basis of positive microscopy, in some cases without requiring lumbar puncture, and which could potentially be taken at home. Healthcare workers interviewed as part of a related study on HAT surveillance capacity in the region were similarly invited to share their views on the introduction of these prospective treatment changes and were included in this analysis.

The study protocol was reviewed and approved by research ethics committees at the University of Edinburgh, Busitema University, and the Ugandan National Council for Science and Technology (UNCST, approval code HS 1876).

2.3. Patient Sample Selection

As only one patient was undergoing treatment at the time of the study, we relied mainly on the accounts of patients who had been treated and discharged within the prior 26 months. The interview sample (25 patients) was drawn from this overall pool (100 patients treated between 01/01/2014 and 28/02/2016, Table 1) and was selected with the assistance of clinical staff responsible for HAT case management at the two treatment centres.

Table 1. Patient characteristics.

	Total	Study Site		Gender		Age (years)	Disease Stage [1]		Attended ≥ 1 Follow-up Appointment [2]	
		Lwala	Dokolo	Male	Female	Median (range)	First	Second	Yes	No
All admitted patients (01/01/2014 – 28/02/2016)	100	69	31	54	46	20 (2–80)	22	75	58	33
Study sample: recent treatment (2014-16)	23	11	12	12	11	30 (12–80)	7	16	11	10
Study sample: historic treatment (2004-6)	2	2	0	1	1	39.5 (29–50)	1	1	2	0

[1] Disease stage information not available for 3 out of 100 patients admitted. [2] Six patients died before completing treatment and three had completed treatment within three months of the study; these patients were thus not eligible for follow-up by the programme.

To collect a wide range of potentially positive and negative treatment experiences, the sampling strategy focused on recruiting a similar number of patients who (a) had returned to the hospital at least once after treatment for a quarterly follow-up appointment or not; (b) were in different disease stages; and (c) had been treated at each facility. One patient was undergoing treatment at the time of the study, so was interviewed there; 22 others were selected and successfully traced at home and invited for interview. Two further respondents who had been treated a decade previously at Lwala (one in 2005, and another in 2004 and again in 2006 after a second infection/relapse) were also invited to interview at the suggestion of other patients or staff to provide a long-term perspective.

Thirteen out of the 25 (52%) patients interviewed were male. The median age of our sample was 30 (range 12–80), which was slightly older than the wider pool of patients. Seventeen patients (68%) were in second stage and were treated with melarsoprol. Three patients relapsed after treatment failures for first stage infections and were later readmitted for second stage treatment. At the time of study, thirteen patients (52%) had attended a follow-up appointment.

2.4. Recruitment and Interviews

Participants were mobilised for interviews at least 2 days prior by telephone and/or in person through village health team workers who had been briefed on the research and could explain the study to them in their own language. For patients under 18 years of age at the time of interview, adult guardians were interviewed instead. Verbal informed consent was obtained from patients on initial contact and written (or witnessed oral consent with the provision of a thumbprint) was recorded before the interview. All those invited into the study consented to participate. Interviews took place at the patient's home or a local health centre per their request. Interviews followed a semi-structured interview guide and took place through consecutive translations to local languages by trained interpreters, as necessary. Discussions were audio-recorded and transcripts were produced shortly afterwards.

2.5. Analysis

Each participant was attributed a unique identification code with accompanying demographic characteristics to aid interpretation. Recurrent themes for each topic were then identified and coded using NVIVO software (version 11), and quotes that articulated these themes were selected to summarise key points. Theoretical concepts from the fields of medical anthropology and social studies of science and innovation were drawn on to understand the social and therapeutic landscape in which HAT medicines were introduced, accessed, and taken up in local context [20–22,28,29,35–43].

This is important in an elimination setting where treatment adherence and outcomes are essential to programme success. We present our findings beginning with the patients' experiences of HAT symptoms, the decision-making that led them to the treatment centre, and how long periods of hospitalisation impacted their lives. We then present patient experiences of suramin and melarsoprol intravenous injections, including the lumbar puncture procedure that guided treatment decisions, alongside accounts of the attentive care of health professionals. We then describe how these experiences informed patients' perceptions of an alternative oral treatment protocol, followed by expectations and concerns about how such a treatment could be delivered in the home setting.

3. Results

3.1. Experiences of Illness and Hospitalisation

Patients described the reputation of HAT as being a "terrible" disease that is widely feared and sometimes attributed to witchcraft; descriptions of this fear are often extended to its medications as well.

> *The people here, the feeling is they fear the disease; [they think] that [it] is so terrible and at times they feel it is caused by some traditional behaviours like witchcraft. The people fear the disease and the medications. People have been tested, but apart from me, no one has been caught with the disease, but they fear it […]. It is even worse than HIV.*

—Patient 8, Dokolo

The symptoms that patients used to illustrate how terrible HAT feels included headaches, fever, an excessive need to sleep, muscle weakness or 'paralysis', and difficulty walking, as well as cognitive impairment.

> *He had a fever, and headache, general body pain, then the muscles on the right side in his calf became so painful that it couldn't allow him to walk. Then eventually he was behaving like someone with mental problems, like he was mentally confused.*

—Parent of Patient 2, Dokolo

> *He had a headache for so long. He would be looking at someone from a distance as if there are two people [as in a hallucination]. The boy complained he would be seeing very big animals with red eyes. And he was talking in an un-coordinated manner.*

—Parent of Patient 9, Lwala

Typical of *rhodesiense* HAT infections, some people's symptoms appeared to progressed very rapidly with escalating severity, which caused great alarm.

> *I started feeling the headache—it moved from one side to the other […] then by late [evening] I started feeling a terrible fever. I became so weak I requested the children to light a fire in my house so I could go and rest. By 10pm, the thing worsened, and it started affecting all the joints, all my joints were paining me. I lost consciousness by that time […] I even went and called the catechist to come and pray for me, I thought I was on my way [going to die].*

—Patient 18, Dokolo

In many cases, previous knowledge of HAT services and high levels of institutional trust in HAT centres were important in ensuring patients sought treatment at hospitals for their symptoms, especially when this involved overriding the advice of others to seek advice from spiritual healers.

> *For example, when I was taking him and he was mentally confused, someone said "is that the sort of thing you take to be treated at the hospital? Take him to the witchdoctor and he will be out with it".*

But I knew that others who had similar symptoms were taken to a health centre, and from there they were treated and improved.

—Parent of patient 2, Dokolo

Almost all patients described difficulty in reaching a hospital for admission. Whether they were brought in an incapacitated state by others or presented themselves, many faced challenges in accessing transport.

The challenge was that I had problems in transport, the place is far and I was very weak so couldn't get myself there. But eventually a woman rode me on a bicycle.

—Patient 4, Dokolo

Most respondents focused heavily on the negative social and economic effects of being admitted to hospital for the duration of treatment. These included having to arrange childcare or help to look after crops, raising funds for food and medical supplies, and finding someone to support and take care of them in hospital. The socio-economic fall-out from HAT was observable in terms of educational absence, transport costs, associated medical costs, and agricultural losses.

Other than distance, there was frequent visiting to the hospital, we had to travel there a lot, we took things like foodstuffs, it was a challenge. It affected his studies so much, he was behind in his studies.

—Parent of patient 6, Apac

I was treated well in terms of treatment, the problem I had was leaving home for one month—I had left rice in the garden and the daughter-in-law was struggling to harvest and had difficulties. Also raising money for the upkeep was difficult.

—Patient 18, Dokolo

3.2. Receptivity Toward an Oral Treatment

A clinician working at Dokolo HC IV described how toxic and painful treatment with melarsoprol can be.

The compound can also cause tissue necrosis, so you must be very careful to get the IV [intravenous] line right, otherwise a patient can even lose an arm […]. Suramin is just fine, there is no problem giving this, but Mel B [melarsoprol] is so, so painful for them because the drug is so viscous and thick. It's like vegetable oil, and it needs a lot of force to push it through the vein, that is why it is so painful for them. Some say it is like having fire in their veins.

Patients liked the idea of an oral administration format because the injections 'burned'. Overall 23/25 (92%) patients reported they would prefer an oral drug regimen over the intravenous injection treatment they experienced (Table 2).

Table 2. Patient preferences for the administration route and setting of human African trypanosomiasis (HAT) treatment.

Protocol Characteristic	Number Who Preferred Existing Protocol	Number Who Preferred Proposed Protocol
Administration route (existing: intravenous injection; proposed: oral tablets)	2 (8%)	23 (92%)
Administration setting (existing: hospital-based; proposed: home-based)	12 (48%)	13 (52%)

The good option would be a tablet because the [melarsoprol] injection, as it is entering, it burns and needs to go just slowly.

—Patient 1, Kaberamaido

If side effects are not there, yes [he would prefer to take the medicine in tablet form]. The pain during [melarsoprol] injection is so painful, I would prefer getting an oral treatment that I can take from home.

—Patient 5, Dokolo

Patient descriptions of pain from the medicine made them feel vulnerable and therefore wished to be under medical supervision, as in this comment from a patient who described falling into an incoherent state while undergoing treatment:

For me, I appreciated that it was good for me to be there [staying in the hospital], because after I got the [melarsoprol] injection, sometimes I could not understand myself, so I think it needed me to be near [to health staff], under supervision

—Patient 1, Kaberamaido

While the experiences described by patients of the treatment itself were unpleasant, the discomfort was nevertheless commonly acknowledged as a necessary side effect of a strong drug working in the body. Some patients, such as Patient 1 felt the oral tablet option would be ineffective as a treatment for such a serious condition, as *"the disease was so terrible that it just needed injection, the tablets could not do it."* However, when asked what they would prefer if an oral treatment could be proven to be safe and effective, these concerns tended to wane alongside the patients' motivation to minimise disruptions to daily activities.

Tablets would be better if they are doing the same thing. I could continue with it [treatment] myself because I need my [social] life.

—Patient 1, Kaberamaido

For those who could remember their diagnosis and treatment experiences in detail, the disease staging procedure was recalled as being particularly uncomfortable and debilitating. An oral treatment that could be given without the need for lumbar puncture was thus an attractive benefit of the new protocol.

I am glad to be cleared of that disease, but I wish to no longer have that needle in my back! I could not bend for a long time, it was so painful.

—Patient 12, Dokolo

In one case, the fear of undergoing the lumbar puncture again, combined with the apparent success of treatment, influenced the patient's decision not to return for follow-up.

They gave a certain period to go back, but during that time I felt so well, and also I was fearing the lumbar puncture, so I didn't go back.

—Patient 4, Lira

3.3. Receptivity Toward Home-Based Treatment Administration

When asked to consider whether they would be receptive to a home-based administration of HAT treatment, patients and their caregivers often discussed the impacts of hospitalisation on their domestic and economic lives.

I am the one looking after him, so home is left behind with my siblings. Feeding is a problem for me for this long. At home we have our cassava garden and vegetables, but here there is no forest here for collecting firewood from. If we go back again we need transport which becomes costly […]. If there was treatment that I could carry home, then I would prefer that.

—Relative of Patient 12, Dokolo

[Home treatment] would be better for me, I would be doing other things at home. If I go away for over one month, when I come home it is a mess.

—Patient 8, Dokolo

I would prefer taking drugs at home because staying at the hospital is expensive and, even going for treatment there, we had to sell land to pay for it.

—Patient 3, Kaberamaido

Health workers also acknowledged the struggles faced by patients during treatment and expressed hope for the benefits of a potential oral treatment that patients could take home:

I think that would be better to manage them from home, because the society we live in and the services we have, I think our community prefer being with their people at home. Staying in hospital is an inconvenience to the patient and the family, but only if the condition can be managed from home.

—Nurse, HCIII, Kaberamaido

Despite the substantial difficulties associated with hospitalisation uniformly expressed by patients, only half of patients 13/25 (52%) claimed that they would prefer a home-based treatment (see Table 2). The remainder expressed a preference to be treated in hospital under close observation throughout their treatment course, regardless of the route of treatment administration.

3.4. The Value of Clinical Monitoring

A key reason that patients expressed discomfort with receiving treatment administered at home was that they imagined their care would not be overseen by health staff. Most patients had felt well cared for when admitted to hospital for HAT treatment, as expressed in comments on the quality of care they received and the trustworthiness and capabilities of the healthcare workers who treated them.

I believed [the diagnosis of HAT given to me] because once a medical person tells you something you cannot deny [...]. I would prefer getting treatment from the hospital like before. It is important [to have] close follow-up by medical workers.

—Patient 19, Dokolo

There [in Lwala Hospital] it was good treatment, I would rather be at the hospital. There you get regular reviews.

—Patient 24, Lwala

Treatment from the hospital [is better], because it's always close to the health workers and the observation is very close [...]. I like the way they handled him at Dokolo, they paid very close attention.

—Parent of Patient 20, Dokolo

At hospital I was given due care perfectly.

—Patient 16, Dokolo

They [hospital staff] are competent, the evidence is how much I have improved, you cannot improve when you are managed by someone who is not competent.

—Patient 8, Dokolo

In some cases, patient preferences for hospital-based administration were coupled with a concern that they might not oversee their own drug administration properly if the onus of treatment was on themselves or their families.

I would rather be at the hospital; it [provides] good treatment because when you are there the people there are full time. There you get regular reviews, because it's always close to the health workers and the observation is very close. At home you might forget your time and take the treatment wrong.

—Patient 21, Dokolo

I would prefer to be given [treatment] at the hospital by the health workers. The oral treatment to be taken, it is possible that I will forget what time and how much I should take, but the health workers at the hospital will give the right drug at the right time. I would trust the health workers.

—Patient 4, Dokolo

Healthcare workers, too, had concerns that patients would not be confident in managing their own treatment or receive appropriate medical support at home, and proposed a model of home-based treatment administration that would be observed by community-based healthcare workers, similar to the directly observed treatment strategy (DOTS) implemented by tuberculosis control programmes in Uganda.

I think the hospital for treatment is good because they [patients] can be constantly and professionally monitored. [The] home might not be a good environment. But if they can be observed at home, like the DOTS, it would be preferred.

—Nurse, HCIII, Lira

I think it is better they stay in hospital where they can be monitored. Also, if you give patients drugs […] they [the drugs] will sit there next to them in the sun. Where is there for people to store drugs properly? […]. Something like DOTs could work, I think. Although if the system of treatment were to change like that then the community would again need to be sensitised beforehand so they understand the new protocol.

—Voluntary Health Team worker, Kobulabulu, Kaberamaido

Although the anxieties associated with painful lumbar punctures and intravenous injections shaped strong preferences for an oral treatment that could avoid such procedures, current treatment modalities, which emphasise inpatient observation, appeared to strengthen the perception of HAT as a serious illness requiring expert clinical management. In such a context, it was evident that the patients' trust in HAT services and the staff providing it was actually stronger than their fear of HAT treatment, itself.

4. Discussion

Fexinidazole is among several promising new tools expected to push HAT elimination 'to the last mile' [27]. Acoziborole (also known as SCYX-7158), which is hypothesized to be capable of curing both stages and forms of HAT in a single oral dose, is currently undergoing Phase 2b/3 clinical trials in the DRC and Guinea [14,44], and has been described as another "game-changer" for elimination efforts [45] (p.14). Admittedly, fexinidazole may not overcome all the problems of HAT patient management. For patients with 'severe' second stage *gambiense* illness who respond better to NECT treatment, for example, lumbar punctures and long-term hospitalisation are likely to remain part of their experience of care, and it is unclear whether, for *rhodesiense* disease, fexinidazole will be able to replace melarsoprol or be delivered in a home-based setting.

Nevertheless, our findings suggest some clear benefits to the introduction of fexinidazole for HAT patients. Patients recalled difficult experiences of treatment and hospital admission where many struggled to pull together the money and social care required to support them through their hospitalisation. Most patients and healthcare workers in this study agreed that a course of oral tablets that could be taken at home would be convenient. Perhaps surprisingly, however, we found less enthusiasm overall for a home-based treatment option than might be expected. Nearly half of patients expressed hesitancy toward taking HAT treatment outside the hospital setting where they could not be monitored closely by medical staff.

Not only are the symptoms of HAT "terrible", they can also be stigmatizing [23]. The frightening experiences of this life-threatening illness, alongside the pain and anxiety associated with lumbar punctures and intravenous injections (particularly for melarsoprol) contributed to the perception of HAT as a serious illness requiring expert medical care. While current treatments are uncomfortable, potentially toxic, and require long hospital stays, the specialist and attentive care they entail has helped to establish melarsoprol and suramin as trusted treatments. The hesitancy expressed by patients about a home-based treatment model were predominantly related less to the prospect of an unknown drug, however, than to satisfaction with the competence and attentiveness of the healthcare workers who cared for them under existing protocols. This can be interpreted not as resistance to a new drug regimen but rather an appreciation of existing HAT services as high-quality care that is comparatively rare in rural areas of Africa where HAT is endemic [46]. Therefore, while it is unlikely that patients with very severe symptoms would be eligible for outpatient or home-based HAT care, programmes may need to offer extensive counselling and monitoring support before even patients in early stage are comfortable accepting care in this way.

5. Conclusions

This study describes the contextual life-worlds that frame the treatment experiences of a sample of *T. b. rhodesiense* HAT patients in Uganda, where a safety and efficacy trial of fexinidazole will shortly begin. Despite the significant impacts that hospitalisation has on the social lives and livelihoods of *rhodesiense* HAT patients, the patient testimonies collected in this study demonstrated the high level of trust patients already have in the existing system of care and the difficulties of changing behaviours in systems more generally.

The roll-out of fexinidazole will be a pivotal moment in the history of HAT care and control. The introduction of an oral treatment would engage with many of the legitimate needs and concerns about current treatment protocols expressed by patients and healthcare workers in this setting. These include painful lumbar puncture and injection procedures, treatment side effects, potentially fatal drug reactions, the economic costs of travel and long stays in hospital. However, meeting elimination goals will require paying close attention to structural and relational elements of health systems and cannot rely solely on the availability of diagnostics and medicines. The reluctance we observed in our study toward home-based management can be interpreted as demonstrating high existing levels of trust in the current system's quality of care, which comprise clinical performances of monitoring and observation as much as the administration of medicines. Inpatient clinical observation appears to be an aspect of existing modes of HAT care that is important to patients. These concerns may be specific to the sample in question but nonetheless raise important considerations for devising locally specific and patient-centred approaches to introducing fexinidazole, which may also be important to patients in other settings.

Programmes introducing the fexinidazole protocol should seek to build on good relations in the existing hospital-based system of HAT treatment delivery and include flexible options for patient management procedures. This is important to ensure that HAT treatment remains patient-centred, both through technological solutions to health system challenges, but also through more relational aspects of interventions, which affect the quality of care.

Author Contributions: Conceptualization, S.J.L. and J.J.P.; methodology, S.J.L. and R.J.A.; software, S.J.L.; validation, S.J.L., J.J.P. and R.J.A.; formal analysis, S.J.L.; investigation, S.J.L.; resources, R.J.A.; data curation, R.J.A.; writing—original draft preparation, S.J.L. and J.J.P.; writing—review and editing, S.J.L., J.J.P. and R.J.A.; supervision, J.J.P.; project administration, S.J.L.; funding acquisition, S.J.L. All authors have read and agreed to the published version of the manuscript.

Funding: This research was funded by the European Research Council (grant no: 295845, http://erc.europa.eu) through a grant for the Investigating Networks of Zoonosis Innovation (INZI) project at the University of Edinburgh, and the Economic and Social Research Council's (ESRC) fieldwork abroad fund.

Acknowledgments: The authors wish to thank George Aroma and Freddie Kansiime for their technical support and supervision during the data collection phase of this study. We also would like to thank Jean-Benoît Falisse and Pete Kingsley for their thoughtful comments on earlier drafts of the manuscript.

Conflicts of Interest: The authors declare no conflict of interest. The funders had no role in the design of the study; in the collection, analyses, or interpretation of data; in the writing of the manuscript, or in the decision to publish the results.

References

1. Mulenga, P.; Lutumba, P.; Coppieters, Y.; Mpanya, A.; Mwamba-Miaka, E.; Luboya, O.; Chenge, F. Passive screening and diagnosis of sleeping sickness with new tools in primary health services: An operational research. *Infect Dis.* **2019**, *8*, 353–367. [CrossRef]

2. Burri, C.; Nkunku, S.; Merolle, A.; Smith, T.; Blum, J.; Brun, R. Efficacy of new, concise schedule for melarsoprol in treatment of sleeping sickness caused by Trypanosoma brucei gambiense: A randomised trial. *Lancet* **2000**, *355*, 1419–1425. [CrossRef]

3. Kuepfer, I.; Schmid, C.; Allan, M.; Edielu, A.; Haary, E.P.; Kakembo, A.; Kibona, S.; Blum, J.; Burri, C. Safety and efficacy of the 10-day melarsoprol schedule for the treatment of second stage rhodesiense sleeping sickness. *PLoS Negl. Trop. Dis.* **2012**, *6*, e1695. [CrossRef]

4. Pépin, J.; Milord, F.; Meurice, F.; Ethier, L.; Loko, L.; Mpia, B. High-dose nifurtimox for arseno-resistant trypanosoma brucei gambiense sleeping sickness: An open trial in central zaire. *Trans. R. Soc. Trop. Med. Hyg.* **1992**, *86*, 254–256. [CrossRef]

5. Priotto, G.; Fogg, C.; Balasegaram, M.; Erphas, O.; Louga, A.; Checchi, F.; Ghabri, S.; Piola, P. Three drug combinations for late-stage trypanosoma brucei gambiense sleeping sickness: A randomized clinical trial in Uganda. *PLoS Clin. Trials* **2006**, *1*, e39. [CrossRef]

6. Priotto, G.; Kasparian, S.; Ngouama, D.; Ghorashian, S.; Arnold, U.; Ghabri, S.; Karunakara, U. Nifurtimox-eflornithine combination therapy for second-stage trypanosoma brucei gambiense sleeping sickness: A randomized clinical trial in Congo. *Clin. Infect. Dis.* **2007**, *45*, 1435–1442. [CrossRef]

7. Chappuis, F.; Udayraj, N.; Stietenroth, K.; Meussen, A.; Bovier, P.A. Eflornithine is safer than melarsoprol for the treatment of second-stage trypanosoma brucei gambiense human African trypanosomiasis. *Clin. Infect. Dis.* **2005**, *41*, 748–751. [CrossRef]

8. Bisser, S.; N'Siesi, F.; Lejon, V.; Preux, P.; Van Nieuwenhove, S.; Miaka Mia Bilenge, C.; Büscher, P. Equivalence trial of melarsoprol and nifurtimox monotherapy and combination therapy for the treatment of second-stage trypanosoma brucei gambiense sleeping sickness. *J. Infect. Dis.* **2007**, *195*, 322–329. [CrossRef]

9. Checchi, F.; Piola, P.; Ayikoru, H.; Thomas, F.; Legros, D.; Priotto, G. Nifurtimox plus eflornithine for late-stage sleeping sickness in Uganda: A case series. *PLoS Negl. Trop. Dis.* **2007**, *1*, e64. [CrossRef]

10. Chappuis, F. Melarsoprol-free drug combinations for second-stage Gambian sleeping sickness: The way to go. *Clin. Infect. Dis.* **2007**, *45*, 1443–1445. [CrossRef]

11. WHO. *Human African Trypanosomiasis: Symptoms, Diagnosis and Treatment*; World Health Organisation: Geneva, Switzerland, 2017.

12. Aksoy, S.; Buscher, P.; Lehane, M.; Solano, P.; van den Abbeele, J. Human African trypanosomiasis control: Achievements and challenges. *PLoS Negl. Trop. Dis.* **2017**, *11*, e0005454. [CrossRef]

13. Kennedy, P.G.E. Update on human African trypanosomiasis (sleeping sickness). *J. Neurol.* **2019**, *266*, 2334–2337. [CrossRef]

14. Deeks, E.D. Fexinidazole: First global approval. *Drugs* **2019**, *79*, 215–220. [CrossRef]

15. WHO. *WHO Interim Guidelines for the Treatment of Gambiense Human African Trypanosomiasis*; World Health Organisation: Geneva, Switzerland, 2019.

16. Clinical Trials Fexinidazole in Human African Trypanosomiasis Due to T.b. Gambiense at Any Stage. Available online: https://clinicaltrials.gov/ct2/show/NCT03025789 (accessed on 9 January 2020).

17. Tilley, H. Ecologies of complexity: Tropical environments, African trypanosomiasis, and the science of disease control in British colonial Africa, 1900–1940. *Osiris* **2004**, *19*, 21–38. [CrossRef]

18. Lachenal, G. *The Lomidine Files: The Untold Story of a Medical Disaster in Colonial Africa*; John Hopkins University Press: Baltimore, MD, USA, 2017.

19. Kovacic, V.; Tirados, I.; Esterhuizen, J.; Mangwiro, C.T.N.; Lehane, M.J.; Torr, S.J.; Smith, H. We remember … elders' memories and perceptions of sleeping sickness control interventions in west Nile, Uganda. *PLoS Negl. Trop. Dis.* **2016**, *10*, e0004745. [CrossRef]

20. Lyons, M. *The Colonial Disease: A Social History of Sleeping Sickness in Northern Zaire, 1900–1940*; Cambridge University Press: Cambridge, UK, 2002; ISBN 978-0-521-52452-0.

21. Mpanya, A.; Hendrickx, D.; Vuna, M.; Kanyinda, A.; Lumbala, C.; Tshilombo, V.; Mitashi, P.; Luboya, O.; Kande, V.; Boelaert, M.; et al. Should I get screened for sleeping sickness? A qualitative study in Kasai province, democratic republic of Congo. *PLoS Negl. Trop. Dis.* **2012**, *6*, e1467. [CrossRef]

22. Lee, S.J.; Palmer, J.J. Integrating innovations: A qualitative analysis of referral non-completion among rapid diagnostic test-positive patients in Uganda's human African trypanosomiasis elimination programme. *Infect. Dis. Poverty* **2018**, *84*, 1–16.

23. Mesu, V.K.B.K.; Kalonji, W.M.; Bardonneau, C.; Mordt, O.V.; Blesson, S.; Simon, F.; Delhomme, S.; Bernhard, S.; Kuziena, W.; Lubaki, J.-P.F.; et al. Oral fexinidazole for late-stage African Trypanosoma brucei gambiense trypanosomiasis: A pivotal multicentre, randomised, non-inferiority trial. *Lancet* **2018**, *391*, 144–154. [CrossRef]

24. Reynolds, C. Going the Last Mile to Eliminate a Long-Neglected Disease: Sleeping Sickness. PATH. Available online: https://www.path.org/articles/going-the-last-mile-to-eliminate-a-long-neglected-disease (accessed on 20 January 2020).

25. Brown, H. "Home-based care is not a new thing" Legacies of domestic governmentality in western Kenya home-based care. In *Making and Unmaking Public Health in Africa: Ethnographic and Historical Perspectives*; Prince, R.J., Marsland, R., Eds.; Ohio University Press: Ascension, OH, USA, 2013.

26. Panter-Brick, C.; Clarke, S.E.; Lomas, H.; Pinder, M.; Lindsay, S.W. Culturally compelling strategies for behaviour change: A social ecology model and case study in malaria prevention. *Soc. Sci. Med.* **2006**, *62*, 2810–2825. [CrossRef]

27. WHO (World Health Organisation) Uganda. Number of New Reported Cases of Human African Trypanosomiasis (T.b. Rhodesiense). 2018. Available online: http://apps.who.int/gho/data/node.main. A1637?lang=en (accessed on 20 January 2020).

28. DNDi. Fexinidazole Study in Adults and Children with HAT Due to T. b. Rhodesiense. Available online: https://www.dndi.org/2016/clinical-trials/clinical-trials-hat/ (accessed on 20 January 2019).

29. Clinical Trials Efficacy and Safety of Fexinidazole in Patients with Human African Trypanosomiasis (HAT) Due to Trypanosoma Brucei Rhodesiensev. Available online: https://clinicaltrials.gov/ct2/show/NCT03974178 (accessed on 9 January 2020).

30. Fexinidazole for T.b. Rhodesiense—DNDi. Available online: https://www.dndi.org/diseases-projects/portfolio/fexinidazole-tb-rhodesiense/ (accessed on 9 January 2020).

31. WHO. *Control and Surveillance of Human African Trypanosomiasis*; World Health Organization Technical Report Series; World Health Organization: Geneva, Switzerland, 2013; pp. 1–237.

32. Gesler, W. Therapeutic landscapes—Medical issues in the light of the new cultural geography. *Soc. Sci. Med.* **1992**, *34*, 735–746. [CrossRef]

33. Winchester, M.S.; Mcgrath, J.W. Therapeutic landscapes: Anthropological perspectives on health and place. *Med. Anthropol. Theory* **2017**. [CrossRef]

34. Winchester, M.S.; McGrath, J.W.; Kaawa-Mafigiri, D.; Namutiibwa, F.; Ssendegye, G.; Nalwoga, A.; Kyarikunda, E.; Birungi, J.; Kisakye, S.; Ayebazibwe, N.; et al. Routines, hope, and antiretroviral treatment among men and women in Uganda. *Med. Anthropol. Q.* **2017**, *31*, 237–256. [CrossRef] [PubMed]

35. Whyte, S.R.; van der Geest, S.; Hardon, A. *Social Lives of Medicines*; Cambridge University Press: Cambridge, UK; New York, NY, USA, 2002; ISBN 0-521-80025-0.

36. Mpanya, A.; Hendrickx, D.; Baloji, S.; Lumbala, C.; da Luz, R.I.; Boelaert, M.; Lutumba, P. From health advice to taboo: Community perspectives on the treatment of sleeping sickness in the democratic republic of Congo, a qualitative study. *PLoS Negl. Trop. Dis.* **2015**, *9*, 1–14. [CrossRef] [PubMed]

37. Atkinson, S.J. Anthropology in research on the quality of health services. *Cad. Saúde Pública* **1993**, *9*, 283–299. [CrossRef]

38. Montgomery, C.M.; Kingori, P.; Sariola, S.; Engel, N. STS and global health. *Sci. Technol. Stud.* **2017**, *3*, 2–12. [CrossRef]

39. Birungi, H. Injections and self-help: Risk and trust in Ugandan health care. *Soc. Sci. Med.* **1998**, *47*, 1455–1462. [CrossRef]

40. Meinert, L. Regimes of homework in AIDS care questions of responsibility and the imagination of lives in Uganda. In *Making and Unmaking Public Health in Africa: Ethnographic and Historical Perspectives*; Prince, R.J., Marsland, R., Eds.; Ohio University Press: Ascension, OH, USA, 2013.

41. van der Geest, S.; Whyte, S.R.; Hardon, A. *The Anthropology of Pharmaceutials: A Biographical Approach*; Annual Review: Palo Alto, CA, USA, 1996; Volume 25, ISBN 0084-6570.

42. Pivotal Clinical Trial to Begin for First Oral Drug Candidate Specifically Developed for Sleeping Sickness—DNDi. Available online: https://www.dndi.org/2015/media-centre/press-releases/pr-scyx-7158/ (accessed on 1 December 2019).

43. DNDi. Newer, Simpler Treatments for Sleeping Sickness. An Update on DNDi R&D Programmes. Available online: https://www.dndi.org/wp-content/uploads/2018/09/DNDi_HAT_2018.pdf (accessed on 20 January 2020).

44. Palmer, J.J. Sensing sleeping sickness: Local symptom-making in South Sudan. *Med. Anthropol.* **2019**. [CrossRef]

45. Palmer, J.J.; Kelly, A.H.; Surur, E.I.; Checchi, F.; Jones, C. Changing landscapes, changing practice: Negotiating access to sleeping sickness services in a post-conflict society. *Soc. Sci. Med.* **2014**, *120*, 396–404. [CrossRef]

46. Varanda, J.; Théophile, J. Putting anthropology into global health: A century of anti-human African trypanosomiasis campaigns in Angola. *Anthropol. Action* **2019**, *26*, 31–41. [CrossRef]

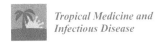

Tropical Medicine and
Infectious Disease

Article

Whose Elimination? Frontline Workers' Perspectives on the Elimination of the Human African Trypanosomiasis and Its Anticipated Consequences

Jean-Benoît Falisse [1,*], Erick Mwamba-Miaka [2] and Alain Mpanya [2,3]

[1]   Centre of African Studies, University of Edinburgh, Edinburgh EH8 9LD, UK
[2]   Programme National de lutte contre la THA (PNLTHA), Kinshasa 2, Democratic Republic of the Congo;
      erickmwamb2002@yahoo.fr (E.M.-M.); mpanya_alain@yahoo.fr (A.M.)
[3]   Faculté des Sciences de la Santé, Université Pedagogique Nationale (UPN), Kinshasa BP 8815,
      Democratic Republic of the Congo
*   Correspondence: jb.falisse@ed.ac.uk; Tel.: +44-131-651-1632

Received: 30 November 2019; Accepted: 25 December 2019; Published: 1 January 2020

Abstract: While academic literature has paid careful attention to the technological efforts—drugs, tests, and tools for vector control—deployed to eliminate Gambiense Human African Trypanosomiasis (HAT), the human resources and health systems dimensions of elimination are less documented. This paper analyses the perspectives and experiences of frontline nurses, technicians, and coordinators who work for the HAT programme in the former province of Bandundu in the Democratic Republic of the Congo, at the epidemic's very heart. The research is based on 21 semi-structured interviews conducted with frontline workers in February 2018. The results highlight distinctive HAT careers as well as social elevation through specialised work. Frontline workers are concerned about changes in active screening strategies and the continued existence of the vector, which lead them to question the possibility of imminent elimination. Managers seem to anticipate a post-HAT situation and prepare for the employment of their staff; most workers see their future relatively confidently, as re-allocated to non-vertical units. The findings suggest concrete pathways for improving the effectiveness of elimination efforts: improving active screening through renewed engagements with local leaders, conceptualising horizontal integration in terms of human resources mobility, and investing more in detection and treatment activities (besides innovation).

Keywords: Human African Trypanosomiasis (HAT); disease elimination; disease eradication; frontline workers; DR Congo; mobile screening; qualitative methods

1. Introduction

Gambiense Human African Trypanosomiasis (HAT), also known as sleeping sickness, is a parasitic tropical infectious disease whose main vector of transmission is the tsetse fly. It is one of the 17 neglected tropical diseases that the World Health Organisation (WHO) put on its 2012 agenda of diseases to be eliminated as a public health problem by 2020, with the additional target of stopping all HAT transmissions by 2030 [1–4]. The abundant literature that has accompanied HAT elimination efforts is primarily focussed on technological innovations, including the development of new drugs, tests, and tools for vector control [4–7]. Only limited attention has been paid to the frontline human and health systems sides of the effort [8–11]. The present article looks at the experiences and perspectives of frontline workers (nurses, doctors, lab technicians and assistants, and clinic and provincial managers) involved in HAT screening and treatment at a time marked by optimistic discourses about and concrete achievements towards the elimination of a disease many frontline workers have dedicated their lives to combatting.

The study is set in the Democratic Republic of the Congo (DR Congo), a country that reportedly sees 80% of the new HAT cases and counts 63% of the at-risk population [12], and revolves around two research questions. The first is: how does elimination look like from the perspective of those doing it in the field? Epidemiologists see the curve of HAT cases dropping, and clinical researchers celebrate more straightforward and more efficient drugs and tests, but what does it mean for those at the frontline? Do they agree that the epidemic is decreasing and the tools are good? Do they think HAT will be eliminated soon? Frontline workers' viewpoints and experiences matter because they are the embodied expression of national and global programmes. The second question relates to the anticipation of life and livelihood 'after the end of the disease' [13,14]: how does elimination affect the prospects of HAT workers? In DR Congo, the fight against HAT is through a vertical programme made of specialised health workers who have often spent their entire career specialising on HAT [15]; HAT elimination would undoubtedly change their work. Do they feel insecure or confident about the future? We believe that these behavioural and organisational aspects are fundamental to comprehend as they can positively or negatively influence the provision of HAT screening and treatment services and are essential to HAT elimination efforts, especially when bearing in mind that periods of low incidence can be vulnerable to a resurgence of the disease (as control efforts ebb away). Our research is also important to help governments prepare their systems for a post-elimination future.

The next section briefly discusses the situation of HAT elimination in DR Congo and explains the institutions and instruments deployed in the field. The methods are then presented; they build on a series of interviews with frontline workers. The results are divided into three sub-sections. The first provides (1) details on HAT careers and the nature of frontline work while the remaining two correspond to the two research questions: one looks at (2) frontline workers perspectives on HAT elimination and the other at (3) perspectives on HAT workers' future. A discussion section puts the results in perspective with the literature on HAT elimination and human resources in the context of disease elimination in general.

2. HAT Elimination in DR Congo

In DR Congo, as in other central African countries, two major HAT epidemics took place during the twentieth century. The first began in 1900 and peaked in the 1930s with over 30,000 new cases annually [15]; it was brought under control by 1960, following the organisation of mass screening campaigns with mobile teams made up of specialised nurses and lab technicians that visited villages and other sites at risk [4,16]. Prevalence levels then reached one case per 10,000 people, and it was believed that the disease would stop spreading [12]. It was an erroneous assumption: as the country entered its turbulent post-independence era and control was somewhat diminished, the number of cases increased again [17]. By 1998, there were 26,318 new cases per year [15].

Over the past twenty years, though, through the efforts of the national HAT control programme, the *Programme National de Lutte contre la Trypanosomiase Humaine Africaine* (PNLTHA), non-governmental organisations, and donors, the number of HAT cases has been reduced to a mere 660 new cases in 2018 [18]. This reduction is readily associated with new technology including (door-to-door) screening tools, treatment, vector control methods, and data collection and data analysis systems [12,19,20]. As in other parts of the world, international actors and the government of DR Congo have embraced the 2020 target, and on 31 January 2018, the government launched the first National HAT Day to celebrate its commitment to the goal. At this occasion, it outlined a new strategy of elimination through "new technologies and an innovative approach to early screening for the disease" [21].

The success of HAT case reduction in DR Congo may, however, come with drawbacks. First, fewer cases may be associated with a demotivation of populations in endemic areas to participate in mass screening campaigns, as HAT is no longer perceived as a threat. Second, rarer cases also affect the health system put in place as there is a risk that staff and funders change interest. The evidence is mostly anecdotal (at this stage), but it invites studies like ours to be careful.

HAT control and treatment in the DR Congo is organised by the PNLTHA, which sits as a vertical programme within the Ministry of Health. The centralisation of expertise inside a vertical programme is possibly stronger than in other countries owing to historical legacies but also the spread of the epidemic that has made HAT careers a reality in the country. The PNLTHA is reliant on external funding for substantial parts of its activities, which does at times put pressure on frontline staff. Besides the vertical programme, which constitutes the bulk of the effort, and similarly to many other countries affected by sleeping sickness, some non-specialised health facilities have integrated HAT-related activities. In this case, the frontline workers would typically have many other responsibilities beyond HAT screening and treatment. The present paper focusses on PLNTHA workers.

Control strategies consist of active early detection, passive detection, and treatment of patients, which are complemented by vector control activities. Early detection through active screening is provided by mobile teams of the PNLTHA. A mobile team consists of 7 to 9 people who travel by vehicle to endemic villages to organise mass screening campaigns. A mobile team has the capacity to examine around 66,000 people per year [22]. There are currently 30 mobile teams and 18 mini-teams on motorbikes, with the latter corresponding to a recent evolution in the mass screening approach [18]. The recent years have also seen new micro-planification strategies with dedicated software to focus efforts according to the recorded prevalence of HAT. Premiums, a form of pay-for-performance, are paid to the mobile teams to incentivise them to identify cases and cover vast areas. The activities of the mobile teams are complemented by passive surveillance with so-called 'fixed' health facilities that are either solely focussed on HAT or include HAT treatment and screening as a part of a broader package of activities. As shown by Mitashi et al. in a 2015 study, it is important to note that the possibility of extending passive screening to all primary healthcare centres is not straightforward: such health facilities typically lack the tools and ability to diagnose HAT [23]. A more recent study by Mulenga et al. is only slightly more optimistic about the potential of passive screening at a wider scale [24]. This has constituted an impetus to the development of new, easier, diagnostic and treatment tools meant to facilitate the integration of HAT activities in endemic areas [5].

HAT screening can be syndromic or serological. Syndromic screening is often late because the signs and symptoms of HAT are not specific enough to allow easy clinical diagnosis of the disease [25,26]. Syndromic screening is typically based on signs of the second stage of the disease and therefore leads to late diagnosis. Serological screening is done on the basis of an agglutination test for Trypanosomiasis (CATT), which is commonly used in mass screening by mobile teams [27]. Significant progress has been made in recent years with the development of a new rapid diagnostic test (RDT) that is individual and easy to use. Patients diagnosed by mobile teams are referred for treatment in health facilities.

The treatment of HAT is stage-dependent. In the first stage, Pentamidine, which appeared in 1940, is still used today [28]. For the second stage, the Nufurtimox-Eflornithine (NECT) combination therapy [29,30] has replaced Melarsopol since 2009. Given the volume of cases it hosts, DR Congo is the focus of ongoing trials and projects to develop HAT innovations that will shape the course of elimination domestically as well as in neighbouring countries. They include two oral drugs, Fexinidazole, which was approved by the Ministry of Health and will soon be used across the country, and Acoziborole.

Finally, HAT control in the field also consists of vector control, which is a complementary strategy to the screening and treatment of patients and is also coordinated by the PNLTHA. The newest technology in this field is the 'tiny targets': small insecticide-impregnated screens that are cheap and easy to use and can be deployed on a large scale [31].

3. Materials and Methods

To understand the perspectives of frontline HAT providers, we conducted semi-structured interviews with officers of the national vertical programme (PNLTHA) who work at the intermediate and peripheral levels of HAT control in the former province of Bandundu. Bandundu has hosted around 50% of all patients diagnosed with HAT in recent years [32,33]. At the time of the interviews in February 2018, HAT screening and treatment activities were carried out by 13 mobile teams doing mass screening in endemic HAT villages, 18 mini-teams that organised home-based HAT screening, 20 'fixed' health facilities specialised in HAT screening and treatment (*Centre de Dépistage, Traitement et Contrôle de la THA* (CDTC)) and several other health centres and general reference hospitals that had integrated passive screening and treatment of patients into their package of activities. Two provincial HAT coordinators (North Bandundu and South Bandundu) were in charge of the mobile teams and treatment and screening centres. The province of Bandundu is now divided into three separate provinces: Kwilu (our fieldwork sites: Bandundu ville, Kikwit, Masinanimba, Bagata, and Yasa Bonga), Maidombe (our fieldwork site: Mushi) and Kwango (our fieldwork site: Kenge).

The research participants worked at the levels of the mobile teams (team leader, secretary, and laboratory technician), at the health facilities that specialise in HAT (nurse in charge of the centre) and at the provincial HAT coordination (coordinating physician and provincial supervisor). It is important to note that our study is only about PLNTHA workers, who are the main responders to the HAT epidemic (but not the only ones, as explained earlier). Sampling was oriented to include participants of different ages and profiles, and the interviews were organised until saturation, which was reached with a total of 21 interviews. Table 1 sums up the profile of the interviewees and includes the interview number that is referenced in the analysis.

Table 1. Profiles of the research participants.

Category	Role	Gender	Experience	Interview Number
mobile unit	2 Community outreach workers 1 Secretary 2 Technicians (lab) 6 Leaders (nurse/technician, *chef d'équipe mobile*)	all males	28 years (SD: 10.9)	1, 2 17 20, 21 3–8
Frontline non-mobile	4 HAT centre (CDTC) chief nurse 2 HAT hospital centre chief nurse	all males	25.8 (6.37)	11–14 15–16
management	2 HAT provincial management (supervisor) 2 HAT provincial management (coordinator)	all males	31 (9.89) 11.5 (2.12)	18, 19 9, 10

The interviews were led by the Congolese co-author (Mpanya) who was already known to some of the interviews (as he has been conducting research in this field for years). Participation was voluntary, and participants were invited for interviews at an agreed location according to their availability. The interviews were conducted in the local language, in Lingala, or in French, depending on the choice of the interviewee. They were recorded on a digital medium with the consent of the interviewee and lasted on average 35 min (the longest took 56 min). The recordings were transcribed and entered in MS Word, and the data were coded and analysed using Nvivo (12.0).

An interview guide was used and is available in Appendix A. The main themes of the guide were directed by our research questions and focussed on the respondents explaining (1) their career in HAT control, (2) the perception of the current efforts vis-à-vis elimination (number of cases, elimination objectives, etc.), and (3) how they perceive their life will be after HAT elimination (if conceivable to them at all). There was no apparent risk to study participants, and the study protocol was approved by the Ethics Committee of the Faculty of Medicine of the University of Lubumbashi and the School of Social and Political Science at the University of Edinburgh. The anonymity and confidentiality of the participants were guaranteed. The consent of the study participants was obtained orally and recorded; written consent would make participants uncomfortable to express themselves easily. Only the two researchers who conducted this research and the assistant who helped with transcription have had access to the collected information.

4. Results

A series of key themes emerged through the coding and analysis of the interviews: many are directly derived from our interview guide, but others were unanticipated such as HAT 'vocations', the preoccupations with vector control, or the expectation that the state will provide future employment after HAT elimination. We identified a total of 12 (key) interrelated topics, which we will present through three sub-section. The first sub-section characterises the profiles, careers, and livelihoods of those involved in frontline HAT control; it shows entire lives devoted to fighting the disease and work conditions that are improving on some aspects and deteriorating on others. The second sub-section shows how HAT workers perceived the announced imminent elimination of the disease; most remain careful and point to two challenges: the coverage of HAT screening activities and difficulties of eliminating the vector. The third sub-section documents the ways in which HAT workers see their lives after elimination and how they are preparing for it.

4.1. Work at the Frontline

Two elements appear central to understanding the experience of frontline workers: the changing nature of their work in recent years and their keen sense of attachment to HAT control.

As touched upon in the background section, HAT control technology has evolved substantially over recent decades. It has deeply affected the work done at the frontline. On the one hand, all our interviewees recognise that new technology such as RDTs and NECT has rendered their work easier. On the other hand, though, the sharp decrease in the number of cases in the last two decades has also had a clear financial and organisational impact on work, especially for mobile units.

In financial terms, fewer cases have meant fewer premiums paid to team members for detecting positive cases. The interviews led to ample discussions about the workers' pay, with mobile unit members complaining that their income has diminished in real terms because of the increased cost of life and the suppression or impossibility to obtain premiums beyond the monthly 'fixed' (*prime fixe*) and 'mobility' (*prime d'itinérance*, premium for being in a mobile team) premiums. For a regular mobile team member, the former is around $100, while the latter is around $200.

The main effect of the progressive elimination of the disease is, however, in terms of workload. Fewer cases typically mean more time spent looking for cases. Mobile teams are asked to spend more extended periods of time in the field. Twenty days per month, which can extend to 22 or 24 days, are the norm. While mobile unit members explain that they are used to spending time in the field, they also explain that 20-day missions lead to complications with family lives and relationships: "it penalises our wives and children" explains a mobile unit member (1, mobile unit). Longer distances also mean that it is harder to come back urgently, with workers reporting cases of colleagues being unable to attend dying partners and children.

Another unanimously reported element that has made work harder is the changing socio-political environment, with the local leaders (customary chiefs, community notables, and community health workers) less inclined to help the teams, sometimes asking to be paid to provide assistance. This is a change from the time when mobile units could automatically count on the support of the chiefs, as explained by a mobile unit veteran:

> "in the time of Mobutu [in the 1970s?] the authorities would fine those who did not come to us, so people came en masse, as they feared to be arrested. But now, the authorities don't do that. […] now it is difficult to get people as the authorities do not get involved" (8, mobile unit)

Against this changing nature of work, a second critical element that stands out in the HAT frontline workers' narratives of their careers is their distinctive attachment to the cause of fighting HAT and to the programme they serve, the PNLTHA. This attachment builds on several entangled elements: long careers, 'vocations' for HAT, comradery and a sense of belonging to a community, and the conviction of being involved in a noble project.

Our study is not a systematic survey of HAT workers, but it is clear from the interviews that many on the frontline spent most if not all of their careers in HAT. Our interviewees often have decades of experience, which is not a coincidence or a sampling anomaly; rather, it signals that careers are being made in HAT. As explained by our participants, when people start working on HAT, they often keep working on HAT. All the mobile unit leaders climbed up the ranks, and so did the coordinators of the treatment centres. The oldest interviewees call themselves the 'second generation' (8, mobile unit) as they came after the first generation of mobile units and dispensaries set up under Belgian rule. Long careers create a sense of attachment and a strong identification with HAT control efforts that are described as a core dimension of people's lives, as one senior interviewee explained:

"When I started working, I was not married yet. I married 'in' [*dans*] sleeping sickness, I got children in sleeping sickness, I schooled my children in sleeping sickness, I built [my house] in sleeping sickness. I could say a good part of my life is built on sleeping sickness" (15, frontline non-mobile)

In around a third of the cases, the interviewees referred to a vocation for HAT control. The origins of such vocation were explained as typically revolving around the traumatic experience of witnessing a patient or a relative dying of HAT or its treatment with Arsobal (*melaprosol*), or around a charismatic mentor. Well-known figures of HAT control in the DR Congo such as Constantin Miaka (former director of PLNTHA) or Herman Bruneel (head of FOMETRO, an NGO that supported the fight against HAT in the 1980s and 1990s) as well as less well-known HAT workers—including, in one case, the father of the interviewed HAT worker—are cited as mentors by workers at all levels of responsibility.

Such a sense of closeness between frontline actors and national level figures such as Miaka naturally leads to discussing another key feature of HAT work: the sense of belonging to a strong community that is clear from all interviews. Such a strong bond is expected in the case of the mobile unit members that spend extensive amounts of time together in hard conditions, but it was also depicted at higher levels of responsibility, at the provincial level (as well as the national level, in a related piece of research we conducted on national level actors). The HAT community, which many described using the word 'family', is primarily but not solely Congolese and includes national and foreign researchers, whom one respondent describes as part of a virtuous circle of information sharing and learning. A senior nurse explained the importance of this community:

"[what I like most about HAT is] the family of the fight against Trypanosomiasis that we have been able to have. Wherever we went, we met people who are in this fight; it really gives us joy; it's really great memory for me, unforgettable because we met a lot of people, of all categories and even some people from foreign countries" (18, management)

Ultimately, this sense of attachment also relates to the idea that HAT workers have of themselves as a specialised unit, which has given them the opportunity to obtain a higher social rank. While staff members regularly complain about their pay, and possibly rightly so, they remain better paid than both public health workers at the same level of qualification and the average Congolese (GDP per capita was $457.58 in 2017), and perhaps more so than in the past as the general job market has deteriorated, as reported by a coordinator (19, management). The sense of HAT control as a form of 'social ladder' is especially visible among older workers of mobile units. When asked what their best memory of HAT control is, two of them spontaneously explained:

"my children have studied, my eldest will soon become a doctor, he is studying in Kinshasa [. . .]. I have also bought a plot of land here in Bandundu." (20, mobile unit)

"well, I can say that with the little they give me at the end of the month, that's what allows me to have my children study [. . .], so, in short, my children study." (2, mobile unit)

A third one explained that the benefit is not only financial. As a doctor, "it was through sleeping sickness that I was able to get this reputation [*heritage*], and sleeping sickness made my name known" (9, management).

Fully understanding that work at the frontline remains hard, albeit in new ways, is crucial to mobilise efforts to achieve HAT elimination. This sub-section has also highlighted the distinctive identity of HAT workers who are characterised by a strong sense of community and common cause and whose professional activity has been, especially for the least qualified, akin to social elevation.

4.2. Perspectives on Elimination

Almost all the interviewees agree that the epidemiological decrease claimed at the national level rings true with their observations as frontline workers—the epidemic is going down. They associate such trends with the efforts of the PNLTHA (but rarely directly cite new technology), and some also identify more systemic change that affects the vector, such as new land use:

"The large forests where tsetse flies used to hide are being pulled up, people are starting to cultivate the fields there, they are making small ponds; and even here in the village, there are no tsetse flies left." (14, frontline non-mobile)

Importantly and interestingly, though, none of the 21 interviewees felt totally comfortable with the year 2020 being selected as the point of elimination of HAT as a public health problem. As we will discuss later, this view contrasts with the view of international and national public health policymakers. The most optimistic of our respondents, around a third of the sample, foresaw the end of the epidemic somewhere between 2022 and 2025, provided that substantial resources go to control. The rest of the respondents were cautiously optimistic; they saw the epidemic as "nearing the end", but they would not risk committing to an end date. Half the respondents did not appear to believe that total elimination was possible; rather they compared the future of HAT to the presence of diseases that have now become very rare in DR Congo, such as leprosy:

"Sleeping sickness can be eliminated, but it will be like leprosy. [They told us it is eliminated but] I saw the people here in Bandundu who don't have toes. When I asked the question, I was told that there was a disease called leprosy, Maba's disease. Even today, we, the mobile unit, have friends who are on the leprosy and tuberculosis programme." (1, mobile unit)

The reason frontline workers are not fully confident that elimination will happen in the short run is related to two aspects: the coverage of their control activities and the work on vectors. It is important to note that none of them questioned the technology. There is no doubt, in the mind of the interviewees, that the tools at their disposal—first and foremost RDT and NECT—are good. However, they do not see further technological progress as absolutely necessary for future progress. The only exception is one interviewee who stressed that finding a way that allows avoiding lumbar punctures would be important (he was apparently unaware of the Fexinidazole trial). Rather, as the two quotes below illustrate, the issue is with the organisation and efficiency of control and sensitisation activities that enable frontline workers to put technology into use:

"to eliminate the disease, two problems need to be solved. First of all, on the molecular side, we have succeeded, we have molecules that are really good. [...] the treatment [NECT] is not as toxic as before [Arsobal]. [The other side is] our explanations in the villages [...] there will be no elimination until everyone understands [can identify] sleeping sickness." (8, mobile unit)

"It is more a question of organisation than just tools. The tools may be there, but if they are not properly used or if the conditions of use of these tools are not met, elimination will not be achieved." (10, management)

The question of the sensitisation of the population is twofold. One issue, as expressed in the quotes above and as alluded to earlier has to do with the difficulty of convincing the population and their leaders to get tested and to report suspicious cases. This is partly a problem of knowledge (people cannot identify the disease) but also a broader issue of trust in the health system:

"Up to now our population, the whole of our population, is not sensitive to active screening. They have their reasons. There are some people who say that sleeping sickness is sometimes transmitted by us, the agents, by evil spirits." (7, mobile unit)

It is also a wider issue of trust in politico-administrative authorities, which echoes the deeper problems of governance in the endemic areas:

"The political-administrative authorities [likely referring to the leaders mentioned earlier] are not so much listened to by the population. [. . .] The population trusts us, but I tell you, the population no longer really trusts the agents of the state [government and administrators], but we greatly need them because the population belongs to them, we must go through their channel to try to take care of their population." (5, mobile unit)

This issue has led, as hinted at earlier, to giving monetary incentives to community leaders. It is seen as tricky by frontline workers who both criticise the situation but also find themselves with no other option than asking the programme and funders to give them such money. This is a change, "in the old days when we went to a village; we gave nothing to the elders" (3, mobile unit) explains a nurse. Another explains how they now have to:

"give people a motivation [understood as a financial incentive in this context] to access people in the villages where we go, because we are dealing with village chiefs, elders, religious leaders and community relays, they are the ones who help us to do our job well. Motivation is one of the realities we encounter in the field in villages" (2, mobile unit)

The question of community involvement and sensitisation, combined with the coverage of active screening activities, leads to the core argument of the frontline workers for why elimination may be farther away than expected: the low level of coverage of the territory by PNLTHA activities. Almost all research participants expressed this concern; some even explained that in their view, such low coverage might hide the real size of the epidemic:

"The decrease in [reported] cases, here I would just like to explain that it is not necessarily related to [a true] decrease in endemicity. So endemicity may still exist, but since the level of control has decreased due to lack of resources, it may also explain the decrease in the number of cases." (18, management)

While many understand that the areas covered are the most at risk of harbouring disease, they refuse to ignore the possibility that cases could be overlooked:

"[When asked about the possibility of elimination by 2020] That is a firm no. We do not yet know how to reach it because, so far, we only have coverage of the population at high risk. We know that currently with the WHO we have categorized the high-risk, medium-risk and low-risk areas, but when we take the areas of active screening together, we do not go well beyond 20% of the population." (9, management)

All our respondents identified coverage as a core issue, "if we don't put the emphasis on coverage, the other ingredients will not kick in" (19, management) explained a manager. The suggestion is to reschedule activities and mobile units to villages not visited in some time (the so-called *reprogrammation*), and put resources "village by village, then we will know whether the disease has been eradicated" (21, mobile unit).

The second objection that was raised to elimination by 2020 is the lack of emphasis on the vector in current efforts: "the strain [trypanosomiasis parasite] must be destroyed, if the tsetse fly continues to multiply, to occur, it is difficult to believe that we can have a total elimination" (13, frontline non-mobile). Half the respondents insisted on the need to engage more substantially with the vector, pointing out to challenges in the current interventions.

"Secondly, in this same population, you will try to set traps wherever there are tsetse flies. We educate them [the population] but these same traps are stolen by the same population [. . .], even if you designate people to monitor these traps and catch tsetse flies [. . .] they ask for money, they must be motivated." (7, mobile unit)

Overall, we see that HAT frontline workers are not as convinced as international actors of the possibility of an imminent elimination of the disease. Based on their experience and practice of HAT control, they explain that such elimination would imply two hard to achieve premises: that PNLTHA activities stretch to all the areas potentially affected by HAT and that the vector is better controlled (they do not explain what this would mean in practice, but agree that not all flies can be eradicated). It is also clear that frontline workers do not see a clear-cut distinction between the elimination and the eradication targets.

4.3. Personal Effects of Elimination

Bearing in mind that many frontline workers do not see elimination as imminent, let's now turn to the workers' perspectives on the effects that elimination would have on them, as individuals.

When asked about their feelings towards the idea of elimination, frontline workers at all levels of responsibility first expressed keen enthusiasm rather than fear for their livelihoods: "I am not worried, I rejoice" explained a mobile unit worker (18, management). The emotional commitment of the HAT workers explained in Section 4.1 should not be underestimated: the interviewees shared a sense of being part of a mission, which is the elimination of the disease, and all personally witnessed the burden of HAT. The primary emotion associated with the possible elimination of HAT was pride, and it was echoed by every research participant: "our objective is not to maintain HAT but to get it out of our country, and if we can eliminate it, that is a source of pride for us. And for our lives" (7, mobile unit).

When seeking to push further on the question of what would happen if the elimination became a reality, different attitudes prevail, sometimes expressed one after the other. The most common was for the frontline workers to mention their status as civil servants and explain that they trust the state to re-allocate them to relevant posts: "the state cannot abandon these people, it will introduce them to the general hospital to treat certain diseases, even in health zones" (16, frontline non-mobile). It is implicitly assumed that it would probably mean a lower level of income: "as we are agents of the state, if the state could pay civil servants properly, we can continue to survive, it is not the end of the world" (5, mobile unit), and the older generations were confident that they would probably not be re-allocated but rather retire with "honourable retirement benefits". In many cases, because the possibility of elimination of HAT is not entertained as a genuine imminent possibility, the sense is that HAT expertise will continue to be needed even if the number of cases is very low, but the work would be slightly different, more related to passive screening:

> "The people in the mobile units are not afraid; they say that the work will not end because the disease will not end. [... even if] the programme (PNLTHA) tends towards the end; the disease will not end; it is since the creation" (16, frontline non-mobile)

Integration in the non-HAT health system is then seen as the main option for many, who also display a sense of confidence in their skills and abilities. It is often doubled with a strong belief in God's will or in one's personal capacity to find an alternative livelihood.

Not all frontline workers are in the same situation, though. Fear is more visible among those who are less qualified or newer and are often not registered on the national level books [*non-mécanisé*], meaning that they were hired locally, or that they are, sometimes at the same time, not on the official payroll [*non-payé*]. Even with them, though, a strong sense of resilience seems to prevail:

> "I am in a new unit without a personnel number [unregistered, *non-mécanisé*], that's something that scares me; I can become unemployed in that sense. But I know that whoever gave me this job knows how he's going to use me. If he is tired of me, I will do agriculture; I will fish if I still have the strength." (2, mobile unit)

> "I'm a registered and 'unpaid' [by the Ministry of Health, *non-payé*] employee, but we'll always go to the inspection [provincial health authorities], or we'll manage. There is always life." (1, mobile unit)

Such a form of (anticipated) resilience is not uncommon in DR Congo, a country which has endured decades of instability and violence. This is not to say that losing the HAT premiums or HAT-related job is not a concern:

"[...] it worries us; it must worry us because where you were able to afford school fees for children, you are stuck with that. [...] As you are given something that is not sufficient enough, you try to find a way, but then you will get used to it." (15, frontline non-mobile)

Managers, even if they share the views that elimination may not happen too soon, have nevertheless been thinking about alternative options for their staff:

"The majority of our service providers, our employees, they are under-qualified, and they will have a lot of difficulties to learn other knowledge. We have a vast project for them that will involve training people, obtaining scholarships [...], on-the-job training for everyone, [...] not specific to sleeping sickness. [...]. And thirdly, we believe that for our staff, as many of them, we must obtain the *mecanisé* status [have them on the ministry books]." (10, management)

Beyond thinking about possible strategies, managers have already had their laboratory technicians and nurses undergo training on malaria, filariasis, and onchocerciasis. As a manager pointed out, "if sleeping sickness is over today, filariasis will not leave today, what would prevent us from continuing to fight communicable diseases with the same teams?" (20, mobile unit). In addition to this, active networking and positioning by staff seem to be taking place as well, as explained by a mobile unit leader:

"We always ask the chief doctors of the zones whether it is the vaccination period and whether they can take people from the mobile units so that they can also immerse themselves in other stories [other contexts] so that when the time comes, they will still be useful to Congolese society." (18, management)

Overall, HAT frontline workers appear to have ambiguous attitudes towards their future in a post-HAT DR Congo. All of them appear genuinely delighted to imagine that such a world may exist, despite the implications it may have for their livelihoods The more experienced and senior workers appear confident that as civil servants, they will be allocated to a new position—which they believe they are qualified and competent for because of their training. Less secure workers seem aware that the risk of unemployment is higher for them but are also confident in their resilience capacity. The sub-section has also shown that managers are already deploying strategies for providing their staff with the best chances of securing alternative positions or livelihoods.

5. Discussion

The interviews reveal frontline workers who form a community of experienced HAT experts who are genuinely dedicated to the elimination of the disease. As it was documented in other cases, their experience is also the local historical memory of HAT research and programmes in the area [34]. The frontline workers form a crucial resource that is trusted by the population and recognised for its capacity. Their value should not be underestimated when operating in the difficult context of the DR Congo; this is for implementing HAT-related innovations, understanding the progress that is being made in the field, but also strengthening the health system in general.

The findings need to be considered in the context of the recent evolution of efforts to fight HAT in the DR Congo, bearing in mind that the mobile units are the ones that feel the most pressure due to the anticipated replacement of mobile units with mini-mobile units and changes in the micro-planification of activities. Overall, the interviewees show some scepticism towards the possibility of a very near elimination of HAT in the DR Congo. It is useful to note that it is only their perspective (and not the perspective of the PNLTHA as a whole), which is informed by their (partial) field experience and work rather than a comprehensive picture of the situation in the whole of DR Congo. On the ground, those working on control think more in terms of the absolute number of cases (that they see) than in terms of incidence rates. There might also be some confusion with the word 'elimination', which is not always used consistently by policymakers and academics alike [35]. The interviewees understand elimination as the elimination of the disease, by which they mean a reduction to zero of the HAT incidence, which is different from WHO's idea of elimination of HAT as a public health problem that still requires "measures to prevent the re-establishment of transmission" [35]. Some of the interviewees also seem to conflate elimination with eradication, which is the situation when no intervention whatsoever is required any longer. Beyond the question of the definition, the issues pointed out by the research participants is that the perceived lack of control of the vector (which was recently reinforced on over 120,000 km^2 with the support of the Liverpool School of Tropical Medicine) and the 'blind spots'—the areas without active screening—are impediments to elimination. Here again, it is useful to remind that the reality seen from the field does not necessarily include a broader level vision of recent efforts to increase data quality, which include projects funded by the Bill and Melinda Gates Foundation and Belgian government since 2015 in the provinces of Kwangu, Maindombe and Kwilu. This caveat aside, the perspectives of the frontline workers align with research pointing to the necessity to properly combine screening, treatment of patients, and vector control to eliminate HAT rapidly [31,36].

The frontline workers also express a discourse that is not necessarily always visible in the policy declarations and academic literature that keenly emphasise technological progress: eliminating HAT requires, in their view, a deeper investment in detection and treatment. They partially echo research that discusses the merits of passive screening [9,26] and suggests difficulties in spreading efficient and easy detection tools such as the combination of RDT with loop-mediated isothermal amplification (LAMP) [5], not so much because it is technically hard to detect cases but rather because of the epidemiological context and the lack of HAT skills in the system (outside PNLTHA) [36]—in other words, the strength of the health system. As one of the interviewees put it: "it is more a question of organisation than just tools".

The changing nature of the work of the frontline health workers, and in particular the difficulties they face enrolling people into active screening [26] and collaborating with the local health authorities [10], points to another set of issues that are not discussed in great length in the literature on HAT elimination. Two dynamics seem to be reinforcing each other. On the one hand, as in all cases of disease elimination, the fact that the disease becomes rarer means that people and their leaders pay less attention to it and are less interested in investing resources in it or endure hardship to fight it. This is similar to what was observed with polio and smallpox campaigns [37–39]. On the other hand, the endemic regions of DR Congo also witnessed profound socio-political changes in recent decades and gaining the trust of communities and their leaders is, according to our findings, harder than before (regardless of the motive). Palmer and colleagues also touch on the issue in a paper on Uganda [40]. The context is slightly different as they look at refugees, but the similarities are clear: populations are seen a 'belonging' to authorities who are their unavoidable gatekeepers, and relations with them seem increasingly monetised. This must also be considered against the background of decades of international aid and changing incentive structures, including the 'culture of per diem' [41,42] that makes it harder for PNLTHA teams to obtain support from community leaders and even health workers without providing monetary incentives. Again, we know from other elimination campaigns that community involvement is absolutely central to elimination [39]. The combination of the difficulty of enrolling people in screening and the difficulty of collaborating with local politico-administrative authorities should be fully considered as it may have an influence on the actual cost [43] and efforts needed to reach elimination.

In answer to our second research question, we found that frontline workers display ambivalent attitudes towards their post-elimination future. Many interviewees doubt that elimination will arise too soon and also appear confident that as civil servants, they will simply be redeployed to other services. Staff of mobile team units, who also have in mind ongoing changes in the organisation of active screening, are probably the most concerned of the interviewees. Polio and smallpox eradication campaigns around the world suggest that such redeployment may happen [13], but the case of HAT in DR Congo and Bandundu may be more complicated for two reasons. First, the level of verticalization or 'siloisation' is very high [44] and workers are very specialised. Contrary to other countries, many HAT frontline nurses and lab technicians mostly, when not only, work on HAT and may not have much experience working on other medical conditions. Managers seem mindful of this issue; they have taken measures to facilitate such redeployment when and if it is needed, for instance they organised the temporary placement of their staff in other units (e.g., in vaccination campaigns), so they gain experience and can demonstrate their usefulness. They also organised refresher courses on non-HAT health issues. Other options are available but were not directly mentioned by the mobile teams and frontline workers; they include maintaining the mobile teams but allocating them to other tasks such as population census, curative healthcare activities (with the mobile unit become a de facto more generalist mobile clinic) in remote areas, or the coordination of preventative healthcare efforts. The second reason redeployment may be challenging is that some frontline workers are hired locally and do not appear in the central level registries. As in other fields of the public service in DR Congo [45], a higher level of struggle is anticipated for those workers.

Beyond the question of the resilience of HAT frontline workers to post-HAT changes in the labour market, a more immediate question is suggested by the research participants. They point out that their expertise may still be useful for quite some time after a 'zero new cases' situation is declared, for monitoring the situation as the local, non-specialised workforce, is not seen as able to do that—an argument that echoes the need for keeping human expertise during the final stages of elimination [36,46]. Such integration, from the perspective of human resources and human expertise rather than tools (e.g., rapid diagnostic tests) and activities, is not really discussed in the emerging literature on integration [24,47]. Future research should explore scenarios of integration that do not only see health facilities as covering new aspects of healthcare but also as integrating practitioners with specific experience. The issue may be DR Congo (or even Bandundu) specific—other countries have a much smaller specialised HAT workforce—but it is worth considering given the place of DR Congo in the HAT epidemic.

There are clear limitations to the present study: it is limited to a few sites, it only collects the views of a few individuals (even if saturation seems reached among them), and it does not address at all issues such as the gendered perspective on HAT (all respondents, as most of the HAT workforce, is male). The article should be considered a preliminary effort towards better understanding frontline realities and livelihoods rather than definitive work on the topic. It is also important to state the exceptionalism of DRC, and especially Bandundu, compared to other contexts: it has high and continuous levels of disease, a culture of incentives, and a history of centralisation of HAT expertise (this is different from many other settings when HAT coordinators are primarily interested in exposing generally skilled health workers to HAT [26]). Replicating the research in other sites, and especially sites that are more peripheral to the HAT elimination efforts would be useful to understand the situation at a more advanced stage of elimination, as would a more systematic review of the concerns expressed by the respondents and in particular communities' and leaders' changing attitude towards HAT and the health system in general and the risks associated with a focus of active screening on only a selected priority endemic areas.

6. Conclusions

The perspectives of frontline workers cast light on aspects of HAT elimination that are not at the forefront of many academic and policy publications: the growing socio-political difficulty of active screening, field perspectives on the coverage of detection and treatment activities, and the strong community of practitioners around HAT. The findings shift the perspective from an emphasis on innovations (drugs, tests, vector targets) to the need to pay sustained attention to the organisation of HAT elimination. While the findings nuance the possibility of an imminent elimination of HAT, they also suggest concrete pathways to improving the efficacy of elimination efforts.

Author Contributions: Conceptualisation, J.-B.F.; methodology, A.M. and J.-B.F.; formal analysis, J.-B.F.; investigation, A.M.; data curation, J.-B.F.; writing—original draft preparation, J.-B.F. and A.M.; writing—review, interpretation, and editing, J.-B.F., A.M. and E.M.-M. All authors have read and agreed to the published version of the manuscript.

Funding: This research was funded by the European Research Council (ERC) under grant agreement 2958450 "Investigating Networks of Zoonosis Innovation (INZI)".

Acknowledgments: The authors would like to thank James Smith for kindly inviting them to his research team as well as Jen Palmer and Michelle Taylor for insightful discussions. Jen Palmer and Shona Lee provided encouraging and constructive feedback on a draft version of the paper. Winnie Mputu and Dora Beya transcribed the interviews. The funders had no role in study design, data collection and analysis, decision to publish, or preparation of the manuscript.

Conflicts of Interest: The authors declare no conflict of interest.

Appendix A. Interview Guide

- Could you briefly tell us about who you are, how and when you started working in sleeping sickness?
- What have been your main responsibilities in the fight against sleeping sickness so far?
- In your role you visit several places where there is sleeping sickness, considering its current evolution, do you think that we will eliminate sleeping sickness
- Currently we are talking about the elimination of the HAT by 2020, do you think this objective is achievable in the DRC?
- What does it mean for you to be on the ground when it comes to the elimination of sleeping sickness in the DRC?
- Some interviewees say that innovations in HAT treatment, diagnosis and new screening approaches are needed to eliminate sleeping sickness. Others, on the other hand, believe that even if there are innovations if the coverage of the population at risk remains low, elimination will not be possible. What are you saying?
- Some interviewees say that you members of the mobile teams and HAT treatment centre are afraid of the elimination of sleeping sickness for fear of losing your job when the disease disappears?
- If tomorrow sleeping sickness were to disappear, what would you do?
- Do you control diseases other than HAT? Is there anything else your team could do that you think your team could do?
- In your opinion, what are the major challenges to eliminating sleeping sickness in the DRC?

References

1. Barrett, M.P. The elimination of human African trypanosomiasis is in sight: Report from the third WHO stakeholders meeting on elimination of gambiense human African trypanosomiasis. *PLoS Negl. Trop. Dis.* **2018**, *12*, e0006925. [CrossRef] [PubMed]
2. Miaka, E.M.; Hasker, E.; Verlé, P.; Torr, S.J.; Boelaert, M. Sleeping sickness in the Democratic Republic of the Congo. *Lancet Neurol.* **2019**, *18*, 988–989. [CrossRef]
3. Akazue, P.I.; Ebiloma, G.U.; Ajibola, O.; Isaac, C.; Onyekwelu, K.; Ezeh, C.O.; Eze, A.A. Sustainable Elimination (Zero Cases) of Sleeping Sickness: How Far Are We from Achieving This Goal? *Pathogens* **2019**, *8*, 135. [CrossRef] [PubMed]
4. Simarro, P.P.; Jannin, J.; Cattand, P. Eliminating human African trypanosomiasis: Where do we stand and what comes next? *PLoS Med.* **2008**, *5*, e55. [CrossRef] [PubMed]
5. Wamboga, C.; Matovu, E.; Bessell, P.R.; Picado, A.; Biéler, S.; Ndung'u, J.M. Enhanced passive screening and diagnosis for gambiense human African trypanosomiasis in north-western Uganda—Moving towards elimination. *PLoS ONE* **2017**, *12*, e0186429. [CrossRef] [PubMed]

6. Mesu, V.K.B.K.; Kalonji, W.M.; Bardonneau, C.; Mordt, O.V.; Blesson, S.; Simon, F.; Delhomme, S.; Bernhard, S.; Kuziena, W.; Lubaki, J.P.F.; et al. Oral fexinidazole for late-stage African Trypanosoma brucei gambiense trypanosomiasis: A pivotal multicentre, randomised, non-inferiority trial. *Lancet* **2018**, *391*, 144–154. [CrossRef]

7. Alirol, E.; Schrumpf, D.; Amici Heradi, J.; Riedel, A.; De Patoul, C.; Quere, M.; Chappuis, F. Nifurtimox-eflornithine combination therapy for second-stage gambiense human African trypanosomiasis: Médecins Sans Frontières experience in the Democratic Republic of the Congo. *Clin. Infect. Dis.* **2013**, *56*, 195–203. [CrossRef]

8. Jamonneau, V.; Bucheton, B. The challenge of serodiagnosis of sleeping sickness in the context of elimination. *Lancet Glob. Health* **2014**, *2*, e306–e307. [CrossRef]

9. Cattand, P.; Jannin, J.; Lucas, P. Sleeping sickness surveillance: An essential step towards elimination. *Trop. Med. Int. Health* **2001**, *6*, 348–361. [CrossRef]

10. Palmer, J.J.; Kelly, A.H.; Surur, E.I.; Checchi, F.; Jones, C. Changing landscapes, changing practice: Negotiating access to sleeping sickness services in a post-conflict society. *Soc. Sci. Med.* **2014**, *120*, 396–404. [CrossRef]

11. Tong, J.; Valverde, O.; Mahoudeau, C.; Yun, O.; Chappuis, F. Challenges of controlling sleeping sickness in areas of violent conflict: Experience in the Democratic Republic of Congo. *Confl. Health* **2011**, *5*, 1–8. [CrossRef] [PubMed]

12. Lumbala, C.; Simarro, P.P.; Cecchi, G.; Paone, M.; Franco, J.R.; Betu Ku Mesu, V.K.; Makabuza, J.; Diarra, A.; Chansy, S.; Priotto, G.; et al. Human African trypanosomiasis in the Democratic Republic of the Congo: Disease distribution and risk. *Int. J. Health Geogr.* **2015**, *14*. [CrossRef] [PubMed]

13. Loevinsohn, B.; Aylward, B.; Steinglass, R.; Ogden, E.; Goodman, T.; Melgaard, B. Impact of targeted programs on health systems: A case study of the polio eradication initiative. *Am. J. Public Health* **2002**, *92*, 19–23. [CrossRef] [PubMed]

14. Kingori, B.P.; Mcgowan, C. After the End of Ebola. *Somatosphere* **2016**. Available online: http://somatosphere. net/2016/after-the-end-of-ebola.html/ (accessed on 28 December 2019).

15. Lutumba, P.; Robays, J.; Bilenge, C.M.M.; Mesu, V.K.B.K.; Molisho, D.; Declercq, J.; Van Der Veken, W.; Meheus, F.; Jannin, J.; Boelaert, M. Trypanosomiasis control, Democratic Republic of Congo, 1993–2003. *Emerg. Infect. Dis.* **2005**, *11*, 1382–1388. [CrossRef]

16. Courtin, F.; Jamonneau, V.; Duvallet, G.; Garcia, A.; Coulibaly, B.; Doumenge, J.P.; Cuny, G.; Solano, P. Sleeping sickness in West Africa (1906–2006): Changes in spatial repartition and lessons from the past. *Trop. Med. Int. Health* **2008**, *13*, 334–344. [CrossRef]

17. Brun, R.; Blum, J.; Chappuis, F.; Burri, C. Human African trypanosomiasis. *Lancet* **2010**, *375*, 148–159. [CrossRef]

18. PNLTHA. *Rapport Annuel 2018 Du Programme National De Lutte Contre La THA En RDC*; Ministry of Health: Kinshasa, Democratic Republic of the Congo, 2018.

19. Franco, J.R.; Simarro, P.P.; Diarra, A.; Jannin, J.G. Epidemiology of human African trypanosomiasis. *Clin. Epidemiol.* **2014**, *6*, 257–275.

20. Franco, J.R.; Cecchi, G.; Priotto, G.; Paone, M.; Diarra, A.; Grout, L.; Mattioli, R.C.; Argaw, D. Monitoring the elimination of human African trypanosomiasis: Update to 2014. *PLoS Negl. Trop. Dis.* **2017**, *11*, e0005585. [CrossRef]

21. Davidson, K. DRC Government Steps Up Commitment to Eliminating Sleeping Sickness by 2020. 2018 (31 Januray). Available online: https://www.path.org/media-center/drc-government-steps-up-commitment-to-eliminating-sleeping-sickness-by-2020/ (accessed on 28 December 2019).

22. PNLTHA. *Rapport Annuel 2016 Du Programme National De Lutte Contre La THA En RDC*; Ministry of Health: Kinshasa, Democratic Republic of the Congo, 2016.

23. Mitashi, P.; Hasker, E.; Mbo, F.; Van Geertruyden, J.P.; Kaswa, M.; Lumbala, C.; Boelaert, M.; Lutumba, P. Integration of diagnosis and treatment of sleeping sickness in primary healthcare facilities in the democratic republic of the congo. *Trop. Med. Int. Health* **2015**, *20*, 98–105. [CrossRef]

24. Mulenga, P.; Boelaert, M.; Lutumba, P.; Vander Kelen, C.; Coppieters, Y.; Chenge, F.; Lumbala, C.; Luboya, O.; Mpanya, A. Integration of Human African trypanosomiasis control activities into primary health services in the democratic republic of the Congo: A qualitative study of stakeholder perceptions. *Am. J. Trop. Med. Hyg.* **2019**, *100*, 899–906. [CrossRef] [PubMed]

25. Jannin, J.; Moulia-Pelat, J.P.; Chanfreau, B.; Penchenier, L.; Louis, J.P.; Nzaba, P.; Elfassi De La Baume, F.; Eozenou, P.; Cattand, P. Trypanosomiase Humaine Africaine: Etude D'Un Score De Presomption De Diagnostic Au Congo. *Bull. World Health Organ.* **1993**, *71*, 215–222. [PubMed]

26. Palmer, J.J. The HAT diagnostic reflex: How do we instil this for elimination? *Trop. Med. Infect. Dis.* submitted.

27. Magnus, E.; Vervoort, T.; Van Meirvenne, N. A card-agglutination test with stained trypanosomes (C.A.T.T.) for the serological diagnosis of T. b. gambiense trypanosomiasis. *Ann. Soc. Belg. Med. Trop. (1920)* **1978**, *58*, 169–176.

28. Büscher, P.; Gilleman, Q.; Lejon, V. Rapid Diagnostic Test for Sleeping Sickness. *N. Engl. J. Med.* **2013**, *368*, 1068–1069. [CrossRef] [PubMed]

29. WHO. Trypanosomiase Humaine Africaine: Lutte Et Surveillance. *Rapports Techniques d'un comité d'experts l'OMS* **2013**, *984*, 1–255.

30. Franco, J.R.; Simarro, P.P.; Diarra, A.; Ruiz-Postigo, J.A.; Samo, M.; Jannin, J.G. Monitoring the use of nifurtimox-eflornithine combination therapy (NECT) in the treatment of second stage gambiense human African trypanosomiasis. *Res. Rep. Trop. Med.* **2012**, *3*, 93. [CrossRef]

31. Mahamat, M.H.; Peka, M.; Rayaisse, J.B.; Rock, K.S.; Toko, M.A.; Darnas, J.; Brahim, G.M.; Alkatib, A.B.; Yoni, W.; Tirados, I.; et al. Adding tsetse control to medical activities contributes to decreasing transmission of sleeping sickness in the Mandoul focus (Chad). *PLoS Negl. Trop. Dis.* **2017**, *11*, e0005792. [CrossRef]

32. Lumbala, C.; Biéler, S.; Kayembe, S.; Makabuza, J.; Ongarello, S.; Ndung'u, J.M. Prospective evaluation of a rapid diagnostic test for Trypanosoma brucei gambiense infection developed using recombinant antigens. *PLoS Negl. Trop. Dis.* **2018**, *12*, e0006386. [CrossRef]

33. Lutumba, P.; Makieya, E.; Shaw, A.; Meheus, F.; Boelaert, M. Human African trypanosomiasis in a rural community, Democratic Republic of Congo. *Emerg. Infect. Dis.* **2007**, *13*, 248–254. [CrossRef]

34. Wenzel Geissler, P.; Lachenal, G.; Manton, J.; Tousignant, N. *Traces of the Future: An Archaeology of Medical Science in Africa*; Intellect: Bristol, UK, 2016.

35. Molyneux, D.H.; Hopkins, D.R.; Zagaria, N. Disease eradication, elimination and control: The need for accurate and consistent usage. *Trends Parasitol.* **2004**, *20*, 347–351. [CrossRef] [PubMed]

36. Mulenga, P.; Lutumba, P.; Coppieters, Y.; Mpanya, A.; Mwamba-Miaka, E.; Luboya, O.; Chenge, F. Passive Screening and Diagnosis of Sleeping Sickness with New Tools in Primary Health Services: An Operational Research. *Infect. Dis. Ther.* **2019**, *8*, 353–367. [CrossRef] [PubMed]

37. Greenough, P. Intimidation, coercion and resistance in the final stages of the South Asian Smallpox Eradication Campaign, 1973–1975. *Soc. Sci. Med.* **1995**, *41*, 633–645. [CrossRef]

38. Bhattacharya, S.; Dasgupta, R. Smallpox eradication's lessons for the antipolio campaign in India. *Am. J. Public Health* **2009**, *99*, 1176–1184. [CrossRef] [PubMed]

39. Larson, H.J.; Ghinai, I. Lessons from polio eradication. *Nature* **2011**, *473*, 446–447. [CrossRef]

40. Palmer, J.J.; Robert, O.; Kansiime, F. Including refugees in disease elimination: Challenges observed from a sleeping sickness programme in Uganda. *Confl. Health* **2017**, *11*, 22. [CrossRef]

41. Closser, S.; Rosenthal, A.; Justice, J.; Maes, K.; Sultan, M.; Banerji, S.; Amaha, H.B.; Gopinath, R.; Omidian, P.; Nyirazinyoye, L. Per diems in polio eradication: Perspectives from community health workers and officials. *Am. J. Public Health* **2017**, *107*, 1470–1476. [CrossRef]

42. Ridde, V. Per diems undermine health interventions, systems and research in Africa: Burying our heads in the sand. *Trop. Med. Int. Health* **2010**, *15*, E1–E4. [CrossRef]

43. Sutherland, C.S.; Tediosi, F. Is the elimination of sleeping sickness' affordable? Who will pay the price? Assessing the financial burden for the elimination of human African trypanosomiasis Trypanosoma brucei gambiense in sub-Saharan Africa. *BMJ Glob. Health* **2019**, *4*, e001173. [CrossRef]

44. Standley, C.; Boyce, M.R.; Klineberg, A.; Essix, G.; Katz, R. Organization of oversight for integrated control of neglected tropical diseases within Ministries of Health. *PLoS Negl. Trop. Dis.* **2018**, *12*, e0006929. [CrossRef]

45. Brandt, C. Teachers' Struggle for Income in the Congo (DRC). Between Education and Remuneration. *SSRN Electron. J.* **2019**. Available online: https://papers.ssrn.com/sol3/papers.cfm?abstract_id=3316289 (accessed on 28 December 2019).

46.   Lee, S.J.; Palmer, J.J. Integrating innovations: A qualitative analysis of referral non-completion among rapid diagnostic test-positive patients in Uganda's human African trypanosomiasis elimination programme. *Infect. Dis. Poverty* **2018**, *7*, 1–16. [CrossRef] [PubMed]

47.   Mulenga, P.; Chenge, F.; Boelaert, M.; Mukalay, A.; Lutumba, P.; Lumbala, C.; Luboya, O.; Coppieters, Y. Integration of human African trypanosomiasis control activities into primary healthcare services: A scoping review. *Am. J. Trop. Med. Hyg.* **2019**, *101*, 1114–1125. [CrossRef] [PubMed]

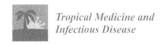

Tropical Medicine and Infectious Disease

Article

Understanding the Role of the Diagnostic 'Reflex' in the Elimination of Human African Trypanosomiasis

Jennifer J. Palmer [1,2,*], Caroline Jones [3], Elizeous I. Surur [4] and Ann H. Kelly [5]

1   Department of Global Health & Development, London School of Hygiene & Tropical Medicine,
    15–17 Tavistock Place, London WC1H 9SH, UK
2   Centre of African Studies, University of Edinburgh, 15a George Square, Edinburgh EH8 9LD, UK
3   Kemri-Wellcome Trust Research Programme, P.O. Box 230, Kilifi 80108, Kenya; cjones@kemri-wellcome.org
4   Independent consultant, Juba, South Sudan; elizeous@gmail.com
5   Department of Global Health & Social Medicine, King's College London, 30 Aldwych, London WC2B 4BG,
    UK; ann.kelly@kcl.ac.uk
*   Correspondence: jennifer.palmer@lshtm.ac.uk

Received: 7 December 2019; Accepted: 26 March 2020; Published: 1 April 2020

Abstract: To successfully eliminate human African trypanosomiasis (HAT), healthcare workers (HCWs) must maintain their diagnostic acuity to identify cases as the disease becomes rarer. HAT experts refer to this concept as a 'reflex' which incorporates the idea that diagnostic expertise, particularly skills involved in recognising which patients should be tested, comes from embodied knowledge, accrued through practice. We investigated diagnostic pathways in the detection of 32 symptomatic HAT patients in South Sudan and found that this 'reflex' was not confined to HCWs. Indeed, lay people suggested patients test for HAT in more than half of cases using similar practices to HCWs, highlighting the importance of the expertise present in disease-affected communities. Three typologies of diagnostic practice characterised patients' detection: 'syndromic suspicion', which closely resembled the idea of an expert diagnostic reflex, as well as 'pragmatic testing' and 'serendipitous detection', which depended on diagnostic expertise embedded in hospital and lay social structures when HAT-specific suspicion was ambivalent or even absent. As we approach elimination, health systems should embrace both expert and non-expert forms of diagnostic practice that can lead to detection. Supporting multidimensional access to HAT tests will be vital for HCWs and lay people to practice diagnosis and develop their expertise.

Keywords: South Sudan; human African trypanosomiasis; diagnosis; symptoms; treatment-seeking; case detection; elimination; embodiment; expertise; serendipity

1. Background

A key area of concern in today's drive towards elimination of human African trypanosomiasis (HAT)—a fatal but curable infectious disease also known as sleeping sickness—is whether healthcare workers (HCWs) in frontline facilities and populations in endemic areas have the necessary "reflex" to suspect HAT when they encounter someone showing characteristics of the disease [1] (p. 36). While important for any elimination campaign, for HAT, this preoccupation with peoples' familiarity with the disease's clinical presentation is an artefact of the particular challenges posed by its diagnosis.

With a variable symptom presentation affecting all parts of the body including the patient's mental capacity, descriptions of HAT have confounded clinical characterization for centuries [2]. Found only in scattered pockets of rural countryside in sub-Saharan Africa, HAT continues to be written about in medical textbooks and infectious disease case reports emphasising its exotic and mysterious character. HAT tends to be described through long lists of strange symptoms, from intermittent fevers to cardiac features, endocrine dysfunction, fertility problems, altered gait and tremors, uncontrollable episodes of sleep, lassitude, hallucinations and excessive sexual impulses [3,4], punctuated with authors' personal observations about other, less tangible ways to recognize the disease such as the "sad or strangely expressionless face" of HAT [5] (p. 150), [6]. "Owing to the many clinical variations of sleeping sickness", experts write, "it is difficult to describe a 'typical' case of the disease" [7] (p. 1310). Provided clinicians have access to the laboratory infrastructure necessary to identify the parasite, "[o]nce thought of, it is not usually a difficult diagnosis to confirm" [8] (p. 681). However, given that HAT infects only 1–2% of a population during outbreaks and is even more rare in places where elimination campaigns are underway [9], both the clinical and laboratory capacity, generally understood as a prerequisite for diagnosis, tend to be limited.

Moreover, 'active screening', the main method adopted by HAT programmes over the last century to detect patients with the most common, *Trypanosoma brucei gambiense* form of the disease, enables programmes to avoid having to consider the best ways to identify cases through clinical questioning. By assembling all people considered at risk of harbouring the infection in an area and asking them to submit a blood sample for analysis, the approach relies on laboratory technology and decision-making algorithms to detect disease rather than direct communication with sick people about their illnesses.

As cases of HAT recede in many areas of Africa today, this more costly active approach to case detection and treatment has given way to 'passive' case detection approaches which test only people with suggestive symptoms and rely on cases being detected during peoples' routine interactions with HCWs in health facilities. The recent development of rapid diagnostic tests (RDTs) for HAT, moreover, has enabled passive detection strategies to be reformed [10]. As with other RDTs, their ease of use means the first screening test in a step-wise algorithm can be taken out of hospital laboratories into primary care settings, broadening the pool of diagnosers able to test patients when they suspect disease.

This shift towards passive detection has stimulated debate in policy circles on how best to engage with the complexities of HAT case presentation and the challenges these pose for detecting the disease. The decision-making processes of HCWs have become a major point of focus. The 'HAT reflex' is a part of this new push towards cultivating frontline providers' syndromic familiarity—also referred to as an "index of suspicion" [11] (p. 192)—which clinicians intimately involved in HAT control say is critical for triggering the HAT reflex.

The importance of the HAT reflex gains amplitude in an elimination setting. The scarcity of cases is believed to pose a particular challenge for passive case detection as HCWs lose their diagnostic expertise due to infrequent contact with the disease. According to this argument, maintaining diagnostic acuity or 'reflexes' is a matter of habitual practice, whether practiced in the clinic among patients or in the lab dealing with samples. This position is captured by a recent World Health Organisation (WHO) guidance document on HAT elimination:

> *"In health centres where transmission of the disease is high, staff deal with gambiense HAT frequently, and clinical [syndromic] suspicion and laboratory work are usually done correctly; but in areas of low transmission, health workers lack the reflex to think about this disease, which has become uncommon, laboratory staff are unfamiliar with HAT tests".* [1] (p. 36)

Contact with the disease is also conceptualised as an important prompt for populations living in an endemic area to think of HAT as an individual risk and a collective public health priority, though medical language such as a 'low index of suspicion' is not explicitly used. Decreasing fear of the disease is often cited as an explanation for decreasing participation in active screening campaigns over time [12–15].

The possibilities of cultivating a diagnostic reflex for HAT among HCWs with minimal clinical training and where health infrastructure is limited provides a promising point of departure to support passive case detection approaches for elimination. However, despite the almost common-sensical importance of enhancing diagnostic acuity, how a reflex operates in practice and how it might be deployed within a programmatic setting remains unclear.

Granular explorations of how HAT diagnosis actually happens in a passive detection context have also been limited. Indeed, despite its contribution to disease control over the last several decades [16], there has been remarkably little research on passive case detection, in general [12]. This empirical gap is perhaps particularly surprising considering the role this approach is expected to play in achieving elimination of HAT in the coming decade.

In this paper, we seek to address what we see as HAT experts' interlinked concerns about a reduction in HCWs' and lay peoples' ability to diagnose HAT in the era of elimination. We ask, what exactly is a 'diagnostic reflex' and could endemic area health systems inculcate one for HAT? To answer these questions, we begin by introducing some key theories about medical diagnosis and case detection. We then present an in-depth study of the diagnostic practices involved in the successful passive detection of 32 cases from a hospital-based HAT programme in South Sudan where HCWs and the public still had relatively frequent contact with the disease. In so doing, we reflect upon what sorts of knowledge, material and social engagements facilitated the exercising of a HAT reflex in this setting and expand on how a HAT reflex could be conceptualised to work in practice. In conclusion, we suggest how such practices may potentially be translated to other settings in preparation for elimination.

The Diagnostic Reflex in Theory

The term, 'reflex', tends to refer to automatic behaviour. Like a neurological reflex which responds to stimuli automatically along pathways that bypass the brain's cognitive reasoning functions, the HAT diagnostic reflex suggests an almost immediate recognition of HAT when presented with a clinical case of the disease. As alluded to in the WHO passage, the skill is not learned through guidelines and training alone, but rather acquired through regular contact with patients and disease—or what medical sociologists term, 'embodied knowledge'.

Practicing medicine combines aspects of both abstract "embrained" and practical "embodied" knowledge [17,18] (p. 490). Whereas embrained knowledge is explicit, objective and depends on abstract cognitive reasoning, embodied knowledge is tacit, intuitive and builds upon 'bodily' or practical experience in a particular context. Embodied knowledge is automatic; its generation and application does not need to be processed through conscious decision-making. One example is the way HCWs learn to gauge a fever by putting their hand to a patient's forehead through cultivating a sensitivity to body temperature.

The transformation of that sense into a 'symptom' is both a cognitive and cultural process, involving integrating medical knowledge on one hand, and judgements about what constitutes normal and abnormal on the other [19–21]. The clinical training HCWs undertake contextualizes a sensibility of illness within biomedical theories of etiology and pathogenesis, enabling them to detect a HAT infection, for example, through the 'look' on a patient face. Their diagnostic expertise, in other words, develops through an integration of formal, codified categories with the social norms and habits associated with particular healthcare settings [22]. This ability to recognise disease is iteratively shaped through routine interactions with patients and colleagues, shared within groups and embedded in working cultures, becoming gradually more automatic and reflex-like through collaborative practice [18,23–27].

An example of this process of integrating embrained and embodied knowledge is the HCW's use of storytelling. To deal with the diagnostic uncertainty they face routinely, HCWs develop internal narrative scripts or templates based on a personal bank of experience with similar patients. Diagnostic scripts help a clinician look backward and forward simultaneously, (re-)telling a patient's syndromic history in a way that fits the narrative and predicts the future prognosis. These stories are shaped by what HCWs think they can do for the patient based on past precedent and by the rules and routines within their healthcare facility using "clinical judgement" [28] (p. 873). Given that diagnostic instruments, such as a microscope or serological agglutination test, do not create meaning independently of the practitioners who use them [29], scripts are what allow HCWs to place test results (as well as symptoms and other forms of evidence) in context. By providing a shortcut through cognitive processes, scripts quickly help a HCW settle on a pathway for action, but can also constrain available options since "knowing where to look strongly affects what clinicians can find" [28] (p. 875).

The diagnostic reflex is not only the province of medical professionals, however. Lay people also routinely rely on embodied knowledge to monitor symptoms and detect illness both before and after 'diagnosis' by a healthcare provider as well as during and after treatment [19,30]. Like that practiced by clinicians, this monitoring involves evaluating different forms of evidence, such as the observations of others or the results of blood tests, which prompts action such as visiting another health facility.

Like clinicians' use of scripts to proscribe practical actions, choosing where to seek a diagnosis can also be seen as involving diagnostic expertise developed through practice. Accessing diagnostic services within a health system requires substantial practical navigational expertise from patients, their families and other lay people within their social networks [31,32]. Sometimes the shortest or most straightforward route to successful care is dependent upon belonging to a social network with established links to clinical providers [33]. Information about HAT symptoms [19] and HAT service availability [34] circulates through cultural and linguistic networks within ethnic and migrant groups which can have widely different knowledge of and experiences with hospital care [34,35].

Seeking HCW expertise when people are uncertain about the meaning of symptoms is, moreover, often only one reason a patient visits a health facility. Patients may access services when they already have a good idea of what the problem is or, on some occasions, to try out new tests and compare results from the facilities where they have been tested previously [31,36]. Patients can prompt HCWs to pursue particular diagnoses [37] or submit to provider-led testing as a means of assisting communication about their illness with HCWs in a way that is acceptable to clinicians [38]. Patient-led testing (also known as voluntary or self-testing), can be seen as a healthcare coping strategy used by patients who have had negative interactions with HCWs in the past or as the behaviour of modern, information-savvy patients fostered in programmes that encourage people to take individual responsibility for their health [31,34,39].

In short, locating the HAT reflex as something that happens solely in HCWs' clinical encounters risks conflating passive case detection with simplistic ideas about treatment-seeking where responsibility for diagnosis is neatly divided between lay people and medical experts, with everything occurring before a patient's first contact with health services under the control of lay peoples' decisions and actions and everything after the responsibility of HCWs [33,40]. Passive case detection, after all, is only a 'passive' act from the perspective of a programme manager considering the additional effort and costs required to implement active screening [41]. Using such terminology tends to obscure the key role of patients and other lay people through the diagnostic process. To arrive at a diagnosis and successfully identify a case requires a great deal of patient engagement with the health system, as they proactively seek out treatment for their illness.

2. Methods

We collected detailed stories of successful case detection about patients identified by the HAT programme in Nimule, South Sudan over eight months in 2008–2009. Our recent work on how diagnostic technologies are integrated into global health research and response have encouraged us to contextualise these insights and reflect on this empirical material anew [42,43].

2.1. Setting

At the time of fieldwork, which happened before the global roll-out of RDTs for HAT, Nimule Hospital supported by the non-governmental organisation, Merlin, was one of only eight sites in the country which could offer HAT detection and treatment. HAT services had been available here and through intermittent active screening campaigns since 2005. During this period, the prevalence of *gambiense* sleeping sickness was around 1% in the public and 2.8% among patients presenting to the HAT service [34]. As the only functioning hospital serving a county population of around 170,000 [44], Nimule hospital was an important focus of general healthcare activity for people living in and far from the town. The HAT service itself was very popular, with 13,815 people screened passively over a five-year period from 2005 to 2010 [34].

HAT patients were diagnosed in the laboratory using a multi-stepped screening algorithm based on the card agglutination test for trypanosomiasis (CATT) (see Supplemental File S1). Like most diagnostic work performed in the laboratory, HAT practices were codified in a hospital protocol based on national programme and World Health Organisation guidance.

At the end of 2009, hospital managers began to draft symptom-based flow-charts for a variety of common patient presentations to aid diagnostic practice in the outpatient department. Their desire for formal guidance on HAT prompted a subsequent study by us on the predictive value of patients' presenting symptoms [45]. For the majority of fieldwork, however, written or visual materials that could have contributed to a material-culture of syndromic diagnosis in the hospital such as algorithms, guidelines and posters, were largely absent. Medical doctors and clinical officers were simply asked to use their discretion to decide when to order a HAT test.

Ordering a test involved requesting lab staff collect a venous blood sample from inpatients in the wards or sending outpatients to a specially demarcated section of the lab for HAT. This section had a separate entrance used to manage screening the large numbers of people who wanted a HAT test when the programme was first introduced and whose demand could not be met by the limited active screening services the programme could offer. Members of the public could request a test for themselves here without referral by a HCW or first discuss their suspicion during an outpatient consultation.

2.2. Data Collection and Analysis

We constructed case studies around 32 patients who were detected at the hospital. Twenty-six were new cases, six had been dismissed by the programme from further follow-up (five who had been treated for HAT 3–7 years earlier and one who had temporarily been considered a serological suspect). These patients represented 61% of cases identified passively during the study period. Between one and three patients per week were followed depending on admission patterns and research team capacity, with patients selected to achieve maximum variation of demographic characteristics (14 females and 18 males aged 11–65 years old, including 16 Dinka, 11 Madi and 1 each of Acholi, Kakwa, Lotuko, Lolubo and mixed Lango-Acholi ethnicities). Nearly all were in the final (second) stage, defined as when parasites can be found in the brain or spinal fluid (27 in stage 2, two in stage 1; three others died between the time when infection was confirmed and disease staging could be carried out).

Case studies were initiated as soon as the research team was notified that a case had been detected, beginning with interviews with hospital staff involved in diagnosis. Research team members were trained in HAT screening procedures and embedded in the lab during weekday mornings to observe many patients' earliest interactions with the programme; team members also observed all medical ward admission interviews required for the initiation of HAT treatment. In-depth research interviews were then conducted with patients or their guardians (if the patient was under 18 years old or had a cognitive impairment that made it difficult to participate fully) on the first or second day of treatment. Extensive field notes were also collected during the patient's hospital stay to capture additional information from patients, their families and friends, health staff and medical observations in patient files.

We explored how a "HAT reflex" comes about by asking patients and family members to narrate their health-seeking activities over the last several years in relation to symptoms that motivated the patient's presentation at the hospital. We asked HCWs (doctors, clinical officers, nurses and laboratory technicians) to recall details of their interaction with patients. Bearing in mind the contributions of lay people to diagnosis and the potentially habitual and iterative nature of HAT diagnostic practices, the focus of enquiries was to identify the critical events that occurred immediately before HAT was identified in the lab, particularly who suggested the patient be tested for HAT and why, considering a range of syndromic experiences and material and social contextual circumstances [46]. Based on analysis of these critical events, qualitative typologies were identified of the diagnostic practices which led to successful detection.

Typologies were initially analysed separately according to the category of person who suggested the diagnosis (the 'diagnoser', either a lay person without biomedical training who advised the patient to seek a HAT test or a HCW who ordered or performed one without a specific prompt from the patient) and brought together in the final presentation of results which focused on understanding the interaction of knowledge and habit in context (see Supplemental File S2). In some key cases, the diagnosis was arrived at in the absence of a decision by any individual who might be classified as a diagnose [47]. What we describe as 'serendipitous' cases, hinged entirely on a series of contingent events which were often set in motion by a willingness or openness to the possibilities of the medical diagnostic process to arrive at a cause for the illness.

Further details of the interviewing and analysis process, including how we addressed some anticipated limitations of interviewing people about the treatment-seeking and diagnostic process are available in Supplemental File S3. Interviewees' detailed experiences of sense-making in relation to HAT symptoms is reported elsewhere [19]. Additional data on patients' treatment-seeking characteristics including the length of time spent seeking treatment and the number of health facilities visited before detection, with methods used to collect it, are available in Supplemental File S4. The alternative diagnoses patients received in relation to their presenting symptoms are available in Supplemental File S5.

All subjects gave their informed consent for inclusion before they participated in the study. The study was conducted in accordance with the Declaration of Helsinki, and the protocol was approved by the London School of Hygiene and Tropical Medicine's ethical review committee (project ID 5507) and the Ministry of Health, Government (now Republic) of South Sudan.

3. Findings

Three typologies of diagnostic practice explained what led patients to be diagnosed with HAT: 'syndromic suspicion', 'pragmatic testing' and 'serendipitous detection' (see Box 1 for definitions of each).

Box 1. Definitions of diagnostic practice typologies which led to successful human African trypanosomiasis (HAT) case detection, highlighting the interplay of knowledge and habit.

Syndromic suspicion: HAT test suggested or ordered based on the diagnosing person's recognition of HAT symptoms. The process of symptom recognition was enabled by embodied knowledge of symptoms accrued through direct exposure to the disease. Closely resembled the idea of an expert HAT reflex.
Pragmatic testing: HAT test suggested or ordered during a process where the diagnosing person was concerned with 'trying' tests for multiple diseases, but their specific suspicion of HAT was ambivalent. While HAT testing was not prompted by an expert syndromic reflex, it was supported through practical knowledge of HAT tests and habitual testing behaviour.
Serendipitous detection: HAT test performed without any specific suspicion of HAT or even a request to test from an individual, with detection based on expertise embedded in the habitual testing practices of the hospital or lay socia network.

A key characteristic which shaped and differentiated these typologies was the degree to which people involved in the case depended on syndromic logic to guide testing decisions. In cases assigned a syndromic suspicion typology, HAT testing decisions appeared deliberative, based on considerations about whether HAT could explain observed symptoms, and often drawing on considerable embodied knowledge suggesting familiarity with the disease presentation. These cases resembled most closely the idea of the HAT reflex in expert discourses. In cases identified through pragmatic testing, HAT-specific suspicion was more ambivalent, emerging only when syndromic suspicion for more common infections failed. Drawing on diagnosers' knowledge of the local testing environment, the logic involved was pragmatic rather than symptomatic. HAT tests were requested to identify new treatment options without necessarily settling on disease labels—a diagnostic openness that enabled a more pragmatic course of therapeutic orientation [48]. Finally, in cases involving serendipitous detection, there appeared to be no specific suspicion of HAT at all and case detection came as a surprise. In these circumstances, no true 'diagnoser' was involved and it was the diagnostic expertise embedded within hospital processes and social networks coupled with peoples' openness towards these institutions which enabled detection in the absence of a HAT reflex in individuals. The typologies therefore suggested that HAT diagnosis happened along a gradient of degrees of suspicion, ranging from diagnostic certainty to surprise, and relying on the diagnostic expertise both embodied in individuals and embedded in systems (Figure 1).

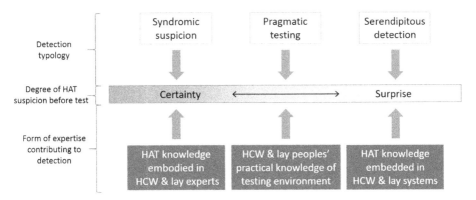

Figure 1. The gradient of certainty versus surprise along which human African trypanosomiasis (HAT) passive case detection happened, indicating the form of expertise which led to diagnosis. (HCW: healthcare worker).

The case studies also highlighted how HAT diagnostic practice was distributed beyond HCWs and healthcare environments to include patients and other lay populations within a wider diagnostic or case detection *system*. Most cases in the series (19/32) were detected after a lay person decided or advised a patient to test for HAT. These included neighbours, teachers, relatives living with patients or visiting on short trips, as well as patients themselves. HCWs were responsible for detecting the remainder (13/32 including 10 from Nimule Hospital and one each from primary healthcare facilities, military barracks and other hospitals), through formal consultations and in informal social interactions with patients. The diagnostic practices lay people engaged in were very similar to HCWs' (Table 1). Both HCWs and lay people successfully diagnosed HAT with an embodied syndromic reflex (nine cases identified by each type of diagnoser). They both also resorted to HAT testing through the pragmatic approach when no syndromic diagnosis was likely, though this was more common in cases where testing was initiated by lay people (eight by lay people vs. two by HCWs). Finally, the systems created by each group also supported HAT diagnosis, whether this was a social network created by lay people to communicate useful information about test availability or the processes and practices instituted by HCWs to manage patients and samples within the hospital. We turn to illustrations of the specific typologies next.

Table 1. Case detection typologies assigned according to the category of diagnoser, for 32 human African trypanosomiasis (HAT) patients.

Case Detection Typology	HAT Test Initiated By	
	Lay Person (# Patients)	Healthcare Worker (# Patients)
Syndromic suspicion	9	9
Pragmatic testing	8	2
Mixed (syndromic; pragmatic)	1	0
Serendipitous detection	1	2
Total	19	13

3.1. Syndromic Suspicion

Cases detected according to this typology closely resembled the idea of the HAT reflex in expert discourses. In the following sections we explore three concepts which help further characterise the HAT reflex: it involves practical, embodied knowledge that emerges from HCW experience with HAT and other diseases and which suits the diagnostic resources available; the habitual prompts or internal narrative 'scripts' that HCWs use to identify HAT frame abnormal behavioural and neurological symptoms as biomedical; and lay people also have a HAT reflex.

3.1.1. Use of Embodied Knowledge

A doctor working on the medical ward recalled how he sensed something strange in the "vacant expression" of a severely ill and febrile pregnant woman. As malaria affects pregnancy so severely, he immediately began her on treatment for cerebral malaria. However, his practical, embodied understanding of what he would expect a critically ill malaria patient to look like prompted him to explore alternatives. He decided that HAT should be included in his differential diagnosis "because these [malaria and HAT] are the diseases that can affect the central nervous system" and ordered both a malaria and a HAT test, successfully identifying the co-infections and her as a case of HAT.

The doctor's explanation of how he identified the differential diagnoses exemplified HCWs' en-skilled understandings of disease, which led them to suspect HAT when faced with complex forms of illness. In this instance, the doctor, who had lived most of his life in the area and managed many HAT patients before, drew from this contextual knowledge on how to manage patients with severe symptoms impairing consciousness which embedded the diagnostic possibility of HAT alongside more common diseases. Given the acute, febrile nature of the patient's condition, the doctor felt an infectious disease was most likely and some of the easiest diseases to test for in this setting (as opposed to, say, bacterial meningitis), were malaria and HAT. Before the test had even been performed, the neurological nature of the condition led the doctor to consider HAT, helping him to make sense of his earlier subtle observation of the patient's vacant expression in light of what he already knew about the disease and label it, prompting syndromic recognition of HAT.

3.1.2. Biomedical Framing

The kinds of symptoms which prompted a HAT reflex among HCW diagnosers were associated with two main narrative scripts: severe illness impairing consciousness as already described and severe mental confusion including hallucinations. Examples of presentations in cases which fit these scripts included intense nightmares in a child, violent paranoia in a woman, convulsions in a man, indications of partial or mild paralysis as well as various degrees of excessive sleeping.

Stemming from their biomedical training, the narrative scripts HCWs developed and used were specifically biomedical, which enabled personnel to suspect HAT when those around patients did not see a medical illness at all. For example, one day in the medical ward, a woman arrived with an abdominal knife wound she had inflicted on herself and a letter from the police. It read:

> To the Medical Officer, Merlin [Nimule] hospital. The above named woman reported to police. She knifed herself alone when her mind got confused. Please help to treat her.

The woman was involved in brewing alcohol for neighbours who were commonly drunk around her and when she became irrationally violent towards them, they taunted her into turning a knife on herself. Unlike the knife wound which needed acute care, family members did not consider this woman's behaviour as symptomatic of an illness that would require hospital consultation itself. Following the script for common causes of mental confusion, however, since the woman did not have a long history of mental illness the clinical officer suspected the event could be explained by a paranoid hallucination induced by an infectious disease such as HAT. Neighbours initially took the woman to the police, reasoning that an expert in security was needed since they framed the problem as dangerous behaviour. It was an expert in medicine, however, who interpreted the behaviour as a medical symptom in need of a biomedical diagnosis which led to her case detection.

3.1.3. Lay Expertise

Our data also suggested that the idea of the HAT reflex should be extended to recognise the expertise of lay people in HAT diagnosis with their own local, social forms of knowledge.

Whereas HCWs gained formal knowledge from preclinical and in-service trainings and practical experience working in HAT screening and treatment programmes, lay people acquired their knowledge of HAT symptoms from non-medical sources which were nevertheless robust. The local population's long experience of living with the disease and interacting with active and passive screening services enabled the development of detailed popular syndromic discourses about HAT as well as practical experience observing patients become sick [19].

In stories about HAT testing initiated by lay people, the incorporation of abstract HAT knowledge was evident from diagnosers' recollections that their suspicion of HAT was prompted by hallmark signs. The husband of one patient, for example, discussed enlarged lymph nodes as such a characteristic symptom of HAT that, when they noticed it, his family knew a HAT test was needed to confirm their suspicion and secure her treatment. He said:

> She was developing lymph nodes around her neck, so some of our family members said why don't I try a sleeping sickness test? If this symptom had appeared earlier, before going to Uganda, I would not have bothered looking for other treatment, I would have come direct for a sleeping sickness test.

A familiar feeling of body pain and weakness while doing agriculture work is the sort of practical HAT knowledge which prompted another patient who had previously been treated to return to the hospital for a HAT test. She recalled, "when it started like that again, I knew nothing else apart from sleeping sickness. That is why even if I was told controls [post-treatment follow-up tests] were over, I didn't go to look for other tests".

A mother's story of how she suspected HAT in her daughter illustrates that popular syndromic knowledge was also incorporated into narrative scripts used by lay people, similarly to HCWs. She said:

> I began to know that she is sick because whenever she came from school she would complain of headache [...] if she failed to get food [...] she would do nothing but sit and begin to close her eyes [...] so I decided, let her come for this test [49] [...] It is good that the sickness is found in an early stage so [...] the child will survive after treatment [...] I heard of a person with sleeping sickness from Uganda. [She] was so sick whereby she had some swellings on her face and some parts of the body and her child was the same [...] this child died.

Reflecting on the 'tools' most available to lay people outside of health facilities, the mother used her senses to observe her daughters' symptoms in the context of domestic life. She empathetically observed the patient's head pains, hunger and sleepiness which were symptoms commonly known to occur in HAT [19]. As "there is no sickness which causes people to eat a lot other than sleeping sickness", a symptom script about eating too much prompted the mother to consider HAT, and the other symptoms supported this. Disease-specific scripts tell the story of a disease's prognosis as well as what can practically be done [28], so once the mother thought of HAT, which had another script of its own, she knew to monitor for swelling. Combining biomedical and ethnophysiological concepts, 'swelling' in HAT was associated with a serious prognosis because of a homologous association with illness progression in magical poisoning [19]. Fear of her daughter developing this symptom was what prompted the mother to take her to Nimule hospital for a HAT test where she was identified as a case.

Lay diagnosers also clearly possessed agency to ensure diagnostic work was done, driven by their syndromic suspicions. This was particularly true of stories about patients who had to work against the habits and rules of the lab's self-testing service for detection to happen. Knowing that patients with negative CATT screening results could not be retested within three months, for example, the families of two cases (both children), returned at quarterly intervals for testing until the children were confirmed. Previously treated patients who had completed their two years of follow-up testing, such as the woman with a familiar feeling of body pain and weakness, also sometimes reported that they were not "allowed" to test for HAT after this point [50]. When she returned for a test, she was twice refused. On the third visit, the patient said she decided to "just keep quiet" and resorted to a small deception by posing as a new tester in the HAT lab queue. This enabled her to be taken through the full diagnostic algorithm used in the lab and confirmed as a case, again. Such stories demonstrated the surprising amount of tenacity involved for some lay people to access tests and achieve test results which matched what they sensed in patient bodies and communicate this to HCWs who could admit them for treatment. Like HCW diagnosers, these lay diagnosers used HAT tests in concerted ways to confirm their suspicions of HAT, unlike in cases belonging to the pragmatic testing typology, discussed next.

3.2. Pragmatic Testing

In diagnostic stories which followed a pragmatic testing typology, knowledge and habit enabled HAT case detection in a way that did not require the people involved to possess strong syndromic suspicion. The following case is illustrative.

The father of a young girl had consulted staff at local clinics and drug shops several times for her recurrent fevers and stomach pains. She was treated sequentially for schistosomiasis, typhoid and brucellosis but she continued to be ill. The patient's father then noticed she was sleeping a lot and that her skin was getting lighter which suggested that she was getting swollen, so he wondered if she could have worms again, or possibly HAT. When he took her to Nimule Hospital to discuss his suspicions, a HCW in the outpatient department enquired about additional HAT symptoms and noted that the patient was also disoriented, incontinent and had difficulty walking. This led the HCW to strongly suspect HAT and he agreed to test the girl for it. After the infection was identified in the lab, her father was more convinced that HAT explained the symptoms but said he would remain sceptical until she was symptom-free. He explained this ambivalent suspicion of HAT as follows:

> Because she is always feeling sleepy, I said [...] maybe it is sleeping sickness which is causing her those other pains [head and muscle aches] [...] since she was treated for those other diseases and didn't recover well. Now I would like to see if it [the correct diagnosis] is sleeping sickness or if there is more pain after treatment for sleeping sickness.

Although a suspicion of HAT on syndromic grounds seemed highly justified to the HCW who was consulted, the lay person's decision-making which led to successful detection depended not only on the father having some syndromic awareness of HAT, but also his willingness to opportunistically try new tests and treatments to identify practical ways to help his daughter.

In contrast to the tenacity involved in accessing HAT tests to confirm syndromic suspicions described in the last typology, in cases characterised by pragmatic testing, energy directed towards HAT testing tended to be obscured by care-seeking for other common infections. In some cases, there was even someone within the patient's therapy management group who recommended a HAT test based on what appeared to be a (syndromic) HAT reflex, but several months nevertheless elapsed before the patient was brought for a test during which the patient received other forms of care. In these situations, the HAT suspicion along with other forms of evidence and circumstantial criteria appeared to get filtered through a decision-maker who ultimately influenced the trajectory of care-seeking and the diagnostic practices pursued (or not).

In the case of the father seeking advice about worms and/or HAT, as well as many others assigned a pragmatic testing typology, finding another test to help explain unresolved symptoms was the narrative focus of peoples' stories, rather than HAT, itself. Recounting how they decided to bring a patient to the hospital, family members might say, for example, "The only test that I forgot to take her for was this sleeping sickness test" or "only sleeping sickness testing and treatment is what she had not done".

As language like "forgetting to test for HAT" would suggest, many people in Nimule had practical experience of HAT tests through exposure to active and passive screening services. Information about HAT tests also circulated through announcements about changes to health services shared at migration meetings, church activities and social events, as well as informal conversations among people enquiring about tests from neighbours, at pharmacies, and within hospital waiting areas [34]. HAT tests contributed to a culture of pragmatic testing that was a commonplace and important health-seeking strategy which helped people manage illness and uncertainty in Nimule. While HAT was usually considered an unlikely diagnosis, people nevertheless arrived at it when syndromic suspicion for more common infections failed through knowledge of the HAT test. Diagnosers—or 'decision-makers', for want of a better word—did not need to commit to a HAT suspicion before (or even after) the HAT test was performed. 'Trying' a HAT test, as patients typically put it, involved settling on a pathway for action but not necessarily a 'diagnosis'. It simply required an openness to various diagnostic options. Thus, it was peoples' practical knowledge and habitual use of HAT tests and other lab services, rather than HAT symptoms, that enabled this sort of detection.

HCWs also pursued HAT testing pragmatically when their other interventions were not working. Faced with a patient experiencing convulsions and disturbances to her gait and speech, for example, one doctor eventually thought to test her for HAT, but only after five days of presumptive treatment for bacterial meningitis and investigations for malaria. Having never treated or even seen a case of HAT before, the doctor had no embodied syndromic knowledge to draw on and said she was unsure if the case could be due to HAT, but she did recall being trained in hospital lab and treatment protocols several months previously, which gave her the idea. This case demonstrated that when a diagnoser's HAT reflexes were weak because of a lack of direct experience with the disease and its symptoms, simply knowing that a HAT test was available could be sufficient to prompt HAT testing in contexts when diagnosers had run out of options.

3.3. Serendipitous Detection

In patient stories featuring serendipity, lay people and HCWs expressed that they had never purposely thought to test for HAT. Rather, it seemed to happen to them in a stroke of luck.

In one story, a lab technician told how he came across trypanosomes while examining a blood film of a man experiencing mood changes, confusion and fevers. The patient had come with a note from a clinician requesting simply that a film be done to identify "any infections that needed to be treated". Not looking for trypanosomes specifically and not using any of the specialised HAT tests normally employed, it was remarkable that he found the parasites by chance. *Gambiense* trypanosomes normally occur at such low levels in the bloodstream that even the most skilled technicians often cannot confirm infections this way; it would be even more difficult for someone not specifically looking for them.

In another story, a patient recalled that he came to Nimule Hospital because it was the biggest hospital he knew of and so must have the biggest selection of tests. With what he thought of as severe malaria symptoms that were not caused by malaria, he knew he wanted to get tested for as many other diseases as possible. He went straight to the hospital lab and joined a queue of people waiting to be tested for HAT. Serendipity seemed to feature in this part of the decision. HAT testing was the only lab service for which patients could self-initiate testing. If he had joined any other queue, lab staff would have sent him to the outpatient department to seek a test order from a clinician who might not have thought to test him for HAT.

In neither story was there a true 'diagnoser' to whom a syndromic HAT suspicion could be attributed or even a 'decision-maker' that actively pursued a HAT test as in the previous typologies. While the HCW who ordered the blood film possessed suspicion for a range of diseases, he did not actually request a HAT test and the lab technician who detected the parasite did not know he was performing a 'HAT test' until he had made the diagnosis. Likewise, having recently moved to Nimule from a non-endemic area, the patient wanting lots of tests had no prior knowledge of HAT or the HAT service. The man he queued behind simply told the patient what test he was waiting for and recommended the patient try this test first because otherwise he would have to wait much longer to be seen in the outpatient department.

Nevertheless, there were HAT diagnostic skills involved: the remarkably practiced eye of the lab technician and the navigational knowledge of the man in the queue who also appreciated the option of a self-testing service and shared it willingly. What enabled these peoples' skills to be practiced was other peoples' openness to the possibilities of the medical diagnostic process to arrive at a cause for the illness, whether this involved placing trust in a big hospital to have a test that could help or trusting a lab technician to identify any infections that needed to be treated. Such expertise was thus not only embodied in the individuals involved, it was embedded in the routines, practices and habits of the hospital lab and its relationships to the HCWs and lay people who used it.

4. Discussion

4.1. Extending the Reflex Metaphor

The importance of embodied knowledge is rarely discussed in public health. Through the idiom of the diagnostic 'reflex', a discourse about embodied knowledge has emerged in the HAT field related to the nature of expertise in the context of disease elimination. While specific to the HAT field, the idea of a reflex nevertheless encapsulates a problem all disease control programmes must address: how to translate abstract diagnostic knowledge into embodied practice.

The vocabulary of the reflex helps us think about how diagnosis happens in places with limited health infrastructure where people rely on their senses and work with the biomedical and laboratory resources available to them to successfully diagnose disease. In discourses about the HAT reflex, curricular training in diagnostic protocols is insufficient to make an expert. Rather, diagnostic expertise develops through HCWs' routine exposures to HAT. This contact acts as stimulation, allowing HCWs to put their knowledge into practice and continually exercise or hone their reflexes. The anatomical origins of the term hints at what else experts know about HAT expertise: that it is something contained within their minds and bodies, accrued through the expert's personal material and social experiences with disease, instantly available to be used by them in context.

Several observations from our study in Nimule help refine our understanding of the reflex metaphor and suggest how it can be extended. First, HCWs here used embodied knowledge to recognise HAT often in the medical ward and in domestic settings outside of working hours but rarely in busy hospital outpatient encounters. This suggested that as much as a HAT reflex is habitual and can appear to happen quickly, time and space help clinicians to respond to a sense that something is abnormal and emphasises the fundamentally creative nature of this reflex [17].

Second, our data suggests that in addition to the minds and bodies of HCWs, a diagnostic reflex is also present in lay people who are familiar with HAT. In Nimule, not only did lay people play an (independent) role in forming diagnoses, they used similar practices as HCWs to do so. Sociologists argue that for self-diagnosis to happen, medical knowledge must escape the walls of a hospital and the bounds of medical authority [17]. In the case of HAT, one could argue that the intermittent accessibility of HAT services through active screening means that successful case recognition through 'passive' means has often relied on the agency of lay people and HAT diagnostic knowledge has never been the sole domain of medical experts. Control programmes should thus avoid misattributing the substantial diagnostic work done by lay people to HCWs; otherwise we risk limiting our expectations about how lay people can and should participate in HAT elimination.

Third, given that expertise can be shared through creation of organizational and social norms [18], HAT diagnosis also appears to happen through the activation of expert knowledge that exists outside of expert bodies, stored in the routine practices of HCWs' and lay peoples' interactions with the hospital lab. Like a neural impulse that becomes apparent as it prompts action while travelling along a network or system of neural connections, our data has encouraged us to think of the HAT reflex as something that is distributed within a healthcare *system*.

4.2. Non-Expert Forms of Practice

According to health systems thinking, people of all sorts—whether HCWs or lay—are at the centre of health systems, mediating them and helping drive them, though they draw on different sorts of experience and operate from different perspectives [51]. Lay people can thus be beneficiaries, advocates, patients, healthcare seekers, or diagnosers. Focusing on the variety of diagnostic practices of lay people helped us identify alternative routes to successful case detection through the system, not captured in expert discourses.

In Nimule, pragmatic testing was a form of non-expert diagnostic practice that led to HAT detection and which, while also sometimes used by HCWs, was particularly suited to lay peoples' needs. In this type of practice, HAT tests were used in ways that seemed casual or tentative—undertaken, at the end of a process rather than in a tenacious, concerted effort to confirm syndromic suspicions as in the expert reflex or to rule out a potentially life-threatening disease as in some HCWs' approaches to their duty of care [52]. In their first steps in the pragmatic testing process, diagnosers did not even consider HAT as a potential diagnosis or test for it. Pragmatic testing was not based on personal experience with the syndromic presentation of HAT, rather it was based on practical knowledge of available tests. In many impoverished healthcare settings, "[diagnostic] uncertainty is so perpetual as to become banal" [48] (p.817). Diagnosers therefore suspend action towards diagnostic 'closure' or categorisation and instead focus on what is practical in the face of imperfect knowledge. In Nimule, for both lay people and HCWs at the hospital, progressive testing through a discrete number of infectious diseases options, including HAT, was an accessible way of solving healthcare problems and engaging with the opportunities of laboratory and biomedical resources. Diagnosis, after all, is not only 'for' the abstract categorization of states of ill health; it is also a means to access treatment [36]. In this circumstance, peoples' pursuit of tests for treatment also had the beneficial effect of leading to case detection.

In our data, the more embodied the HAT reflex was, the more certain people were of a HAT diagnosis based on syndromic criteria. Patients in this case series were mostly in stage 2, so it generally took patients in Nimule a long time to achieve a correct diagnosis of HAT (an average of 9.7 months (median 6) on 2.8 visits seeking healthcare before being tested for HAT, Supplemental File S4). While our study was not designed to explore reasons for diagnostic delay or opportunities for missed diagnosis, it may be reasonable to assume that patients detected later had later or less contact with an expert HAT diagnoser. Descriptive quantitative analysis of our small sample supports this idea, suggesting that when a diagnoser with an embodied syndromic reflex was involved, cases tended to be identified more quickly, whether this was a HCW or a lay person (an average of 6.1 months on 1.8 visits for people identified using syndromic suspicion compared to 9.8 months on 3.2 visits using a pragmatic testing approach, Supplemental File S4).

Case detection not only happened along a *decreasing* 'index' or gradient of certainty, however. We also saw it happening along an *increasing* gradient of serendipity, given that the more open and familiar people were with the hospital systems, the more chances they had to arrive at a diagnosis by surprise. While patients and other people involved in detection of serendipitous cases saw the un-sought diagnosis as unexpected good fortune, dismissing such events as simply the result of chance underappreciates how interpreting serendipity as a "mix of accident and sagacity" contributes to an analysis [53] (p.139). For us, given that we were seeking to uncover the implicit structures, behaviours and conditions which led to HAT diagnosis, paying attention to apparently serendipitous cases enabled us to identify unexpected ways that the HAT reflex could be seen as translated across and embedded within a system.

4.3. Preparing Health Systems for HAT Elimination

Can a HAT reflex based on embodied knowledge be cultivated in contexts with less disease? As long as HAT transmission continues and at least some of the cases in a population continue to be detected, diagnostic expertise can be expected to develop, albeit at a slower rate. As suggested by HAT expert fears of the threat of elimination to their reflexes, we should nevertheless treat HAT case detection events as important opportunities for learning. Moreover, an inclusive approach to health systems development in which diagnostic learning by many different types of actor is encouraged means that many peoples' reflexes will be primed, ready to identify the final cases of HAT for elimination.

Hospitals in endemic areas, for example, could use admitted patients to purposely—and practically—teach the symptoms of HAT to other clinicians in their facility. Patients and the lay people involved in their detection can also be given feedback on their diagnostic skills and offered opportunities to further develop their expertise through trainings or participate in volunteer HAT detection or community surveillance programmes.

HAT RDTs will also be part of the solution to maintaining people's diagnostic reflexes, particularly if we resist seeing them as magical technology that enable us to by-pass untrusted local expertise [54]. HCWs in a primary health care context are familiar with using RDTs to diagnose other diseases and may have practical knowledge of HAT from living in endemic areas. With HAT expertise historically concentrated in hospitals, however, many of the HCWs who are being asked to use the HAT RDTs will need to do so without much embodied knowledge of the disease's clinical presentation. HAT programmes deploying RDTs in these settings should thus ensure that supervisors use monitoring visits to discuss specific patient histories that primary care staff have thought (or think) could be HAT cases to regularly stimulate development of their HAT reflexes. Supervisors could also confidentially discuss the patient syndromic profiles of new cases found elsewhere within the endemic area.

Importantly, our observations from Nimule have also shown that other forms of diagnostic practice can still lead to HAT case detection when an embodied HAT reflex is not present. 'Novice' diagnosers can precipitate detection through pragmatic testing strategies and detection can happen serendipitously through the skills of experts which have been embedded in systems. Health systems should embrace all such practices not only for their contributions to detection today, but also for their potential contributions to the creation of embodied expertise for tomorrow. No matter how people arrive at HAT diagnoses, reflecting on how a lab diagnosis fits a patient's syndromic presentation even after detection is an important part of the personal *experience* of diagnosis which helps embody diagnostic knowledge of HAT that can be used to identify new cases in the future.

To encourage use of HAT tests in pragmatic testing strategies, health systems should take care not to inadvertently exclude lay people from engaging with HAT tests on their own terms and acknowledge that HCWs and lay people alike always make decisions to test for HAT in relation to alternative diagnostic possibilities.

Decoupling diagnosis from particular diseases is a key aim of patient-centred approaches in public health because of the way HCWs in primary care often diagnose and manage *types* of presenting symptoms or syndromes rather than pathologically-defined disease [55]. As in some other elimination programmes for neglected tropical skin diseases [56], HCWs in HAT elimination settings should be trained to consider a broad differential diagnosis when confronted with patient presentations that fit both typical and atypical presentations of HAT. How best to conceptualise HAT diagnosis in relation to HCWs' existing engagements with presenting syndromes such as neurological disorders, psychiatric problems or persistent fevers, however, remains underexplored in discussions of HAT integration and the HAT reflex [12,57,58] (see also the range of medical, social and other conditions patients in our study were diagnosed with before HAT detection, Supplemental File S5).

We can also imagine situations where well-equipped systems create the possibility for serendipity. In our data, the conditions that enabled serendipitous detection involved a well-resourced laboratory with skilled staff offering a range of tests as well as a highly-engaged patient population. The lively engagement of lay people with Nimule Hospital's HAT service related to the easy accessibility of HAT screening through the self-referral option at the lab. Not only did people enjoy bypassing outpatient systems to access it, its popularity created a physical presence in outpatient areas of the hospital through the regular formation of queues. Just as crowds and generators involved in active screening draw people in to test for HAT, the queues associated with passive screening in Nimule contributed to the test's—and therefore the disease's—visibility. As substantial things, diagnostic tests, like medicines, help make illnesses tangible and communicable in the collective imaginary by creating an aura of facticity [59]. RDT deployments should thus consider where, when and how we want to stimulate people's diagnostic reflexes in a health system [60].

As we approach HAT elimination and cases of disease become more rare, our HAT diagnostic reflexes may indeed slacken as experts fear. As a living entity, however, diagnostic expertise is born and grows through practice. Treating HAT detection events as important learning opportunities and ensuring multidimensional access to HAT tests will thus be vital to provide HCWs and lay people with opportunities to practice HAT diagnosis and develop their reflexes for elimination.

Supplementary Materials: The following are available online at http://www.mdpi.com/2414-6366/5/2/52/s1, Supplementary File S1: Laboratory algorithm used to screen for and diagnose cases of HAT in Nimule Hospital, Supplementary File S2: Patient typology classifications, Supplementary File S3: Interview and analysis process, Supplementary File S4: Patient healthcare-seeking characteristics, Supplementary File S5: Alternative diagnoses given to patients.

Author Contributions: Conceptualization, J.J.P., C.J. and A.H.K.; Formal analysis, J.J.P.; Investigation, J.J.P. and E.I.S.; Methodology, J.J.P., C.J., E.I.S. and A.H.K.; Project administration, J.J.P.; Writing—original draft, J.J.P.; Writing—review and editing, J.J.P., C.J., E.I.S. and A.H.K. All authors have read and agree to the published version of the manuscript.

Funding: This work was funded by the Canadian Institutes for Health Research (grant number DPH-88,226), the Sir Halley Stewart Trust and the European Research Council through grants for the Investigating Networks of Zoonosis Innovation (INZI) (grant number 295,845) and Investigating the Design and Use of Diagnostic Devices in Global Health (DiaDev) (grant number 715,450) projects at the University of Edinburgh. The views expressed are those of the authors and not necessarily those of the funders.

Acknowledgments: We thank all study participants and the following people who collected data: Augustine Severino, Duku James Marino, Garang William Goch, Mangar Abraham Mayen and Sisto Aluma. The Ministry of Health and local authorities in South Sudan kindly authorised this research. Many staff within the UK and South Sudan offices of Merlin, which employed E.I.S. at the time of fieldwork, facilitated and supported this work. Thank-you to Chris Whitty and Francesco Checchi for providing supervision of data collection and for insightful discussions on early drafts of this article. Clare Chandler, Shona Jane Lee, Michelle Taylor and Jean-Benôit Falisse also reviewed this manuscript and two anonymous peer reviewers provided useful insights. Thank-you to James Smith and Alice Street for providing leadership of the INZI and DiaDev projects which provided stimulus for this data to find new life.

Conflicts of Interest: The authors declare no conflict of interest.

References and Notes

1. WHO. *Report of the Second WHO Stakeholders Meeting on Gambiense Human African Trypanosomiasis Elimination, Geneva, Switzerland, 21–23 March 2016*; World Health Organisation: Geneva, Switzerland, 2016.
2. Steverding, D. The history of African trypanosomiasis. *Parasites Vectors* **2008**, *1*, 3. [CrossRef] [PubMed]
3. Kennedy, P.G. Clinical features, diagnosis, and treatment of human African trypanosomiasis (sleeping sickness). *Lancet Neurol.* **2013**, *12*, 186–194. [CrossRef]
4. Blum, J.; Schmid, C.; Burri, C. Clinical aspects of 2541 patients with second stage human African trypanosomiasis. *Acta Trop.* **2006**, *97*, 55–64. [CrossRef] [PubMed]
5. Gill, G.; Beeching, N. African Trypanosomiasis. In *Lecture Notes on Tropical Medicine*, 6th ed.; Blackwell Science Ltd.: Hoboken, NJ, USA, 2009.
6. Stich, A.H. African Trypanosomiasis. In *Principles of Medicine in Africa*, 4th ed.; Mabey, D., Parry, E., Gill, G., Al, E., Eds.; Cambridge University Press: Cambridge, UK, 2012.
7. Burri, C.; Brun, R. Chap 73: Human African Trypanosomiasis. In *Manson's Tropical Diseases*, 21st ed.; Cook, G., Zumla, A., Eds.; Elsevier Sciences: London, UK, 2003; pp. 1303–1323.
8. Apted, F. Chapter 35: Clinical Manifestations and Diagnosis of Sleeping Sickness. In *The African Trypanosomiases*; Mulligan, H., Ed.; George Allen and Unwin Ltd.: London, UK, 1970.

9.   Checchi, F.; Chappuis, F.; Karunakara, U.; Priotto, G.; Chandramohan, D. Accuracy of five algorithms to diagnose gambiense human African trypanosomiasis. *PLoS Negl. Trop. Dis.* **2011**, *5*, e1233. [CrossRef]

10.   Wamboga, C.; Matovu, E.; Bessell, P.R.; Picado, A.; Biéler, S.; Ndung'u, J.M. Enhanced passive screening and diagnosis for gambiense human African trypanosomiasis in north-western Uganda–Moving towards elimination. *PLoS ONE* **2017**, *12*, e0186429. [CrossRef]

11.   WHO. *Control and Surveillance of Human African Trypanosomiasis: Report of a WHO Expert Committee*; World Health Organisation: Geneva, Switzerland, 2013.

12.   Mulenga, P.; Chenge, F.; Boelaert, M.; Mukalay, A.; Lutumba, P.; Lumbala, C.; Luboya, O.; Coppieters, Y. Integration of Human African Trypanosomiasis Control Activities into Primary Healthcare Services: A Scoping Review. *Am. J. Trop. Med. Hyg.* **2019**, *101*, 1114–1125. [CrossRef]

13.   Checchi, F.; Cox, A.P.; Chappuis, F.; Priotto, G.; Chandramohan, D.; Haydon, D.T. Prevalence and under-detection of gambiense human African trypanosomiasis during mass screening sessions in Uganda and Sudan. *Parasites Vectors* **2012**, *5*, 157. [CrossRef]

14.   Falisse, J.-B.; Mpanya, A. Whose elimination? Frontline workers' perspectives on the elimination of the Human African Trypanosomiasis and its anticipated consequences. *Trop. Med. Infect. Dis.* **2020**, *5*, 6. [CrossRef]

15.   Other authors recommend programmes not invest resources in passive detection through primary healthcare systems if disease prevalence is too low [10,12]. This advice primarily relates to a cost effectiveness argument about the chances of finding cases, rather than reflecting whether frontline HCWs can reliably identify HAT suspects when HAT is very rare.

16.   Checchi, F.; Funk, S.; Chandramohan, D.; Chappuis, F.; Haydon, D.T. The impact of passive case detection on the transmission dynamics of gambiense Human African Trypanosomiasis. *PLoS Negl. Trop. Dis.* **2018**, *12*, e0006276. [CrossRef]

17.   Nettleton, S.; Burrows, R.; Watt, I. Regulating medical bodies? The consequences of the 'modernisation'of the NHS and the disembodiment of clinical knowledge. *Sociol. Health Illn.* **2008**, *30*, 333–348. [CrossRef]

18.   Lam, A. Tacit knowledge, organizational learning and societal institutions: An integrated framework. *Organ. Stud.* **2000**, *21*, 487–513. [CrossRef]

19.   Palmer, J. Sensing sleeping sickness: Local symptom-making in South Sudan. *Med. Anthropol.* **2019**. [CrossRef] [PubMed]

20.   Andersen, R.S.; Nichter, M.; Risør, M.B. Sensations, symptoms and healthcare seeking. *Anthropol. Action* **2017**, *24*, 1. [CrossRef]

21.   Nichter, M. Coming to our senses: Appreciating the sensorial in medical anthropology. *Transcult. Psychiatry* **2008**, *45*, 163–197. [CrossRef] [PubMed]

22.   Kleinman, A. Concepts and a model for the comparison of medical systems as cultural systems. *Soc. Sci. Med. Part B Med. Anthropol.* **1978**, *12*, 85–93. [CrossRef]

23.   Hazlehurst, B.; McMullen, C.; Gorman, P.; Sittig, D. How the ICU follows orders: Care delivery as a complex activity system. *AMIA Annu. Symp. Proc.* **2003**, *2003*, 284–288.

24.   Gardner, J.; Williams, C. Corporal diagnostic work and diagnostic spaces: Clinicians' use of space and bodies during diagnosis. *Sociol. Health Illn.* **2015**, *37*, 765–781. [CrossRef]

25.   Moreira, T. Coordination and Embodiment in the Operating Room. *Body Soc.* **2004**, *10*, 109–129. [CrossRef]

26.   Svenaeus, F. *The Hermeneutics of Medicine and the Phenomenology of Health: Steps Towards a Philosophy of Medical Practice*; Springer Science & Business Media: Berlin, Germany, 2013; Volume 5.

27.   Hutchins, E. *Cognition in the Wild*; MIT Press: Cambridge, MA, USA, 1995.

28.   Davenport, N. Medical residents' use of narrative templates in storytelling and diagnosis. *Soc. Sci. Med.* **2011**, *73*, 873–881. [CrossRef]

29.   Schubert, C. Making sure: A comparative micro-analysis of diagnostic instruments in medical practice. *Soc. Sci. Med.* **2011**, *73*, 851–857. [CrossRef]

30.   Williams, H.; Jones, C. A critical review of behavioural issues related to malaria control in sub-Saharan Africa: What contributions have social scientists made? *Soc. Sci. Med.* **2004**, *59*, 501–523. [CrossRef] [PubMed]

31.   Yellapa, V.; Devadasan, N.; Krumeich, A.; Pant Pai, N.; Vadnais, C.; Pai, M.; Engel, N. How patients navigate the diagnostic ecosystem in a fragmented health system: A qualitative study from India. *Glob. Health Action* **2017**, *10*, 1350452. [CrossRef] [PubMed]

32. Samerski, S. Health literacy as a social practice: Social and empirical dimensions of knowledge on health and healthcare. *Soc. Sci. Med.* **2019**, *226*, 1–8. [CrossRef] [PubMed]

33. Coast, E.; Murray, S. These things are dangerous: Understanding induced abortion trajectories in urban Zambia. *Soc. Sci. Med.* **2016**, *153*, 201–209. [CrossRef] [PubMed]

34. Palmer, J.J.; Kelly, A.H.; Surur, E.I.; Checchi, F.; Jones, C. Changing landscapes, changing practice: Negotiating access to sleeping sickness services in a post-conflict society. *Soc. Sci. Med.* **2014**, *120*, 396–404. [CrossRef]

35. Bell, S. Interpreter assemblages: Caring for immigrant and refugee patients in US hospitals. *Soc. Sci. Med.* **2019**, *226*, 29–36. [CrossRef]

36. Jutel, A. Sociology of diagnosis: A preliminary review. *Sociol. Health Illn.* **2009**, *31*, 278–312. [CrossRef]

37. Chandler, C.; Mangam, L.; Njei, A.; Achonduh, O.; Mbacham, W.; Wiseman, V. As a clinician, you are not managing lab results, you are managing the patient: How the enactment of malaria at health facilities in Cameroon compares with new WHO guidelines for the use of malaria tests. *Soc. Sci. Med.* **2012**, *74*, 1528–1535. [CrossRef]

38. Ansah, E.K.; Reynolds, J.; Akanpigbiam, S.; Whitty, C.J.M.; Chandler, C.I.R. Even if the test result is negative, they should be able to tell us what is wrong with us: A qualitative study of patient expectations of rapid diagnostic tests for malaria. *Malar. J.* **2013**, *12*, 258. [CrossRef]

39. Copelton, D.A.; Valle, G. You don't need a prescription to go gluten-free: The scientific self-diagnosis of celiac disease. *Soc. Sci. Med.* **2011**, *69*, 623–631. [CrossRef]

40. Brandner, S.; Stritter, W.; Müller-Nordhorn, J.; Fotopoulou, C.; Sehouli, J.; Holmberg, C. Taking responsibility: Ovarian cancer patients' perspectives on delayed healthcare seeking. *Anthropol. Action* **2017**, *24*, 41–48. [CrossRef]

41. Kegels, G. Vertical Analysis of Human African Trypanosomiasis. In *Studies in Health Services Organisation and Policy*; ITG Press: Antwerp, Belgium, 1997; Volume 7.

42. INZI. Investigating Networks of Zoonosis Innovation (INZI). Available online: http://www.cas.ed.ac.uk/research/grants_and_projects/investigating_neglected_zoonosis_innovation_inzi (accessed on 6 December 2019).

43. DiaDev. Investigating the Design and Use of Diagnostic Devices in Global Health. Available online: http://www.diadev.eu/ (accessed on 6 December 2019).

44. SSCCSE. *Statistical Yearbook for Southern Sudan 2010*; Southern Sudan Centre for Census, Statistics and Evaluation: Juba, South Sudan, 2010.

45. Palmer, J.; Surur, E.; Goch, G.; Mayen, M.; Lindner, A.; Pittet, A.; Kasparian, S.; Checchi, F.; Whitty, C. Syndromic algorithms for detection of gambiense human African trypanosomiasis in South Sudan. *PLoS Negl. Trop. Dis.* **2013**, *7*, e2003. [CrossRef]

46. For patients with previous interactions with the HAT programme as cases or suspects, typologies were identified based on events occurring after they had been dismissed by the programme for follow-up.

47. These cases were assigned to the HCW or lay diagnoser category based on which population's distributed knowledge and practice led to a patient being tested.

48. Street, A. Artefacts of not-knowing: The medical record, the diagnosis and the production of uncertainty in Papua New Guinean biomedicine. *Soc. Stud. Sci.* **2011**, *41*, 815–834. [CrossRef]

49. "Let her come" was a common and polite way of saying "she should go"; it was the mother who thought of testing for HAT and, with the support of her family, decided she would take her daughter to the hospital.

50. Some members of staff possibly interpreted protocols incorrectly by believing HAT tests should not be offered to anyone after they had completed their two years of follow-up. Alternatively, staff may not have given patients a chance to explain that they were symptomatic so that a message such as "you do not need to be tested" was interpreted as a refusal to perform tests.

51. De Savigny, D.; Adam, T. *Systems Thinking for Health Systems Strengthening*; Alliance for Health Policy and Systems Research; WHO: Geneva, Switzerland, 2009.

52. Chandler, C.; Jones, C.; Boniface, G.; Juma, K.; Reyburn, H.; Whitty, C. Guidelines and mindlines: Why do clinical staff over-diagnose malaria in Tanzania? A qualitative study. *Malar. J.* **2008**, *7*, 53. [CrossRef]

53. Shaw, I. One-eyed mules and social work: An essay on serendipity. *Qual. Soc. Work* **2016**, *15*, 136–149. [CrossRef]

54. Street, A. The Testing Revolution: Investigating Diagnostic Devices in Global Health. In Somatosphere. 2018. Available online: http://somatosphere.net/2018/testing-revolution.html/ (accessed on 12 December 2019).

55. Armstrong, D. Diagnosis and nosology in primary care. *Soc. Sci. Med.* **2011**, *73*, 801–807. [CrossRef]

56. Hay, R. Skin NTDs: An opportunity for integrated care. *Trans. R. Soc. Trop. Med. Hyg.* **2017**, *110*, 679–680. [CrossRef]

57. Mukendi, D.; Lilo Kalo, J.R.; Mpanya, A.; Minikulu, L.; Kayembe, T.; Lutumba, P.; Barbe, B.; Gillet, P.; Jacobs, J.; Van Loen, H.; et al. Clinical Spectrum, Etiology, and Outcome of Neurological Disorders in the Rural Hospital of Mosango, the Democratic Republic of Congo. *Am. J. Trop. Med. Hyg.* **2017**, *97*, 1454–1460. [CrossRef]

58. Alirol, E.; Horie, N.S.; Barbe, B.; Lejon, V.; Verdonck, K.; Gillet, P.; Jacobs, J.; Buscher, P.; Kanal, B.; Bhattarai, N.R.; et al. Diagnosis of Persistent Fever in the Tropics: Set of Standard Operating Procedures Used in the NIDIAG Febrile Syndrome Study. *PLoS Negl. Trop. Dis.* **2016**, *10*, e0004749. [CrossRef]

59. Van der Geest, S.; Whyte, S.R. The charm of medicines: Metaphors and metonyms. *Med. Anthropol. Q.* **1989**, *3*, 345–367. [CrossRef]

60. Palmer, J.; Robert, O.; Kansiime, F. Including refugees in disease elimination: Challenges observed from a sleeping sickness programme in Uganda. *Confl. Health* **2017**, *11*. [CrossRef] [PubMed]

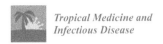 *Tropical Medicine and Infectious Disease*

Article

An Active Follow-up Strategy for Serological Suspects of Human African Trypanosomiasis with Negative Parasitology Set up by a Health Zone Team in the Democratic Republic of Congo

Matthieu Nkieri [1,†], Florent Mbo [2,3,*,†], Papy Kavunga [1], Pathou Nganzobo [2], Titus Mafolo [4], Chalet Selego [4] and Eric Mwamba Miaka [2]

1   Bagata Health Zone, Avenue Kalanganda N 10, Mwendo Bagata,32 Kwilu Province,
     Democratic Republic of the Congo; drmathieu.nkieri@gmail.com (M.N.); plukula@dndi.org (P.K.)
2   National Sleeping Sickness Control Program (PNLTHA) (PNMLS building), Boulevard Triomphale Crossing
     Av. 24 November, 10 Kinshasa, Democratic Republic of the Congo; drnganzobo@yahoo.fr (P.N.);
     erickmwamb2002@yahoo.fr (E.M.M.)
3   HAT Platform, Avenue Milambo N 4 Quartier Socimat, Gombe, 10 Kinshasa,
     Democratic Republic of the Congo
4   Provincial Health Ministry of Kwilu, Aviation/Ifuri/Bandundu town, Bandundu,
     Democratic Republic of the Congo; titusmafolotitu@gmail.com (T.M.); selegochalenda2005@yahoo.fr (C.S.)
*   Correspondence: fmbo@dndi.org or docflorentmbo@yahoo.fr; Tel.: +243-814313838
†   These authors contributed equally.

Received: 6 January 2020; Accepted: 2 April 2020; Published: 4 April 2020

Abstract: Background: The World Health Organization aims for the elimination of Human African Trypanosomiasis (HAT) as a public health problem by 2020 and for full elimination (absence of new cases) by 2030. One of strategies to achieve this is the active follow-up of all HAT serological suspects found during passive screening who have never been re-tested for parasitology. This is important because these cases can maintain HAT transmission and may be responsible for reemergence of the disease. **Methods:** In order to improve case finding at low cost in the targeted population, a general recall was transmitted to aparasitemic serological suspects about the availability of confirmation services at the general referral hospital. Transport was facilitated for re-testing. The initial examinations were carried out in Health Centers from Bagata Health Zone (HZ) in the Democratic Republic of the Congo between January 2017 and April 2019. This strategy of using a HZ team has not been previously documented. **Results:** From a total sample of 74 serological suspects listed by the health centers, 36 cases were re-examined at the general reference hospital; 19% (7/36) self-presented and 81% (29/36) were actively followed up by HZ personnel. Of those re-examined at the general reference hospital, 39% (14/36) resulted in a parasitologically confirmed case. Of the 14 people diagnosed with HAT, 14% (2/14) self-presented and the remaining 86% (12/14) were diagnosed in suspects who were actively followed up. This new strategy of facilitating transport from the villages added value by contributing to the detection of 12 HAT cases, compared to the passive approach, waiting for self-reference, which resulted in the detection of 2 new HAT cases. The cost per detected patient was 70 USD from the group of 7 suspects who self-presented for testing at the hospital and 346 USD per detected case for the group of 29 patients who were actively followed up by health zone staff. **Conclusion:** Targeted active follow-up of aparasitemic serological suspects by HZ teams is a cost-effective and promising approach to identifying additional cases of HAT in areas of very low prevalence, which would contribute to the HAT elimination goal set by the World Health Organization.

Keywords: CATT positive serological suspects; active follow-up strategy; human African trypanosomiasis

1. Background

WHO set the goal of eliminating HAT as a public health problem by 2020 and full elimination (absence of new cases) by 2030. To achieve elimination, all HAT cases will need to be detected using adapted strategies in the field. However, there are unexpected issues to resolve. One of these is tracing all HAT serological suspects who have never been tested for parasitology. Another is specifically targeting HAT serological suspects who had negative parasitology during active screening performed by traditional mobile teams and passive screening done at selected health facilities.

National sleeping sickness control programs (NSSCP) list, but rarely actively follow-up, subjects with positive serology but negative parasitology, who then remain untreated. Some will progress to the disease because the parasite was not detected for various reasons (including parasite fluctuation, technician performance, and lack of sensitive laboratory techniques).

There are two types of serological tests: The Card agglutination test for trypanosomiasis (CATT) and rapid diagnostic tests (RDT), which identify a large number of positive serological suspects. However, in order to positively define a HAT case and trigger treatment, parasitological confirmation is currently required.

In this article we focus on CATT positive serological suspects with negative parasitology, defined as aparasitemic serological suspects, which may be detected by two different approaches:

1. CATT positive aparasitemic serological suspects detected during active screening conducted by NSSCP mobile teams, which are unconfirmed despite using sensitive parasitological techniques (including mini anion exchange centrifugation technique (m-AECT)).

2. CATT positive aparasitemic serological suspects detected after spontaneously coming for passive screening conducted by health facilities with integrated HAT activities (which may include sensitive diagnostic techniques or only direct microscopy). This second group was the specific target of the activity.

General reference hospitals and reference health centers in endemic foci can perform sensitive diagnostic concentration techniques such as m-AECT or capillary tube centrifugation (CTC) but other health centers only perform microscopy on samples such as thick film, fresh blood, or lymph node puncture, which are less sensitive.

Usually, follow-up of CATT positive serological suspects with negative parasitology should be conducted by mobile teams during their annual active screening activities. During active screening in endemic villages, the mobile teams produce a report listing all aparasitemic serological suspects, which includes their addresses to facilitate follow-up.

These unconfirmed CATT positive serological suspects receive a recommendation during passive and active screening to go back to health facilities with HAT diagnostic capacity near their village every three months. Most suspects do not return to the recommended health facilities for follow-up because they are a long way from the village. They may not have the means to travel or may not feel very sick. During active screening, mobile teams can look for the remaining aparasitemic serological suspects from the previous year, but many of them do not participate in the screening visit for different reasons (absence from the village, fear of lumbar puncture, lack of confidentiality) [1].

According to the DRC Programme de Lutte contre la Trypanosomiase Humaine Africaine (National Sleeping Sickness control program, PNLTHA) data, over 20,000 aparasitemic serological suspects were reported in 2018 (unpublished data from the PNLTHA DRC, 2018 Annual report: Page 37, Table 5.2). In the three months before the beginning of the targeted active follow-up for passively detected aparasitemic serological suspects in Bagata health zone (HZ), no HAT patients had been diagnosed by Bagata mobile team and health centers.

Other authors have attempted to explain the number of HAT *T.b. gambiense* patients that remain undiagnosed. First, not all infected people are reached by screening activities [2]. Second, current diagnostic techniques do not pick up all *T.b. gambiense* infections due to lack of sensitivity of serological screening tests, of molecular techniques, or of the parasitological confirmation tests [3]. These undiagnosed, yet infected, people may act as a human reservoir of the parasite and might sustain transmission, forming a maintenance population [4]. Another potential human reservoir may be latent infections, also called 'healthy carriers', who do not always progress to clinical disease, although the relative contribution of these individuals to parasite transmission still needs to be documented. This last category was only recently described in Ivory Coast and consists of latently infected people that may carry trypanosomes for years or even decades [5].

In Guinea, patients with asymptomatic or latent infections were found to have consistently high titres in CATT/*T.b. gambiense* and positive results in the immune trypanolysis test, although no parasites could be detected in blood or lymph node fluid during a 2-year follow-up period [6]. This observation is in line with the fact that trypanosomes may survive in the extravascular spaces of diverse organs such as the heart, the central nervous system, and the skin [7,8]. Some projects conducted reactive searches using mobile teams to reach previously detected CATT or RDT positive serological suspects who had not responded to follow-up appointments for parasitology set up by mobile teams or health facilities.

Reactive searches have been implemented by specialized mobile teams and extended RDT detection centers supported by FIND (Foundation for Innovative New Diagnostics) tested with RDT 50 percent of HAT serological suspects (228/457) in the Province of Kongo Central in DRC between August 2015 and July 2016. Using parasitological methods, 111 cases were confirmed; this was 24 percent of all seropositive (111/457) or 49 percent of those examined (111/228) [9]. This is an important contribution to finding the remaining HAT cases, but an alternative simpler targeted approach could also contribute, such as active follow-up of aparasitemic serological suspects found during passive screening.

We describe here an alternative approach to reaching the aparasitemic serological suspects found during passive screening by permanent health staff that involves health workers and community health workers. After sensitization by health workers and community health workers, HZ teams used their means of transport (motorbike, car) to take all aparasitemic suspects, who had not previously independently returned, to the reference general hospital for follow-up appointments. This approach has not been used before.

2. Materials and Methods

2.1. Project Objective

To assess the added value of having HZ personnel actively following up and facilitating transport for aparasitemic serological suspects, who had been previously identified passively, for re-testing in order to improve case finding at low cost in a targeted population.

2.2. Strategy Used by the Health Zone Team

The aim of the HZ team was to organize active follow-up of aparasitemic serological suspects who would not return to the referral general hospital for re-testing by themselves after sensitization by health workers and community health workers. Most aparasitemic serological suspects found through passive screening do not respond to the follow-up appointments for re-testing, which are fixed at every three months according to PNLTHA recommendations. After three months, the aparasitemic serological suspect is considered as non-attendant. In our intervention, there was a two-week window after sensitization for all aparasitemic serological suspects to return spontaneously for re-testing to the referral general hospital. After this time, they were actively sought out by HZ staff.

2.3. Place of Work: Bagata Health Zone

The Bagata HZ, located at 535 km East of Kinshasa, in Kwilu province in the Democratic Republic of the Congo, is endemic for HAT. The Health Zone has eighteen health centers and one general reference hospital. Five of these health centers, and the general reference hospital, offer a package of HAT management activities: screening, diagnosis, and treatment. Six health facilities, including the general reference hospital, use CATT as the screening test; it is performed with fresh blood and not with serum. The general reference hospital diagnostic algorithm for serologically positive cases starts with lymph node palpation, and aspiration if enlarged cervical nodes are detected. The hospital performs sensitive diagnostic techniques such as m-AECT, modified simple centrifugation and CTC to search for HAT parasites. Parasite detection is confirmed under an LED microscope with a camera with 5 s video capture of the parasites for quality control. This general reference hospital was equipped as part of a clinical trial. The five health centers perform other less sensitive parasitological tests such as lymph node examination, and direct examination of thick blood film and fresh blood under the microscope.

2.4. Programmatic Follow-up of Activities

Before organizing this active follow-up approach, the HZ team retrospectively collected information about CATT positive serological suspects with negative parasitology from the five health centers and the referral general hospital described above from January 2017 to April 2019 using a PNLTHA data collection form. Suspects' data were collected in register books as follows: initials of patient, age, address, sex, date of previous examination, signs and/or symptoms of HAT during the previous examination, CATT result, and results of any other parasitological diagnostic test. This initial data was completed, when available, with follow-up visits 1 and 2, including date, CATT result, diagnostic result, signs, and/or symptoms of HAT and the distance in kilometers between the home location of each aparasitemic serological suspect and the reference hospital. To the form we added additional information about whether the suspect reached the hospital by him- or herself or whether the hospital staff brought him/her with a car or motorbike. HZ teams started with sensitization sessions with health workers and community health workers during meetings at the five health centers with capacity to do serological testing. Community health workers then proceeded to locate the aparasitemic serological suspects to inform them about the importance of respecting their follow-up appointments. The HZ team mapped the home locations of CATT-positive serological suspects with negative parasitology, including a schedule for their active follow-up. Active follow-up by HZ staff of all aparasitemic serological suspects who had not spontaneously attended the recommended visits started after a two-week lag period. Bagata HZ vehicles were used to transport suspects who, after sensitization, were unable or unwilling to come by themselves to the reference general hospital. Transportation was also organized to return patients to their villages. Suspects living far from the referral hospital could stay overnight at the hospital without paying a fee. Food was provided at the hospital. Active follow-up of suspects was combined with supervisory visits by the HZ team to minimize costs, as the supervisory budget included accommodation and a per diem for health zone staff.

2.5. Ethical Aspects

Ethical approval was not needed as passive follow-up of aparasitemic serological suspects is included in the recommended routine activities of the PNLTHA in DRC.

2.6. Data Analysis

A simple descriptive analysis was performed. The target population is presented according to availability, showing the number and proportion of aparasitemic serological suspects re-tested, their sex and age, and whether they came spontaneously or were transported to the reference hospital; the parasitological results for all those re-tested are also mentioned. The institutional marginal cost data directly attributed to this additional activity were examined, without including the basic costs of provision of general health care. We included in the calculation: transport linked costs (fuel/oil + maintenance of the vehicles); training and motivation of the community health workers, direct supervision by the HZ staff food for the patients during their time in the hospital, and the cost of the m-AECT tests performed. No administrative costs or salaries have been considered as they would have existed anyway without the additional activity. Treatment was donated.

3. Results

3.1. Population Examined

In the lists gathered by Bagata HZ staff from 5 health centers and the reference hospital with capacity for HAT case detection, 74 persons were identified between January 2017 and April 2019 as aparasitemic serological suspects (Table S1). Of these, 36 were found and tested using parasitological techniques. The small number of detected individuals that could be effectively followed up (36/74, 49% of suspects) shows the limits of this case search process with the available funds.

The average age was 30 years for selected suspects and 34 for detected cases; 54% (40/74) of suspects and 36% (5/14) of detected cases were female. 9% (7/74) travelled to the hospital by their own means for follow-up examinations and 39% (29/74) were actively recovered by the HZ team, see Figure 1.

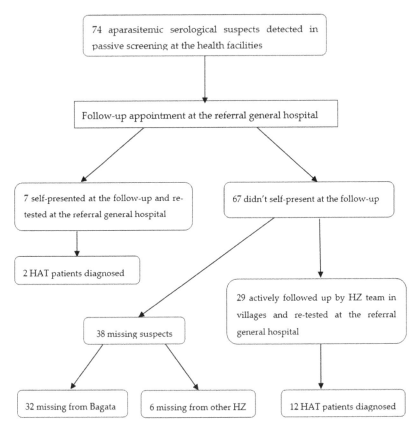

Figure 1. Flow diagram including passive approach (spontaneous visits after sensitization) and active follow-up strategy.

51% (38/74) of aparasitemic serological suspects were not followed by HZ staff for re-testing and remained untested (Table 1). Of these, 6 had been detected in Bagata, but lived in other HZ.

Trop. Med. Infect. Dis. **2020**, *5*, 53

Table 1. Achievements of passive and active follow-up approaches with parasitology results.

Category of Suspects	N	CATT Result at Follow-Up	Parasitology Result at Follow-Up
Suspects who self-presented	7	6 positives 1 negative	2 HAT patients
Suspects actively followed-up	29	19 positives 10 negatives	11 HAT patients 1 HAT patient
Suspects not re-examined	38	N/A	N/A

N/A: Not available.

3.2. Cases Detected

Of the aparasitemic serological suspects who self-presented (passive approach), 14% (2/14) were diagnosed with HAT. The remaining 86% of all confirmed HAT cases (12/14) were diagnosed in suspects who HZ personnel actively followed up. Overall, 39% (14/36) of CATT-positive suspects with negative parasitology coming from health centers were confirmed positive with sensitive diagnostic techniques such as m-AECT, CTC and modified simple centrifugation performed in the reference general hospital, although two of them required a second visit (Table S2). Two confirmed cases had a negative CATT test during the first visit, one was confirmed after a second positive CATT test in a supplementary visit and the other may have been a manipulation error and was confirmed in the parasitological exam at the same visit when the negative serology was found, and 42% (6/14) of new HAT cases were in the first stage of the disease and 58% (8/14) in the second stage. The positive predictive value of the screening test increased to 52% for the 36 CATT positive suspects with negative parasitology who responded to one or two follow-up visits at the reference general hospital for parasitology examination. Of the CATT positive suspects with negative parasitology who were followed, 30% (11/36) were found to be CATT negative during the follow-up visit at the reference general hospital.

3.3. Cost Assessment of the Strategy

We calculated the additional institutional cost to organize and execute the new activities.

The active follow-up strategy implemented by the HZ team had an additional cost of 306 USD per new case detected, taking into consideration all 14 new cases, including those that came spontaneously after the community health workers' sensitization visits (Table 2). Dividing the attributable costs between the patients that came spontaneously (their proportion of food, sensitization, and m-AECT) and those that had to be transported (adding all transport and supervision costs to this group), the cost per detected patient is 70 USD from the group of 7 suspects who self-presented for testing at the hospital and 346 USD per detected case for the group of 29 patients who were actively followed up by health zone staff.

Table 2. Marginal direct cost of active search strategy from January 2017 to April 2019.

Materials Activities	Quantity	Unit Cost (USD)	Total Cost (USD)	Observation
Diesel + Gasoline + Oil	800 + 420 + 23 L	1.5/1.8/5	2071	Transportation and river crossing
Maintenance (vehicle and motorbike)	-	-	900	-
Supervision cost	-	-	600	Health zone team
Food for the suspects	36	10	360	Hospital stay
Sensitization of Community agents	50	5	250	Location of suspects
m-AECT	36	3	108	-
Total	-	-	4289	-

4. Discussion

Despite the fact that almost half of the identified suspects missed the follow-up examination and possible confirmation by sensitive parasitological testing, these data show that this new active follow-up strategy improved detection of HAT cases. It also shows that with the existing economic means at

Trop. Med. Infect. Dis. **2020**, *5*, 53

the time of the investigation, the passive approach will have a limited impact on the interruption of HAT transmission up to 2030. Four suspects that self-referred to the health structure and nine of those examined via the active follow-up strategy, who remained CATT positive, could not be confirmed. These 13 cases, along with the 38 missing individuals, fall into the category of unconfirmed suspects who may contribute to re-emergence of the disease. The HZ staff should continue to follow them until their serology becomes negative or parasites are detected. The present strategy, while only covering a single HZ and a limited number of seropositive suspects, seems to be cost effective as it targets a high-risk subgroup of the population. We believe that to maximize the detection of HAT cases, this strategy should be generalized and that it must be combined with a continued extension of serological testing and follow-up of positive cases in known endemic areas.

In Uganda, in a low prevalence environment, Lee and Palmer discovered the limitations of a surveillance strategy that used RDT to progress to the next step of confirming serological suspects. Patient misunderstanding of the referral rationale was a key structural weakness due to poor provider communication about the possibility of discordant HAT test results. The biggest difficulty was how to communicate the concept of possible false positives in the serological test and the need to find parasites microscopically in order to be able to treat; this may lead the patients to distrust the whole system. Transport and possible health services costs were an additional deterrent [10].

The high proportion of new cases detected corroborates the usefulness of sensitive techniques, as described by Robays et al., 2004 [2], who examined the diagnostic process used in active screening performed by mobile teams in the field in DRC stating that, once a sensitive algorithm is in place, the attendance rate is a critical factor.

Pepin et al., 1989 [11], showed that passive screening followed by an active follow-up strategy at health facilities level is likely to improve case detection. The same authors also showed that in the Nioki health zone, Democratic Republic of the Congo in 1987 health centers and the general referral hospital could detect 71.5% of all patients after re-training personnel and updating equipment.

Penchenier et al., 1991, reported that 30.6% of 193 suspected positives to either blood or serum (discordant) became negative after one month, mentioning the possibility of false positivity or cross-reaction problems, with another cause being blood hemagglutination, and pointing at possible contact with animal trypanosomes in case of a previously positive serum sample [12]. In our sample we found 10/36 (28 percent) became negative for CATT in blood and parasitology.

The active follow-up strategy of previously CATT positive parasitologically unconfirmed suspects in our analysis in Bagata allowed the identification of 43% (6/14) of new cases in the early stage of the disease, thus breaking the transmission chain and stopping the evolution towards the advanced stage.

By comparison, an analysis in a context with higher prevalence by Lutumba et al., 2007, showed that the best cost-effectiveness of a confirmation strategy after screening with CATT was the combination with lymph node puncture and two concentration methods (CTC and m-AECT). It was calculated as 265.46€ per life saved. [13]. The costs of performing the two tests (m-AECT and CTC) of the current study in the field have not been elucidated yet. The cost per patient detected would increase if more suspects were searched via an active follow-up strategy by motorbike or vehicle, as those not examined tended to live further away and were more difficult to find. In a low prevalence context, the active follow-up strategy would be more efficient compared with traditional active screening performed by mobile teams; Bagata mobile teams did not detect any HAT cases in the same area for the three months before starting this strategy.

The remaining CATT positive suspects with negative parasitology after screening at the hospital may suggest, according to other authors, the existence of non-virulent or non-pathogenic trypanosome strains and/or human susceptibility that may lead to long-term seropositivity without detectable parasitemia [14]. This may also suggest the possibility or existence of a human reservoir of trypanosomes that can contribute to the maintenance or periodic resurgence of HAT in endemic foci, often attributed to an animal reservoir [15–18].

A recent cost analysis has shown a disproportionate increase in the cost per case detected by mobile teams using traditional methods, which is directly related to the reduction in prevalence. According to this analysis, the average cost per case detected for 10 mobile teams in DRC climbed from 1,789 USD in 2014 to 21,324 USD in 2018 [19]. Mini mobile teams acting door to door resulted in a lower cost per individual examined (1.67 vs 1.89) when compared with the full mobile teams, but screening the general population still cost 110,994 USD per mini mobile team and 122,932 per traditional mobile team in DRC per year [20]. To improve the effectiveness of the active search strategy, a door-to-door method has been the targeted option, which involves looking for previously identified cases or seropositive individuals and people in their immediate environment [21].

These observations indicate that we must combine several strategies, adapted to the local epidemiology, to maintain cost-effectiveness [22]. They need to include active follow-up of suspects in a low prevalence context in order to detect the last cases of sleeping sickness.

An active follow-up strategy can be extended to the remaining CATT or RDT positive suspects with negative parasitological results found during active screening, who were not considered for this investigation. Health facilities that are able to perform serological testing would need to be included in a network with the health centers and general reference hospitals able to perform sensitive diagnostic tests. To make this network functional, several aspects need to be considered and developed: training of laboratory technicians, a regular supply of laboratory equipment and consumables, sensitization of community agents and health workers, and transport of serologically positive suspects.

5. Conclusions

An active follow-up strategy that targets CATT-positive or RDT-positive serological suspects by implementing a HZ team would be a cost-effective and promising approach to identifying the last cases of HAT in areas of very low prevalence, which would contribute to the HAT elimination goal set by the World Health Organization. The integration of this strategy in the activities of the general health system would allow for sustainability.

Supplementary Materials: The following are available at http://www.mdpi.com/2414-6366/5/2/53/s1. Table S1: Number of CATT positive serological suspects collected in Bagata Health Zone (HZ), Table S2: Signs and test results of 36 CATT positive serological suspects at previous exam at health centers and at the follow-up visits at the hospital.

Author Contributions: Conceptualization, F.M. and M.N.; Methodology, F.M.; Validation, E.M.M.; Formal Analysis, F.M.; Investigation, M.N.; Resources, M.N.; Writing – Original Draft Preparation, F.M.; Writing – Review & Editing, M.N., F.M., P.K., P.N., T.M., C.S. and E.M.M.; Supervision, E.M.M.; Project Administration, F.M.; Funding Acquisition, M.N. All authors have read and agreed to the published version of the manuscript.

Funding: This research received no external funding.

Acknowledgments: We would like to acknowledge all laboratory technicians, health workers and HZ staff from Bagata who were involved in this operational study. We thank Olaf Valverde and Louise Burrows from DND*i* for their careful review of the text.

Conflicts of Interest: The authors declare no conflict of interest.

References

1. Mpanya, A.; Hendrickx, D.; Vuna, M.; Kanyinda, A.; Lumbala, C.; Tshilombo, V.; Mitashi, P.; Luboya, O.; Kande, V.; Boelaert, M.; et al. Should I Get Screened for Sleeping Sickness? A Qualitative Study in Kasai Province, Democratic Republic of Congo. *PLoS Negl. Trop. Dis.* **2012**, *6*, e1467. [CrossRef] [PubMed]

2. Robays, J.; Bilengue, M.M.C.; Stuyft, P.V.D.; Boelaert, M. Effectiveness of active population screening and treatment from sleeping sickness Control in the Democratic Republic of Congo. *Trop. Med. Int. Health* **2004**, *9*, 542–550. [CrossRef] [PubMed]

3. Ngoyi, D.M.; Ekangu, R.A.; Kodi, M.F.M.; Pyana, P.P.; Balharbi, F.; Decq, M.; Betu, V.K.; van der Veken, W.; Sese, C.; Menten, J.; et al. Performance of parasitological and molecular techniques for the diagnosis and surveillance of gambiense sleeping sickness. *PLoS Negl. Trop. Dis.* **2014**, *12*, e2954. [CrossRef]

4.   Viana, M.; Mancy, R.; Biek, R.; Cleaveland, S.; Cross, P.C.; Lloyd-Smith, J.O.; Haydon, D.T. Assembling evidence for identifying reservoirs of infections. *Trends. Ecol. Evol.* **2014**, *29*, 270–279. [CrossRef] [PubMed]

5.   Jamonneau, V.; Ilboudo, H.; Kaboré, J.; Kaba, D.; Koffi, M.; Solano, P.; Garcia, A.; Courtin, D.; Laveissière, C.; Lingue, K.; et al. Untreated human infections by *Trypanosoma brucei gambiense* are not 100% fatal. *PLoS Negl. Trop. Dis.* **2012**, *6*, e1691. [CrossRef] [PubMed]

6.   Ilboudo, H.; Jamonneau, V.; Camara, M.; Camara, O.; Dama, E.; Léno, M.; Ouendeno, F.; Courtin, F.; Sakande, H.; Sanon, R.; et al. Diversity of response to *Trypanosoma brucei gambiense* infections in the Forecariah mangrove focus (Guinea): Perspectives for a better control of sleeping sickness. *Microbes. Infect.* **2011**, *13*, 943–952. [CrossRef] [PubMed]

7.   Blum, J.A.; Schmid, C.; Burri, C.; Hatz, C.; Olson, C.; Fungula, B.; Kazumba, L.; Mangoni, P.; Mbo, F.; Deo, K.; et al. Cardiac alterations in human African trypanosomiasis (*T.b. gambiense*) with respect to the disease stage and antiparasitic treatment. *PLoS Negl. Trop. Dis.* **2009**, *3*, e383. [CrossRef] [PubMed]

8.   McGovern, T.W.; Williams, W.; Fitzpatrick, J.E.; Cetron, M.S.; Hepburn, B.C.; Gentry, R.H. Cutaneous manifestations of African trypanosomiasis. *Arch. Dermatol.* **1995**, *131*, 1178–1182. [CrossRef] [PubMed]

9.   Lumbala, C.; Kayembe, S.; Makabuza, J.; Picado, A.; Bessell, P.; Bieler, S.; Ndung'u, J. Intensive passive screening and targeted active screening for human African trypanosomiasis detects most patients in first stage disease. In Proceedings of the Unpublished Oral Communication, 4th Joint EANETT-HAT Platform Scientific Meeting, Conakry, Guinea, 21 September 2016.

10.   Lee, S.J.; Palmer, J.J. Integrating innovations: A qualitative analysis of referral noncompletion among rapid diagnostic test-positive patients in Uganda's human African trypanosomiasis elimination programme. *Infect. Dis. Poverty* **2018**, *7*, 1–16. [CrossRef] [PubMed]

11.   Pepin, J.; Guern, C.; Milord, F.; Bokelo, M. Integration of African Human Trypanosomiasis control in a network of multipurpose health centers. *Bull. WHO* **1989**, *67*, 301–308. (In French) [PubMed]

12.   Penchenier, L.; Jannin, J.; Moulia-Pelat, J.P.; de la Baume Elfassi, F.; Fadat, G.; Chanfreau, B.; Eozenou, P. The problem of interpretation of the CATT (Card Agglutination Trypanosomiasis Test) in mass screening for *Trypanosoma brucei gambiense* sleeping sickness. *Ann. Soc. Belg. Med. Trop.* **1991**, *71*, 221–228. (In French) [PubMed]

13.   Lutumba, P.; Meheus, F.; Robays, J.; Miaka, C.; Kande, V.; Büscher, P.; Dujardin, B.; Boelaert, M. Cost Effectiveness of algorithms for confirmation test of human African trypanosomiasis. *Emerg. Inf. Dis.* **2007**, *13*, 1484–1490. [CrossRef] [PubMed]

14.   Koffi, M.; Solano, P.; Denizot, M.; Courtin, D.; Garcia, A.; Lejon, V.; Büscher, P.; Cuny, G.; Jamonneau, V. Aparasitemic serological suspects in *Trypanosoma brucei gambiense* human African trypanosomiasis: A potential human reservoir of parasites? *Acta Trop.* **2006**, *98*, 183–188. [CrossRef] [PubMed]

15.   Njiokou, F.; Laveissière, C.; Simo, G.; Nkinin, S.; Grébaut, P.; Cuny, G.; Herder, S. Wild fauna as a probable animal reservoir for *Trypanosoma brucei gambiense* in Cameroon. *Infect. Genet. Evol.* **2006**, *6*, 147–153. [CrossRef] [PubMed]

16.   Noireau, F.; Gouteux, J.P.; Frézil, J.L. Sensibilité du test d'agglutination sur carte (Testryp CATT) dans les infections porcines à Trypanosoma (Nannomonas) congolense en Republique Populaire du Congo. *Ann. Soc. Belg. Med. Trop.* **1986**, *66*, 63–68. [PubMed]

17.   Noireau, F.; Gouteux, J.P.; Toudic, A.; Samba, F.; Frézil, J.L. Importance épidémiologique du réservoir animal à *Trypanosoma brucei gambiense* au Congo. 1. Prévalence des trypanosomoses animales dans les foyers de maladie du sommeil. *Trop. Med. Parasitol.* **1986**, *37*, 393–398. [PubMed]

18.   Mehlitz, D.; Zillmann, U.; Scott, C.M.; Godfrey, D.G. Epidemiological studies on the animal reservoir of gambiense sleeping sickness. Part III: Characterization of Trypanozoon stocks by isoenzymes and sensitivity to human serum. *Tropenmed. Parasitol.* **1982**, *33*, 113–118. [PubMed]

19.   Valverde Mordt, O. Human African trypanosomiasis: The challenge of continuing active case detection in an elimination context. In Proceedings of the Oral Presentation at the ISCTRC Biannual Conference, Abuja, Nigeria, 25 September 2019.

20.   Rian, S.; Alain, F.; Yves, C.; Epco, H.; Alain, M.; Erick, M.; Pascal, L.; Filip, M.; Marleen, B. *Comparison of Costs between Two Strategies of Active Case Finding of Sleeping Sickness in the Democratic Republic of the Congo*; ASTMH: New Orleans, LA, USA, 2018.

21. Koffi, M.; N'Djetchi, M.; Ilboudo, H.; Kaba, D.; Coulibaly, B.; N'Gouan, E.; Kouakou, L.; Bucheton, B.; Solano, P.; Courtin, F.; et al. A targeted door-to-door strategy for sleeping sickness detection in low-prevalence settings in Côte d'Ivoire. *Parasite* **2016**, *23*, 51–56. [CrossRef] [PubMed]
22. Simarro, P.P.; Franco, J.R.; Diarra, A.; Postigo, J.R.; Jannin, J. Diversity of human African trypanosomiasis epidemiological settings requires fine-tuning control strategies to facilitate disease elimination. *Res. Rep. Trop. Med.* **2013**, *4*, 1–6. [CrossRef] [PubMed]

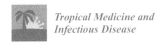

Tropical Medicine and Infectious Disease

Article

Haemoparasitic Infections in Cattle from a *Trypanosoma brucei* Rhodesiense Sleeping Sickness Endemic District of Eastern Uganda

Enock Matovu [1], Claire Mack Mugasa [1,*], Peter Waiswa [1], Annah Kitibwa [1], Alex Boobo [1] and Joseph Mathu Ndung'u [2]

[1] College of Veterinary Medicine, Animal Resources and Biosecurity, Makerere University Kampala, P.O. Box 7062 Kampala, Uganda; matovue@covab.mak.ac.ug (E.M.); pwaiswa@covab.mak.ac.ug (P.W.); kitty.ann34@yahoo.com (A.K.); alexboobo@yahoo.com (A.B.)

[2] Foundation for Innovative New Diagnostics, Campus Biotech, Chemin des Mines 9, CH 1202 Geneva, Switzerland; joseph.ndungu@finddx.org

* Correspondence: claire1mack@covab.mak.ac.ug

Received: 13 January 2020; Accepted: 3 February 2020; Published: 7 February 2020

Abstract: We carried out a baseline survey of cattle in Kaberamaido district, in the context of controlling the domestic animal reservoir of *Trypanosoma brucei rhodesiense* human African trypanosomiasis (rHAT) towards elimination. Cattle blood was subjected to capillary tube centrifugation followed by measurement of the packed cell volume (PCV) and examination of the buffy coat area for motile trypanosomes. Trypanosomes were detected in 561 (21.4%) out of 2621 cattle screened by microscopy. These 561 in addition to 724 apparently trypanosome negative samples with low PCVs ($\leq$25%) were transported to the laboratory and tested by PCR targeting the trypanosomal Internal Transcribed Spacer (ITS-1) as well as suspect Tick-Borne Diseases (TBDs) including Anaplasmamosis, Babesiosis, and Theileriosis. PCR for *Anaplasma* sp yielded the highest number of positive animals (45.2%), followed by *Trypanosoma* sp (44%), *Theileria* sp (42.4%) and *Babesia* (26.3%); multiple infections were a common occurrence. Interestingly, 373 (29%) of these cattle with low PCVs were negative by PCR, pointing to other possible causes of aneamia, such as helminthiasis. Among the trypanosome infections classified as *T. brucei* by ITS-PCR, 5.5% were positive by SRA PCR, and were, therefore, confirmed as *T. b. rhodesiense*. Efforts against HAT should therefore consider packages that address a range of conditions. This may enhance acceptability and participation of livestock keepers in programs to eliminate this important but neglected tropical disease. In addition, we demonstrated that cattle remain an eminent reservoir for *T. b. rhodesiense* in eastern Uganda, which must be addressed to sustain HAT elimination.

Keywords: Haemoparasites; human African trypanosomiasis; elimination; animal reservoirs

1. Introduction

African trypanosomes transmitted by tsetse flies (*Glossina* sp.) cause the zoonotic human African trypanosomiasis (HAT; also known as sleeping sickness) as well as animal African trypanosomiasis (AAT; nagana). AAT is a major hindrance to livestock productivity in tsetse infested areas of sub-Saharan Africa. This disease was reported to affect various animal productivity parameters, including growth, mortality, calving rate, draft power, meat, and milk production by up to 20% in susceptible animals [1]. The economic losses attributable to AAT were estimated at US$4.5bn per annum [2]. On the other hand, the human disease (HAT) was for many years among the leading causes of death in rural areas. HAT is caused by two subspecies of *T. brucei* that are able to resist the naturally occurring trypanolytic factor (APOL I) and establish infections in humans. The chronic form of HAT associated with *T. b. gambiense* (gHAT) occurs in central and western Africa (including parts of northwestern Uganda), while the acute *T. b. rhodesiense* (rHAT) is found in eastern and southern Africa, in a belt presently stretching from eastern Uganda through Tanzania to Malawi and Zambia. In the past 5 decades, the number of HAT cases ranged between 50,000 and 70,000, dropped to below 10,000 in 2009, and continued to drop to 6743 cases by 2011 [3]. This reduction in HAT incidence was as a result of campaigns spearheaded by the World Health Organization (WHO) working together with non-governmental organizations [4] as well as National control programs. Consequently, in 2012, the WHO included HAT on the list of diseases set for elimination, first as a public health problem by 2020 followed by complete interruption of transmission by 2030 [5].

The role of animal reservoirs in rHAT transmission was recognised by pioneer researchers [6,7] and was the basis for game destruction as a method of sleeping sickness control during colonial times. In Uganda, research carried out during the 1980s and 1990s singled out cattle, pigs and dogs as the domestic animal reservoirs of rHAT [8–11]. According to Simarro et al. (2010) [12], eastern Uganda contributed over 50% of *T. b. rhodesiense* reported cases in Africa between 2000 and 2009; many of these were of livestock reservoir origin. Indeed, the latest outbreak that spilled over to Teso and Lango regions was attributed to cattle movement from the southerly endemic areas [13,14]. In line with the above facts, Uganda embraces a control strategy that involves surveillance and treatment of all detected HAT cases, vector control to supress tsetse populations, thereby limiting transmission, as well as control of the animal reservoir by chemotherapy. However, full implementation of this strategy is hampered by limited resource availability such that some aspects cannot be consistently executed.

In this baseline survey to support elimination of HAT by targeting the animal reservoir, we aimed to identify the major haemoparasites particularly associated with the typically low packed cell volume (PCVs) of less or equal to 25% of cattle blood observed both in the presence and absence of the motile trypanosomes in buffy coats following capillary tube centrifugation.

2. Materials and Methods

2.1. Study Area and Study Population

The livestock survey was carried out in Kaberamaido district (approximate latitudes 1.5500 to 2.3834 and longitudes 30.0167 to 34.3000), in Eastern Uganda (Figure 1). A total of 15 parishes (Ochuloi, Opilitok, Kaberikole, Omoru, Amukurat, Anyara, Kalaki, Ariamo, Abalang, Palatau, Achan-pii, Kamuk, Omarai, Aperkina and Abalkweru) in five sub-counties (Otuboi, Kalaki, Alwa, Kaberamaido and Kobulubulu) were included in the survey. The main occupation in the entire study area is subsistence agriculture. Cattle are the major livestock and communal grazing is usually practiced.

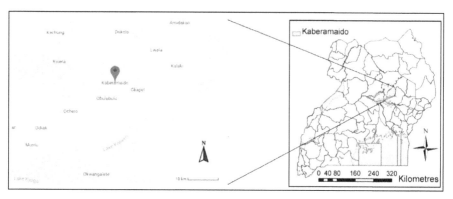

Figure 1. Regional map of Uganda showing the location of the study area. (https://www.google.com/maps/place/Kaberamaido).

2.2. Study Design and Field Surveys

This was a cross-sectional study carried out in the above-mentioned parishes. Cattle were screened by a mobile team at a designated site per parish, selected with assistance from the District Veterinary Officer (DVO) and local leaders. Cattle blood was drawn by venipuncture into EDTA-coated vacutainer tubes and subjected to Haematocrit Centrifugation Technique (HCT) [15]. Packed cell volume (PCV) readings were taken for all the samples using a manual micro-haematocrit reader (Thomas Scientific, Swedesboro, NJ, USA) [16]. This was followed by examination of the buffy coat area of the centrifuged capillary tubes under the microscope (Leica Microsystems, Wetzlar, Germany) at 100× magnification for the presence of motile trypanosomes. Aliquots of blood from cattle with low PCVs, regardless of whether they had detectable trypanosomes or not, were transported in liquid nitrogen to the laboratory for further analysis. In addition, representative thin smears from apparently trypanosome-negative samples were made and fixed with methanol, then stored in slide boxes and transported to the laboratory in slide boxes for staining and examination for possible presence of other haemoparasites.

The animals were treated with either diminazene aceturate (3.5 mg/kg body weight) or isometamidium chloride (1 mg/kg body weight) as per design of the mother project for which this was the baseline study. In addition, deltamethrin pour-on as a tsetse control tool was applied superficially on all the cattle to control tsetse flies.

3. Laboratory Procedures

3.1. Staining of Blood Smears

The thin blood smears were stained with acridine orange following protocols developed by the Foundation for Innovative New diagnostics (FIND) [17] and examined for the presence of tick-borne pathogens under a fluorescence microscope (Carl Zeiss Microscopy, Jena, Germany) at 400× magnification.

3.2. Extraction of Genomic DNA

Genomic DNA was extracted from 100 μL of whole blood samples using a commercial Quick gDNA mini prep kit (Zymo Research, Irvine, CA, USA) following the manufacturer's instructions. It was eluted in 50 μL PCR water and stored frozen at −20 °C until use in the PCR reactions.

3.3. Identification Trypanosome Species by PCR

All PCRs in this study were done using the My Taq Mix® (Bioline, London, UK) (https://cn.bioline.com/mytaq), while primers were ordered from Microsynth company (The Swiss DNA company, Bern, Switzerland).

The infecting trypanosome species were identified by PCR using primers targeting the Internal Transcribed Spacer-1 (ITS-1) region of the rDNA as described by Njiru et al. [18]. PCR reactions were performed in a volume of 25 μL, containing 1x My Taq Mix polymerase enzyme, the primer pair ITS1-CF (5′ CCG GAA GTT CAC CGA TAT TG 3′) and ITS1-BR (5′ TTG CTG CGT TCT TCA ACG AA 3′) each at 0.5 μM. Amplification was performed under the following conditions; 94 °C for 5 min (initial denaturation) followed by 35 cycles of 94 °C, 1 min (denaturation), 60 °C, 1 min (annealing), 72 °C, 1 min (extension) and a final extension of 72 °C for 5 min. Three microlitres of genomic DNA was added to each PCR reaction as template. A positive control (*Trypanosoma brucei brucei* GVR-35 strain) and a negative control (double distilled water) were included alongside the test samples. Ten microlitres of each amplicon was subjected to electrophoresis on a 2% agarose gel containing ethidium bromide (0.5 μg/mL). The amplified products were visualized using an ultra violet transilluminator (Waghtech international) and the band sizes estimated by comparison with a standard DNA marker (www.Finnzymes.com).

The DNA samples that were negative with the single step ITS-PCR described above were thereafter subjected to nested ITS-PCR as described by Cox et al. [19] to rule out negativity due to limiting quantities of trypanosomal DNA in the samples. The primary PCR reaction mixture was 25 µL total volume, with the primer pair ITS-1 (5' GAT TAC GTC CCT GCC ATT TG 3') and ITS-2 (5' TTG TTC GCT ATC GGT CTT CC 3') each at 0.5 µM. Five microlitres of genomic DNA was added to each PCR reaction as template and amplification cycle included 98 °C for 1 min (initial denaturation) followed by 25 cycles of 98 °C, 5 s (denaturation), 64 °C, 30 s (annealing), 72 °C, 30 s (extension) and a final extension of 72 °C for 10 min. This was followed by the second PCR reaction where the primer pair ITS3 (5' GGA AGC AAA AGT CGT AAC AAG G 3') and ITS4 (5' TGT TTT CTT TTC CTC CGC TG 3') each at 0.5 µM concentration and 5 µL of primary PCR product as the template were used. The amplification was performed under similar conditions, with controls included as above. Gel electrophoresis was done in 1% agarose alongside a 1 kb standard DNA size marker (Bioline, London, UK).

3.4. Identification of Trypanosoma brucei Bub-Species by PCR

The DNA samples that were positive for *Trypanosoma brucei* species by single step or nested ITS-PCR were also subjected to a nested PCR using sub-species-specific primers that target the Serum Resistance Associated (SRA) gene [20] that is specific to *T. b. rhodesiense* (*T.b.r*). In the first run, amplification of three microlitres of template DNA was performed in a 25 µL reaction volume with the primer pair, SRA outer-s 5' CCT GAT AAA ACA AGT ATC GGC AGC AA 3' and SRA outer-as 5' CGG TGA CCA ATT CAT CTG CTG CTG TT 3' each at 0.5 µM concentration. The thermocycling conditions were as follows; 98 °C for 1 min (initial denaturation) followed by 25 cycles of 98 °C, 5 s (denaturation), 64 °C, 30 s (annealing), 72 °C, 2 min (extension) and a final extension of 72 °C for 1 min. In the second run, three microlitres of product from first run was amplified under similar conditions as in the first run but using primer pair, SRA inner-s 5' ATA GTG ACA TGC GTA CTC AAC GC 3' and SRA inner-as 5' AAT GTG TTC GAG TAC TTC GGT CAC GCT 3' also at 0.5 µM. A negative control, double distilled water (with no template DNA added) and a positive control, *T.b.r* 729 strain (Molecular biology laboratory, MUK-COVAB) were included in the PCR amplification. Electrophoresis was done in 2% agarose gels.

3.5. PCR Amplification for Anaplasma Species

In the first screen of stained blood smears, *Anaplama* sp., *Babesia* sp., and *Theileria* sp. were detected in some of the slides. This informed us of the choice tick-borne parasites to screen for in the entire set of low PCV samples using previously published specific PCRs.

PCR amplification for *Anaplasma* species was with specific primers targeting the 16S rRNA [21]. The thermo cycling profile was 95 °C for 5 min (initial denaturation) followed by 45 cycles of 95 °C, 30 s (denaturation), 51 °C, 30 s (annealing), 72 °C, 45 s (extension) and a final extension of 72 °C for 10 min. A positive control, (bovine field isolate confirmed with *Anaplasma* species) and a negative control (double distilled water with no template DNA added) were included in the PCR amplification; electrophoresis was in a 1.5% agarose gel alongside a 100 bp standard DNA marker (Bioline, London, UK).

3.6. PCR Amplification for Babesia Species

For *Babesia* species, PCR using a primer pair that target 18S rRNA gene [22] was performed in 25 µL PCR mixture containing 5 µL of DNA template, and the primer pair Bab-1s 5' CAA GAC AAA AGT CTG CTT GAA AC 3' and Bab-s 5' GTT TCT GAC CCA TCA GCT TGA C 3'. Amplification was under the following conditions; 95 °C for 5 min followed by 45 cycles of 94 °C, 30 s (denaturation), 63 °C, 30 s (annealing), 72 °C, 45 s (extension) and a final extension of 72 °C for 10 min. A positive control, (bovine field isolate confirmed with *Babesia* species) and a negative control (double distilled water with no template DNA added) were included in the PCR amplification. Electrophoresis was in a 1.5% agarose gel alongside a 100 bp standard DNA marker (Bioline, London, UK).

3.7. PCR Amplification for Theileria Species

Amplification was carried out by PCR targeting the small subunit (SSU) rRNA which is common to *Theileria* species [23]. All PCR reactions were performed in a volume of 25 µL with the primer pair, F (989) 5' AGT TTC TGA CCT ATC AG 3' and R (990) 5' TTG CCT TAA ACT TCC TTG 3' each at 3.2 µM. Five microlitres of genomic DNA was added to each PCR reaction as the template. The PCR conditions were 95 °C for 5 min (initial denaturation) followed by 35 cycles of 94 °C, 1 min (denaturation), 60 °C, 1 min (annealing), 72 °C, 1 min (extension) and a final extension of 72 °C for 10 min. A negative control (double distilled water with no template DNA added) and a positive control (bovine field isolate confirmed with *Theileria* species) were included in the PCR amplification. Ten microlitres of each amplicon was subjected to electrophoresis in a 1.5% agarose gel alongside a 100 bp standard DNA marker (Bioline, London, UK).

4. Results

In all, 2621 cattle were screened using the HCT, of which 561 were positive for trypanosomes, translating into a parasitological prevalence of 21.4%. We took representative smears from HCT negative, low PCV (≤25%) cattle for iLED microscopy to look for trypanosomes and other haemoparasites. This was in order to determine which hemoparasites to search for by PCR executed on the entire collection, in addition to *Trypanosoma* species. None of these smears had detectable trypanosomes but we identified *Babesia* sp., *Anaplasma* sp. and *Theileria* sp. DNA was therefore prepared from the 1285 low PCV samples to perform species specific PCRs for *Trypanosoma* sp., *Babesia* sp., *Anaplasma* sp. and *Theileria* sp., (Supplementary material, Figures S1–S5) to show to what extent each might have contributed to the low PCVs.

Of the 561 HCT positive cattle as well as 724 cattle with no detectable trypanosomes but with low PCV, trypanosomal ITS-PCR was positive in 473 and 94 samples respectively, consequently missing 15.7% of the samples in which trypanosomes had been detected by microscopy. The ITS-PCR results are summarized in Table 1. *T. brucei* was the most abundant species, present in 254 of the 567 (44.8%) positive samples, followed by *T. congolense* (38.1%), the benign trypanosome *T. theileri* (22.6%) and *T. vivax* (20.3%). In this analysis, 14 out of 254 *T. brucei* positive cattle (5.5%) were SRA positive, indicating that they were the human infective *T. b. rhodesiense*.

Table 1. ITS1-PCR results and the identified trypanosome species. Samples classified as trypanosmoe positive or negative by the HCT were tested by PCR to detect and identify the respective trypanosome species.

Infection Status	Total	ITS +ve	T. brucei	SRA +ve	T. congolense	T. vivax	T. theileri
Trypanosome positive	561	473	204	14	178	92	128
Trypanosome negative	724	94	50	0	38	23	0
Grand Total	1285	567	254	14	216	115	128

Considering the low PCV animals (1285, of which 561 were HCT positive and 724 negative; Table 1), and combining positive results from both HCT and ITS-PCR (composite reference; total 655 cases), 51% of these cattle had trypanosomiasis, and as such, the anaemia in 49% of them could have been associated with other causes.

Of the 567 ITS-PCR positive samples 146 (25.7%) were infected with more than one *Trypanosoma* species, the majority with two species, mainly *T. brucei* and *T. congolense* as shown in Table 2.

Table 2. Trypanosome species identified in cattle samples. Mixed infections were a common feature.

Infection Status	ITS +ve	T. b./T. c.	T. c./T. v.	T. t./T. v.	T. b./T. v.	T. b./T. c./T. v.
Trypanosome positive	473	107	11	8	5	1
Trypanosome negative	94	6	1	0	4	3
Total	567	113	12	8	9	4

(T. b. = T. brucei; T. c. = T. congolense, T. v. = T. vivax; T. t. = T. theileri).

Considering trypanosomiasis in relation to the tick-borne haemoparasites whose PCRs were done in this analysis (Table 3), it was revealed that 492 of the 1285 low PCV cattle (38.3%) had both trypanosomes and any of the tick-borne haemoparasites. Infection with *Anaplasma* was highest (45.2%) among the cattle with low PCV, followed by *Theileria* (42.4%), and least was *Babesia* infection that accounted for 26.3%. Co-infection of trypanosomes with *Babesia* occurred in 19.5% of animals with low PCV.

Table 3. Results for trypanosomiasis and tick-borne-diseases (TBD) in cattle with PCV.

Infection Status	PCR						
	Total	Theil	Bab	Ana	Tryp + Any TBD	Tryp + Bab	None
Trypanosome positive	561	406	234	401	447	234	NA
Trypanosome negative	724	139	104	180	45	16	373
Total	1285	545	338	581	492	250	373

Theil = *Theieria*; Bab = *Babesia*; Ana = *Anaplasma*; Tryp = trypanosomes.

Finally, from Table 3, it is noteworthy that among tested cattle with low PCV (n = 1285), no trypanosomes or any of the 3 tick-borne infections were detected in 373 cattle blood samples (29%).

5. Discussion

Despite its continued decline in incidence over the past decade, rHAT remains an important disease, with potential to re-emerge if relevant control measures are not sustained. rHAT is a zoonotic disease involving mainly cattle and wild animals in the transmission cycle; therefore, its control requires a multi-sectoral approach. This study aimed to identify the major haemoparasites affecting cattle in Kaberamaido district as a basis to devise appropriate strategies to accelerate and sustain elimination of rHAT. Kaberamaido is one of the districts in the cattle corridor in eastern Uganda where the latest rHAT outbreak in Uganda occurred since 2005 [24]. Since then, over 500 cases were treated at Lwala hospital alone, which serves the Kaberamaido-Lango focus. The outbreak was attributed to influx of cattle infected with *T. b. rhodesiense* from active rHAT foci in the south [13,25]. Interventions, including tsetse control and mass treatment of cattle, led to a decline in incidence recorded since the late 2000s [26].

Haemoparasitic infections have globally been documented to cause immense production losses in the livestock sector [27,28]. In Uganda, Rubaire-Akiiki et al. [29] reported the sero-prevalence of *Theileria parva* among communally grazed cattle in low lands to be as high as 70% while those of *Babesia* and *Anaplasma* were 65% and 15%, respectively. Later, in 2011, Angwech et al. [30] assessed the prevalence of tick-borne parasites in relation to different livestock production systems in Gulu district in northern Uganda and found that the prevalence of *Theileria* was highest in cattle (28.1%), that of *Anaplasma* was highest in goats (19.0%), while the prevalence of *Babesia* was highest in sheep (3.64%) under the open grazing system [30]. In yet another study conducted in central and western Uganda, the prevalence of haemoparasites was reportedly 47.4%, 6.7%, 1.9% and 14.4% for *Theileria parva*, *Babesia* spp., *Trypanosoma brucei*, *Anaplasma* spp respectively. Generally, previous studies ahave shown that livestock that are grazed openly have high prevalence rates of haemoparasites [29–32].

Thus, even in this study, which was addressing the animal reservoir of rHAT, it was important to identify other hemopasitic challenges in the district, in order to consider appropriate interventions.

In this study, a considerable proportion of trypanosome-positive samples (15.7%) were not detected by PCR. This could partly have been due to the loss of DNA quality during field collection or processing of the blood samples, a usual challenge of molecular investigations. It is also plausible that the undetected samples could have been with triple and quadruple trypanosome species infections, in which case the ITS PCR has a markedly low sensitivity, as was previously reported by Njiru et al. [33]. The scenario of double infection is common in animals, as is shown in this study as well as by Mugittu et al. [34]; however, triple and quadruple trypanosome infections, although rare, occur in animals as well as the tsetse fly vector [33,35]. Another possible explanation is that the undetected samples could have been infected with *T. vivax* strain variants that have changes in regions where the primers anneal; as was observed by Njiru et al., [18]. In that study, field samples from Kenya were analyzed using ITS-1 and gave differing sizes (250, 249, 248 base pairs) of the ITS region. Similarly, Malele et al. [36], while analyzing tsetse flies in Tanzania, reported such variation in *T. vivax* strains. Indeed, earlier in 2001, it was reported that the evolution rate of the 18S rRNA gene of *T. vivax* was significantly faster than that of other trypanosomes and specifically evolved 7 to 10 times that of non-salivarian trypanosomes [37]. Because of these changes, the primer annealing capacity may be compromised, thus the false negative results in the current study.

The current study demonstrated that only 4.5% (58) of the 1285 cattle with low PCV were infected with trypanosomes alone, 38.2% (492) had both trypanosomes and tick-borne parasites, while 29% (375 cattle) were infected with the latter in the absence of trypanosomes. Thus, based on these results, any intervention targeting trypanosomes alone would benefit less than half of the anaemic animals. This could conceal the benefits of block trypanocidal treatment campaigns from the point of view of general improvement in herd health. The implication of this is that livestock farmers might need to see a considerable improvement of herd health in order to appreciate and fully participate in control operations.

Another observation in the current study that might be of importance to policy is that 250 of the 655 composite reference positive animals (38.2%) had both trypanosomiasis and babesiosis. Thus, it might be a tough decision to make in such a scenario, whether to use isometamidum that clears the trypanosomes and offer protection for 3 months or to use diminazene aceturate that clears both parasites (trypanosomes and *Babesia*) and could lead to better (short-term) improvement in general herd health but offers no prophylaxis against trypanosomiasis [38]. The latter may call for more frequent interventions, translating into more cost and time inputs. These arguments all point to the need to fully analyse the situation and formulate relevant interventions that are likely to be readily acceptable to the animal owners, while maintaining the rational use of the trypanocides to delay the emergence of drug resistance.

The role of social science will be very crucial in this era of near-to-complete elimination or HAT, as we need innovative ways to sustain the gains accrued from the recent outbreak "fire-fighting" situations. It is clear that we need to go to the field with a more open mind and approach since there are many other challenges than trypanosomiasis alone, even though we primarily move in with rHAT control objectives. For example, the chemicals to consider for animal bait tsetse control should be those that equally affect ticks so that the pastoralists get maximum benefit from the intervention. Similarly, restricted application of insecticide to cattle [39], though indisputable with regard to effective tsetse control, should be carefully designed in order not to leave some equally important tick-borne diseases co-existing in the control areas unattended to.

Of the cattle that were positive for the trypanosomal ITS-PCR, 44.8% were infected with *T. brucei* while 5.5% of these had the human infective *T. b. rhodesiense* circulating in the animal reservoir. The significance here is that since *T. brucei* is not the most pathogenic species to cattle in absence of harsh environmental conditions such as droughts, the clinical presentation might not be so striking, to the extent that the farmers may fail to seek veterinary attention for apparently healthy looking animals.

Therefore, these clinically healthy animals may continue to harbor human infective trypanosomes for long without raising suspicion. This scenario poses eminent challenges in the control of sleeping sickness in livestock farming communities, such as in this study area, and may require regular testing and treatment of the cattle reservoirs irrespective of their clinical status. To our observation, *T. brucei* tends to dominate cattle infections in active rHAT foci.

In addition to the known pathogenic trypanosomes detected in the study area, we also demonstrated the presence of the benign *T. theileri*. This implies that the nuisance biting flies are active in the area, adding to the livestock productivity constraints faced by the livestock farmers.

As outlined above, samples from cattle with low PCV were analyzed using PCR to detect DNA of trypanosomes and any of three tick-borne parasites (*Babesia*, *Theileria* and *Anaplasma*); however, 29% of these animals were negative for any of these infections. Thus, we could not attribute the low PCV values to trypanosomiasis or any of the three TBDs tested for. We suggest that other contributors to the low PCV could include helminth infections that are common in the field where no control measures are practiced, as is the case among many subsistence livestock farmers. It is thus equally important to control helminths for maximum livestock production. In other words, there might be need for a complete package to deliver to the communities in order to sustainably control rHAT; again, the important role of social scientists or social economists cannot be ignored.

6. Conclusions

This study revealed various haemoparasites infecting cattle in Kaberamaido, including *Theileria*, *Babesia*, *Anaplasma* and *Trypanosoma*, and suggests that trypanosomiasis (though high on the list) might not necessarily be the number one problem faced by the livestock farmers. Noteworthily, without a vigorous community engagement and education campaign, the farmers might fail to fully appreciate the contribution of domestic animals to rHAT transmission. Any rHAT elimination effort should therefore come as a package that not only secures human health but leaves behind a population with better livelihoods and economic empowerment arising from improved animal productivity. Multi-sectoral, multi- and trans-disciplinary teams shall definitely be required to address and sustain rHAT elimination. We perhaps presently need social scientists more than ever before, in the face of diminishing rHAT incidence, bearing in mind that a resurgence can happen if no properly thought out measures against this zoonosis are implemented. The notable presence of *T. b. rhodesiense* in cattle in this area reminds us that the domestic animal reservoir is still around and should be sustainably addressed.

Supplementary Materials: The following are available online at http://www.mdpi.com/2414-6366/5/1/24/s1, Figure S1: Electrophoretic analysis of Trypanosoma ITS PCR products, Figure S2: Electrophoretic analysis of SRA PCR products, Figure S3: Electrophoretic analysis of Theileria PCR products, Figure S4: Electrophoretic analysis of Babesia PCR products, Figure S5: Electrophoretic analysis of Anaplasma PCR products.

Author Contributions: Conceptualization, E.M. and J.M.N.; Formal analysis, C.M.M., P.W., A.K., A.B. and J.M.N.; Funding acquisition, E.M.; Investigation, C.M.M., A.K. and A.B.; Methodology, C.M.M., P.W., A.K. and A.B.; Project administration, E.M.; Supervision, E.M.; Writing—original draft, P.W. and A.B.; Writing—review & editing, E.M., C.M.M., A.K.; and J.M.N.; E.M., C.M.M., J.M.N. designed the study, undertook data analysis and wrote the manuscript; P.W., C.M.M., A.K., A.B. conducted field work, undertook lab experiments and contributed to data analysis and manuscript writing. All authors have read and agreed to the published version of the manuscript.

Funding: This study was funded UBS Optimus under the grant number 3223.

Acknowledgments: We acknowledge the District Veterinary Officer of Kaberamaido District, local council leaders in the study area as well as the livestock farmers who participated in the study. We acknowledge UBS Optimus for funding the research work.

Conflicts of Interest: The authors declare that they have no financial or personal relationship(s) that may have inappropriately influenced them in writing this article.

Ethical Approval: The study received approval from the School of Biosecurity, Biotechnical and laboratory, Sciences IRB: under the protocol number SBLS/REC/14/011.

Trop. Med. Infect. Dis. **2020**, *5*, 24

References

1. Swallow, B.M. *Impacts of Trypanosomiasis on African Agriculture*; PAAT Technical and Scientific Series 2; Food and Agriculture Organization of the United Nations: Rome, Italy, 2000.
2. Budd, L.T. *DFID-Funded Tsetse and Trypanosomiasis Research and Development since 1980 (V. 2. Economic Analysis)*; Department for International Development: London, UK, 1999.
3. Simarro, P.P.; Cecchi, G.; Franco, J.R.; Paone, M.; Diarra, A.; Antonio Ruiz-Postigo, J.; Fèvre, E.M.; Mattioli, R.C.; Jannin, J.G. Estimating and mapping the population at risk of sleeping sickness. *PLoS Negl. Trop. Dis.* **2012**, *6*, e1859. [CrossRef]
4. Aksoy, S. Sleeping sickness elimination in sight: Time to celebrate and reflect, but not relax. *PLoS Negl. Trop. Dis.* **2011**, *5*, e1008. [CrossRef]
5. Franco, J.R.; Simarro, P.P.; Diarra, A.; Ruiz-Postigo, J.A.; Jannin, J.G. The journey towards elimination of gambiense human African trypanosomiasis: Not far, nor easy. *Parasitology* **2014**, *141*, 748–760. [CrossRef]
6. Kinghorn, A. Human Trypanosomiasis in the Luangwa Valley, Northern Rhodesia. *Ann. Trop. Med. Parasitol.* **1925**, *19*, 283–289. [CrossRef]
7. Heisch, R.B.; McMahon, J.P.; Manson-Bahr, P.E.C. The isolation of *Trypansoma rhodesiense* from a bushbuck. *Br. Med. J.* **1958**, *32*, 1203–1204. [CrossRef] [PubMed]
8. Okuna, N.M.; Mayende, J.S.; Guloba, A. *Trypanosoma brucei* infection in domestic pigs in a sleeping sickness epidemic area of Uganda. *Acta Trop.* **1986**, *43*, 183–184. [PubMed]
9. Enyaru, J.C.K.; Odiit, M.; Gashumba, J.K.; Carasco, J.F.; Rwendeire, A.J.J. Characterization by isoenzyme electrophoresis of Trypanozoon stocks from sleeping sickness endemic areas of south-east Uganda. *Bull. World Health Organ.* **1992**, *70*, 631–636. [PubMed]
10. Hide, C.; Welburn, S.C.; Tait, A.; Mudlin, I. Epidemiological relationships of Trypanosoma brucei stocks from south East Uganda: Evidence for different population structures in human infective and non-human infective isolates. *Parasitology* **1994**, *109*, 95–111. [CrossRef] [PubMed]
11. Waiswa, C.; Olaho-Mukani, W.; Katunguka-Rwakishaya, E. Domestic animals as reservoirs for sleeping sickness in three endemic foci in south-eastern Uganda. *Ann. Trop. Med. Parasitol.* **2003**, *97*, 149–155. [CrossRef]
12. Simarro, P.P.; Cecchi, G.; Paone, M.; Franco, J.R.; Diarra, A.; Ruiz, J.A.; Fèvre, E.M.; Courtin, F.; Mattioli, R.C.; Jannin, J.G. The Atlas of human African trypanosomiasis: A contribution to global mapping of neglected tropical diseases. *Int. J. Health Geogr.* **2010**, *9*, 57. [CrossRef]
13. Fèvre, E.M.; Coleman, P.G.; Odiit, M.; Magona, J.W.; Welburn, S.C.; Woolhouse, M.E.J. The origins of a new *Trypanosoma brucei rhodesiense* sleeping sickness outbreak in eastern Uganda. *Lancet* **2001**, *358*, 625–628. [CrossRef]
14. Selby, R.; Bardosh, K.; Picozzi, K.; Waiswa, C.; Welburn, S.S. Cattle movements and trypanosomes: Restocking efforts and the spread of *Trypanosoma brucei rhodesiense* sleeping sickness in post-conflict Uganda. *Parasites Vectors* **2013**, *6*, 281. [CrossRef] [PubMed]
15. Woo, P.T.K. The haematocrit centrifugation technique for the diagnosis of African Trypanosomiasis. *Acta Trop.* **1970**, *27*, 384–386. [PubMed]
16. Brown, B. *Hematology-Principles and Procedures*, 5th ed.; Lea & Febiger: Philadelphia, PA, USA, 1988; p. 83.
17. Biéler, S.; Matovu, E.; Mitashi, P.; Ssewannyana, E.; Bin Shamamba, S.K.; Bessell, P.R.; Ndung'u, J.M. Improved detection of *Trypanosoma brucei* by lysis of red blood cells, concentration and LED fluorescence microscopy. *Acta Trop.* **2012**, *121*, 135–140. [CrossRef] [PubMed]
18. Njiru, Z.K.; Constantine, C.C.; Guya, S.; Crowther, J.; Kiragu, J.M.; Thompson, R.C.; Davila, A.M. The use of ITS1 rDNA PCR in detecting pathogenic African trypanosomes. *Parasit. Res.* **2005**, *95*, 186–192. [CrossRef] [PubMed]
19. Cox, A.; Tilley, A.; McOdimba, F.; Fyfe, J.; Eisler, M.; Hide, G.; Welburn, S. A PCR based assay for detection and differentiation of African Trypanosome species in blood. *Exp. Parasitol.* **2005**, *111*, 24–29. [CrossRef] [PubMed]
20. Maina, N.W.N.; Oberle, M.; Otieno, C.; Kunz, C.; Maser, P.; Ndungu, J.M.; Brun, R. Isolation and propagation of *Trypanosome brucei gambiense* from sleeping sickness patients in south Sudan. *Trans. R. Soc. Trop. Med. Hyg.* **2007**, *101*, 540–546. [CrossRef]

21. Goodman, J.L.; Nelson, C.; Vitale, B.; Madigan, J.E.; Dumler, J.S.; Kurtti, T.J.; Munderloh, U.G. Direct cultivation of the causative agent of human granulocytic ehrlichiosis. *J. Med. Res.* **1996**, *334*, 209–215. [CrossRef]

22. Hilpertshauser, H.; Deplazes, P.; Schnyder, M.; Gern, L.; Mathis, A. Babesia spp. identified by PCR in ticks collected from domestic and wild ruminants in southern Switzerland. *Appl. Environ. Microbiol.* **2006**, *72*, 6503–6507. [CrossRef]

23. D'Oliveira, C.; Van der Weide, M.; Habela, M.A.; Jacquiet, P.; Jongejan, F. Detection of *Theileria annulata* in blood samples of carrier cattle by PCR. *J. Clin. Microbiol.* **1995**, *33*, 2665–2669. [CrossRef]

24. Berrang-Ford, L.; Odiit, M.; Maiso, F.; Waltner-Toews, D.; McDermott, J. Sleeping sickness in Uganda: Revisiting current and historical distributions. *Afr. Health Sci.* **2006**, *6*, 223–231. [PubMed]

25. Hutchinson, O.C.; Fèvre, E.M.; Carrington, M.; Welburn, S.C. Lessons learned from the emergence of a new *Trypanosoma brucei rhodesiense* sleeping sickness focus in Uganda. *Lancet Infect. Dis.* **2003**, *3*, 42–45. [CrossRef]

26. Selby, R. Limiting the Northerly Advance of *Trypanosoma brucei* rhodesiense in Post Conflict Uganda. Ph.D. Thesis, University of Edinburgh, Edinburgh, UK, 2011.

27. Uilenberg, G. International collaborative research: Significance of tick-borne hemoparasitic diseases to world animal health. *Vet. Parasitol.* **1995**, *57*, 19–41. [CrossRef]

28. Jongejan, F.; Uilenberg, G. The global importance of ticks. *Parasitology* **2004**, *129*, S3–S14. [CrossRef]

29. Rubaire-Akiiki, C.; Okello-Onen, J.; Nasinyama, G.W.; Vaarst, M.; Kabagambe, E.K.; Mwayi, W.; Musunga, D.; Wandukwa, W. The prevalence of serum antibodies to tick-borne infections in Mbale District, Uganda: The effect of agro-ecological zone, grazing management and age of cattle. *J. Insect Sci.* **2004**, *4*, 8. [CrossRef]

30. Angwech, H.; Kaddu, J.B.; Nyeko, J.H.P. Tick-Borne Parasites of Domestic Ruminants in Gulu District, Uganda: Prevalence Varied with the Intensity of Management. *Vet. Res.* **2011**, *4*, 28–33.

31. Muhanguzi, D.; Picozzi, K.; Hatendorf, J.; Thrusfield, M.; Welburn, S.C.; Kabasa, J.D.; Waiswa, C. Prevalence and Spatial Distribution of *Theileria parva* in Cattle under Crop-Livestock Farming systems in Tororo District, Eastern Uganda. *Parasites Vectors* **2014**, *7*, 91. [CrossRef]

32. Kasozi, K.I.; Matovu, E.; Tayebwa, D.S.; Natuhwera, J.; Mugezi, I.; Mahero, M. Epidemiology of increasing hemo-parasite burden in Ugandan cattle. *Open J. Vet. Med.* **2014**, *4*, 220–231. [CrossRef]

33. Njiru, Z.K.; Makumi, J.N.; Okoth, S.; Ndungu, J.M.; Gibson, W.C. Identification of trypanosomes in *Glossina pallidipes* and *G. longipennis* in Kenya. *Infect. Genet. Evol.* **2004**, *4*, 29–35. [CrossRef]

34. Mugittu, K.N.; Silayo, R.S.; Majiwa, P.A.O.; Kimbita, E.K.; Mutayoba, B.M.; Maselle, R. Application of PCR and DNA probes in the characterization of trypanosomes in the blood of cattle in farms in Morogoro Tanzania. *Vet. Parasitol.* **2000**, *94*, 177–189. [CrossRef]

35. Mwandiringana, E.; Gori, E.; Nyengerai, T.; Chidzwondo, F. Polymerase chain reaction (PCR) detection of mixed trypanosome infection and blood meal origin in field-captured tsetse flies from Zambia. *Afr. J. Biotechnol.* **2012**, *11*, 14490–14497.

36. Malele, I.; Craske, L.; Knight, C.; Ferris, V.; Njiru, Z.; Hamilton, P.; Lehane, S.; Lehane, M.; Gibson, W.C. The use of specific and generic primers to identify trypanosome infections of wild tsetse flies in Tanzania by PCR. *Infect. Genet. Evol.* **2003**, *3*, 271–279. [CrossRef]

37. Stevens, J.; Rambaut, A. Evolutionary rate differences in trypanosomes. *Infect. Genet. Evol.* **2001**, *1*, 143–150. [CrossRef]

38. Magona, J.W.; Mayende, J.S.P.; Okiria, R.; Okuna, N.M. Protective efficacy of isometamidium chloride and diminazene aceturate against natural Trypanosoma *brucei*, *Trypanosoma congolense* and *Trypanosoma vivax* infections in cattle under a suppressed tsetse population in Uganda. *Onderstepoort J. Vet. Res.* **2004**, *71*, 231–237. [CrossRef] [PubMed]

39. Muhanguzi, D.; Picozzi, K.; Hatendorf, J.; Thrusfield, M.; Welburn, S.C.; Kabasa, J.D.; Waiswa, C. Improvements on restricted insecticide application protocol for control of Human and Animal African Trypanosomiasis in eastern Uganda. *PLoS Negl. Trop. Dis.* **2014**, *8*, e3284. [CrossRef] [PubMed]

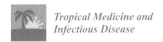

Case Report

The Flipside of Eradicating a Disease; Human African Trypanosomiasis in a Woman in Rural Democratic Republic of Congo: A Case Report

Junior Mudji [1,2], Jonathan Benhamou [3,4], Erick Mwamba-Miaka [5], Christian Burri [3,4] and Johannes Blum [1,3,4,*]

[1] Hôpital Evangélique de Vanga, Vanga Mission, B.P. 4728 Kinshasa 2, Congo; mudjijunior@gmail.com
[2] Unit of Clinical Pharmacology and Pharmacovigilance, Protestant University of Congo, B.P. 4745 Kinshasa 2, Congo
[3] Swiss Tropical and Public Health Institute, 4002 Basel, Switzerland; jonathan.benhamou@hotmail.com (J.B.); christian.burri@swisstph.ch (C.B.)
[4] University of Basel, 4001 Basel, Switzerland
[5] Programme National de Lutte contre la Trypanosomiase Humaine Africaine (PNLTHA), Kinshasa 2, Congo; erickmwamb2002@yahoo.fr
* Correspondence: johannes.blum@swisstph.ch

Received: 18 November 2019; Accepted: 7 December 2019; Published: 11 December 2019

Abstract: Human African Trypanosomiasis (HAT) is a neglected disease caused by the protozoan parasites Trypanosoma brucei and transmitted by tsetse flies that progresses in two phases. Symptoms in the first phase include fever, headaches, pruritus, lymphadenopathy, and in certain cases, hepato- and splenomegaly. Neurological disorders such as sleep disorder, aggressive behavior, logorrhea, psychotic reactions, and mood changes are signs of the second stage of the disease. Diagnosis follows complex algorithms, including serological testing and microscopy. Our case report illustrates the course of events of a 41-year old woman with sleep disorder, among other neurological symptoms, whose diagnosis was made seven months after the onset of symptoms. The patient had consulted two different hospitals in Kinshasa and was on the verge of being discharged from a third due to negative laboratory test results. This case report highlights the challenges that may arise when a disease is on the verge of eradication.

Keywords: Human African Trypanosomiasis (HAT); mydriasis; neurological signs; eradication; re-emergence

1. Background

Human African Trypanosomiasis (HAT) is a neglected disease that progresses in two phases. Symptoms in the first phase include fever, headaches, pruritus, lymphadenopathy, and, in certain cases, hepato- and spleno- megaly. Neurological disorders such as sleep disorder, aggressive behavior, logorrhea, psychotic reactions, and mood changes are signs of the second stage of the disease [1,2]. Laboratory tests are needed for a definitive confirmation of the diagnosis. Our case report illustrates the case of a 41-year old woman with sleep disorder, among other neurological symptoms, whose diagnosis was made seven months after onset of symptoms. The patient had consulted two different hospitals in Kinshasa and was on the verge of being discharged from the third due to negative laboratory test results and an alarming lack of knowledge concerning this very treatable disease. This case report attempts to highlight the problems that may arise when a disease is on the verge of eradication.

2. Clinical presentation

A 41-year old woman working as a teacher presented to the emergency department of Vanga Hospital with sleep and behavioral disorders, along with tremors in both upper limbs. Her next of kin reported that she had been sick for seven months. Symptoms started with headaches, and one month later, sleep disorder, aggressive behavior, and mood changes appeared. In addition, her husband reported unquantified weight loss, sporadic fever episodes, logorrhea, and urinary incontinence in the past two months. The patient had no known medical history of mental illness. She is married and lives with her husband and two children. Tobacco, alcohol, or illicit drug use were denied. Until 2007, the patient had lived in a village in western Democratic Republic of Congo (DRC), where HAT is endemic. Since then, the family has moved to a part of Kinshasa, which, incidentally, is also endemic for HAT. Before consulting Vanga Hospital, the patient had been to two different hospitals in Kinshasa, both of which had treated her for malaria without any improvement in symptoms.

Upon arrival, her vital parameters were as follows: pulse rate was 76 beats per minute (bpm), blood pressure was 80/60 mmHg, respiratory rate was 16 breaths per minute, and corporeal temperature was 36.7 °C. The patient's consciousness level teetered between fast asleep and wide awake. When awake, she was fully oriented and had no loss of memory. The results of the physical examination were as follows: respiratory excursions were full and symmetrical, lungs resonant to percussion, and a normal, vesicular breath sound in all fields; no rales, rhonchi, wheezes, or rubs were present. A cardiovascular examination showed a regular rate and rhythm with no extra sounds or murmurs; jugular venous pressure was normal. Concerning the abdomen, bowel sounds were normal. Superficial and deep palpation did not reveal any organomegaly or masses, and no evidence of direct or rebound tenderness was found. Neurological examination showed clear and fluent speech. No nuchal rigidity was found, and Kernig's and Brudzinski's signs were negative. Cranial nerve examination showed no abnormalities aside from an areflexic bilateral mydriasis (see Figure 1). While cranial nerve palsies and ocular nerve symptoms have been described in the past [3], an isolated areflective bilateral mydriasis has, to our knowledge, never been reported in HAT patients. Fundoscopy was normal without signs of elevated intracranial pressure or inflammation. Slight symmetrical muscle weakness (4/5) was seen in both the upper and lower limbs with flexors, extensors, abductors, and adductors all being affected; muscle tone, however, was normal. Sensory function was intact in the fingers and toes. Her reflexes were 1+ and symmetric at the biceps, triceps, and ankles, and 3+ and symmetric at the patella; Babinski's sign was negative. The patient showed a slow and uneven gait, without any signs of asymmetry, dragging of toes on the ground, or loss of balance. Trendelenburg sign was negative. An examination of her coordination showed normal diadochokinesia, a negative Romberg's sign, and a slightly slow and uncoordinated Finger-to-Nose-Test without any signs of tremor.

The first laboratory tests showed negative thick drop and blood smear for malaria and trypanosomiasis, a thrice negative Card Agglutination Test for Trypanosomiasis (CATT), and a positive Rapid Plasma Reagin (RPR) for syphilis. The attending physician confirmed the diagnosis of neurosyphilis and a treatment with ceftriaxone was planned. The differential diagnosis of syphilis and HAT is challenging, because both diseases have a broad clinical spectrum of neurological and psychiatric findings, and false positive results of RPR have been reported. Being that the patient had spent several days in hospital without receiving proper treatment, the family wanted to remove her from the hospital's care. Had the staff doctor not intervened at that moment, asking for a lumbar puncture, the patient would have been sent home without a certain diagnosis, and therefore, without receiving adequate treatment. Examination of the spinal fluid showed 105 white blood cells per mm^3 and the presence of live trypanosomes, confirming the diagnosis of stage-2 HAT.

Treatment with albendazol and nifurtimox-eflornithine combination therapy (NECT) was immediately started. Following a full 10-day cycle of treatment, the patient was re-evaluated. She reported a drastic improvement in her general state of health. The behavioral disorders, somnolence, and tremor in both upper limbs had disappeared. Upon physical examination, the patient showed clear signs of improvement. The areflexic bilateral mydriasis had disappeared under treatment (see Figure 2), as did the muscle weakness in all four limbs. Her reflexes were 2+ and symmetric at the biceps, triceps, and ankles, and remained at 3+ at the patella. Gait and coordination exams, including a Finger-to-Nose-Test, showed no signs of impairment.

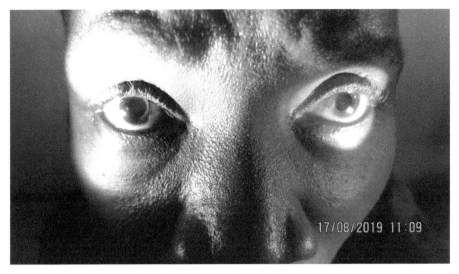

Figure 1. Areflective bilateral mydriasis in HAT patient.

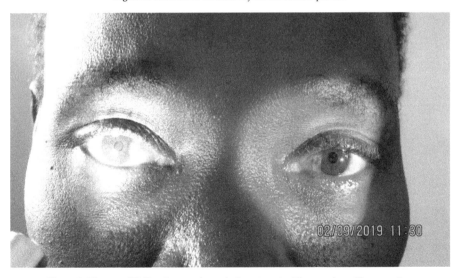

Figure 2. The same HAT patients at the end of treatment with normal pupillary reaction.

3. Discussion

What is alarming about this case, is the number of misdiagnoses within the three hospital stays the patient had. Thanks to numerous efforts during colonial times, HAT was nearly eradicated in the DRC (see Figure 3). Following the DRC's independence, political unrest and the interruption of the Belgian-Zairois cooperation led to a drastic increase in new cases. Thanks to national and international efforts following the re-emergence of HAT as a major health concern in the DRC, the prevalence of new cases decreased from 26,318 in 1998 to 660 in 2018. This success brings with it one main downside, namely, that with decreasing prevalence of HAT, younger doctors and nurses do not see many cases, and therefore, lack appropriate awareness and knowledge about the disease. The thrice false negative CATT is worrying. There are two possible explanations: First, CATT is only available in kits with 50 aliquots of reagents, which remain stable for 3–5 days, and it is possible that an expired reagent was used. Second, with the decreasing number of patients, laboratory personnel do not frequently see HAT cases, and are therefore, more error prone. In the three months following the diagnosis and treatment of the aforementioned patient, four more cases were diagnosed in Vanga Hospital, all in the second stage of the illness. All four patients consulted numerous hospitals before coming to Vanga. More worryingly, one of the four patients was kept in a psychiatric clinic and put on an antipsychotic treatment for two months.

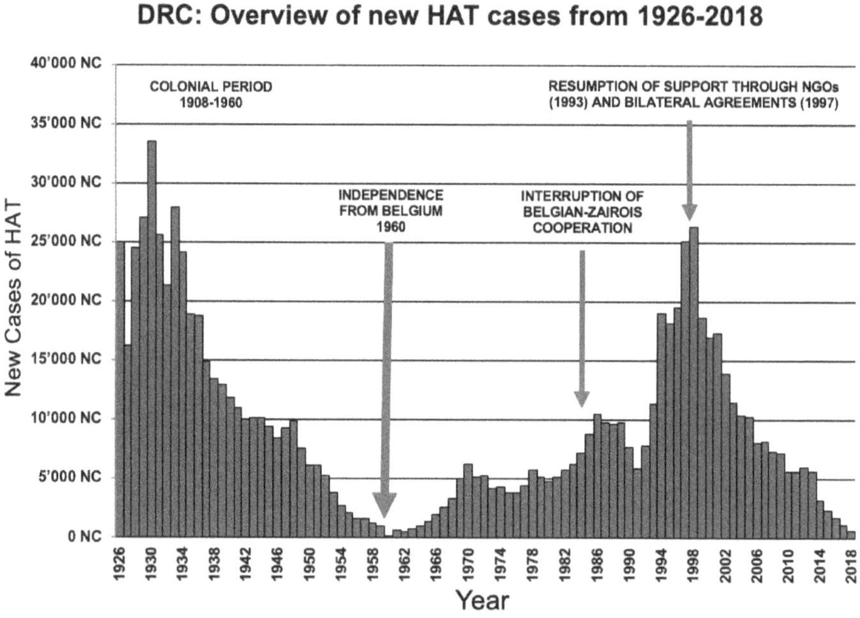

Figure 3. Overview of new HAT cases in the DRC from 1926-2018. Figure from the Programme National de Lutte contre la Trypanosomiase Humaine Africaine (PNLTHA), Kinshasa, DR of Congo, 2018.

4. Conclusions

HAT was almost eradicated in the DRC in the 1960s, but a civil war and a lack of attention to and funding for the disease led to a resurgence. To prevent this from happening again, young hospital personnel, especially in a country like the DRC, where HAT is endemic, require proper education, repetition training, and adequate funding. Continued public information is paramount to maintaining awareness of this disease. In this respect, the National Day of Commemoration of Human African Trypanosomiasis in the DRC on 30 January 2020, with the participation of the Head of State and the Minister of Health, is an important and commendable example.

We received written informed consent from the patient to use the pictures above as well as write about and publish her case.

Author Contributions: Attending physician: J.M., Writing: J.B. (Jonathan Benhamou), Epidemiological data: E.M.-M., Writing/Editing: C.B., Supervision/Staff Doctor/Diagnosed the patient: J.B. (Johannes Blum).

Funding: This research received no external funding.

Conflicts of Interest: The authors declare no conflict of interest.

Trop. Med. Infect. Dis. **2019**, *4*, 142

References

1. Blum, J.; Schmid, C.; Burri, C. Clinical aspects of 2541 patients with second stage human African trypanosomiasis. *Acta Trop.* **2006**, *97*, 55–64. [CrossRef] [PubMed]
2. Buscher, P.; Cecchi, G.; Jamonneau, V.; Priotto, G. Human African trypanosomiasis. *Lancet* **2017**, *390*, 2397–2409. [CrossRef]
3. Mwanza, J.C.; Kazumba, L.; Plant, G.; Tylleskär, T. Neuro-ophthalmologic manifestations of human African Trypanosomiasis. *Afr. J. Neurol. Sci.* **2004**, *23*, 1.

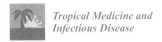

Article

Gambiense Human African Trypanosomiasis Sequelae after Treatment: A Follow-Up Study 12 Years after Treatment

Junior Mudji [1,2,†], **Anna Blum** [3,4,†], **Leticia Grize** [3,4], **Rahel Wampfler** [3,4], **Marie-Thérèse Ruf** [3,4], **Lieselotte Cnops** [5], **Beatrice Nickel** [3,4], **Christian Burri** [3,4] and **Johannes Blum** [3,4,*]

1   Hôpital Evangélique de Vanga, Vanga Mission, B.P. 4728 Kinshasa 2, Democratic Republic of the Congo; mudjijunior@gmail.com
2   Department of family medicine and primary care, Protestant University of Congo, B.P. 4745, Kinshasa 2, Democratic Republic of the Congo
3   Swiss Tropical and Public Health Institute, 4002 Basel, Switzerland; blumdocdoc@gmail.com (A.B.); let.grize2015@gmail.com (L.G.); rahel.wampfler@swisstph.ch (R.W.); therese.ruf@swisstph.ch (M.-T.R.); beatrice.nickel@swisstph.ch (B.N.); christian.burri@swisstph.ch (C.B.)
4   University of Basel, 4001 Basel, Switzerland
5   Institute of Tropical Medicine, 2000 Antwerp, Belgium; lcnops@itg.be
*   Correspondence: johannes.blum@swisstph.ch
†   These authors contributed equally to the manuscript.

Received: 8 November 2019; Accepted: 8 January 2020; Published: 11 January 2020

Abstract: The clinical presentation of Human African Trypanosomiasis (HAT) due to *Trypanosoma brucei gambiense* is well known, but knowledge on long-term sequelae is limited. In the frame of studies conducted between 2004 and 2005 in the Democratic Republic of the Congo (DRC), the prevalence of HAT related signs and symptoms were evaluated before the start of treatment and at the end of treatment. To explore possible long-term sequelae, the same clinical parameters were assessed in 2017 in 51 first stage and 18 second stage HAT patients. Signs and symptoms 12–13 years after treatment were compared to before and immediately after treatment and to controls matched for sex and age (±5 years). In first stage HAT patients, the prevalence of all signs and symptoms decreased compared to before treatment but were still higher after 12–13 years than immediately at the end of treatment and in the control group. In second stage HAT patients, all HAT-specific findings had continuously decreased to the point where they were in the range of the healthy control group. In a selection of oligosymptomatic first stage HAT patients, no trypanosomes were detected in the blood by microscopic examination or PCR. An oligosymptomatic presentation of HAT due to the persistence of parasites in compartments, where first stage HAT medications do not penetrate, could not be ruled out.

Keywords: human African trypanosomiasis; sequelae; serology; treatment; oligosymptomatic HAT

1. Introduction

Human African trypanosomiasis (HAT) is caused by the protozoan parasites *Trypanosoma brucei gambiense (T.b. gambiense)* and *Trypanosoma brucei rhodesiense (T.b. rhodesiense)*, which are transmitted by tsetse flies. Whereas the *T.b. gambiense* form is characterized by a progressive course typically lasting three years [1], the *T.b. rhodesiense* form is usually acute, and death occurs within weeks or months of infection.

T.b. gambiense is endemic in foci in Western and Central Africa and today causes more than 98% of reported cases of HAT. The disease occurs in two stages, the first, or hemolymphatic, stage without invasion of the central nervous system (CNS) and the second, or neurological, stage with invasion of the CNS by the trypanosomes.

According to the last WHO report (WHO interim guidelines for treatment of gambiense human African trypanosomiasis, August 2019) [2], the worldwide number of *T.b. gambiense* HAT cases dropped from over 25,000 in the year 2000 to below 1000 reported cases worldwide in 2018 [2].

Fever, headache, pruritus, lymphadenopathy, and, to a lesser extent, hepato-splenomegaly are the leading signs and symptoms of the first stage but may also be present, to a lesser degree, in the second stage. During the second stage, neuro-psychiatric disorders such as lethargy, aggressive behaviour, logorrhoea, psychotic reactions, mood changes, and sleep disturbances/disorders dominate the clinical presentation. The neurological symptoms include tremor, general motor weakness, paralysis of an extremity, epilepsy, akinesia, and abnormal movements (dyskinesia, unspecific movement disorders, Parkinson-like movements, speech disorders) [3–8]. Sleep disorder with somnolence and short interposed sleeping episodes during the day and at night are imposing clinical symptoms from which "sleeping sickness" derives its name. Total sleep duration, however, remains normal [9].

HAT had always been perceived and described as inevitably fatal if untreated. However, oligosymptomatic forms of HAT with few symptoms, non-detectible parasites, and persistent serological titers were recently described along with their potential role for transmission of HAT [10,11]. The clinical presentation of *T.b. gambiense* HAT has been well documented, but studies on long-term sequelae of HAT have not been performed. The present observational case control study describes the clinical signs and symptoms of HAT patients before treatment and 12–13 years after.

2. Materials and Methods

2.1. Study Design and Setting (See also Flowcharts below)

The present study assessed the prevalence of HAT related long-term clinical sequelae (signs and symptoms 12–13 years after treatment) and compared signs and symptoms of the HAT patients before, immediately after, and 12–13 years after treatment. Patients at follow-up time were also compared with controls matched by sex and age (±5 years).

This follow-up study was conducted in two phases from 19 July to 14 September 2017 and from 3 May to 30 May 2019 at the Hôpital Evangélique de Vanga, located in the Kwilu province of the Democratic Republic of the Congo (DRC). The area is rural; villages are very remote and only accessible with major efforts by very difficult roads.

2.2. Participants

In a clinical study carried out in 2004 on endocrinological changes and the involvement of the heart in second stage HAT (detection of parasite, pathological cerebrospinal fluid), clinical parameters from 29 patients were assessed before treatment, at the end of treatment, and after a follow-up of three months [12–14]. Additionally, in the framework of clinical trials carried out between 2004 and 2005, clinical parameters were documented before and after treatment (but without a follow-up of three months) in 96 first stage HAT patients (parasitology confirmed) in Vanga. In these trials, the safety and efficacy of the newly developed drug pafuramidine was compared to the standard treatment with pentamidine for first stage HAT [15,16].

A list of all formerly recruited patients in the above-mentioned studies was compiled, and their place of residence (village) was traced. The villages for the recruitment of study participants were chosen according to the number of eligible patients living there and the accessibility of the villages (distance to Vanga hospital, navigability of roads, and distance between affected villages). According to these parameters, visits were planned, starting with a visit that allowed the enrollment of the largest possible number of patients. Accessible persons were included in the study after informed consent with the exception of patients with one of the following exclusion criteria: history of severe chronic diseases such as tuberculosis, HIV, cancer, liver cirrhosis, and diabetes mellitus. In patients who died or were not accessible, a third-party history by a family member or friend was taken. These patients were not included in the analysis but were discussed separately.

2.3. Sample Size

Different clinical parameters of HAT have largely different frequencies. The calculation of a sample size yielding 80% power ($\alpha = 0.05$) was, e.g., 11 patients for sleeping disorders versus 485 patients for abnormal behavior. It was therefore decided to aim at a minimum 60 patients, which would be sufficient to allow the covering of the major signs and symptoms. Due to the limited number of available patients, the sample size calculation was only performed for the first stage HAT patients. Ninety-six first stage and 29 second stage patients who participated in the former studies lived in the perimeter of the Vanga hospital.

2.4. Study Procedure/Clinical Examination

The study was conducted in two parts—a site visit to the villages as described above, followed by a laboratory assessment at the hospital for the first stage HAT patients with clinical signs and symptoms (see below). The original working hypothesis was that no or only rare sequelae or signs of continued infection would be found in treated HAT patients revisited more than 10 years after treatment. Therefore, the study focused on clinical signs and symptoms of HAT patients 12–13 years after treatment. The second part of the study emerged from the findings, which had revealed a significant number of first stage HAT patients with continued or returning complaints. The resulting follow-up study, comprising blood examinations, could only be done with about two years of delay, due to the necessary protocol amendment, time-consuming ethical clearance, and challenges of accessibility and free movement in the election period in the DRC.

For each former patient (=a case), a control person matched by age (±5 years) and sex was enrolled. Family members were preferred and, if not available, hospital personnel or patients with minor surgical problems (i.e., herniotomy) were enrolled instead.

In all HAT patients and controls, a short history and physical examination was established. Questions regarding the symptoms of HAT were asked in the same manner as in the former original study and trials, and the case report form used to compare signs and symptoms was based on those used in the previous trials. The data collected were compared to those before treatment and after treatment from the former studies.

2.5. Additional Blood Examination on Patients with Symptoms

For the second part of the study, 15 first stage HAT patients who were still oligosymptomatic and had shown clinical signs or symptoms such as headache, sleep disorders, pruritus, or minor neurological problems during the village visits were invited to report to the hospital for additional tests. The following laboratory tests were performed: Microscopic examination of the blood and the aspiration fluid of enlarged lymphatic glands (if present) for the presence of trypanosomes, serologic testing for trypanosomiasis (CATT/*T.b.gambiense*, Institute of Tropical Medicine, Antwerp, Belgium;IFA, in-house test, Swiss Tropical and Public Health Institute, Basel, Switzerland), and PCR from blood samples. CATT was performed immediately after blood withdrawal in the DRC, and EDTA-blood and serum samples for IFA and PCR were stored in aliquots at −20 °C at the study site until transfer on dry ice to Switzerland.

2.6. T.b. gambiense Card Agglutination Test for Trypanosomiasis (CATT)

The CATT is a direct agglutination test using lyophilized bloodstream forms of *T.b. gambiense* variable antigen type LiTat 1.3. It detects specific antibodies in the blood, serum, or plasma of patients infected with *T.b. gambiense* [17]. The test was performed according to the kit manual. For each participant, one CATT test was performed on undiluted whole blood.

The CATT exhibits a sensitivity of 87%–98% [17,18] and a specificity of 95.9% on undiluted whole blood. Cross reactivity with antibodies generated against *Plasmodium* spp. and other parasites is possible.

2.7. Trypanosoma brucei IFA, Malaria IFA, and Leishmania IFA Serological Tests

Immunofluorescence staining was performed with bloodstream forms of *T.b. brucei* (strain STIB 345) in addition with *Plasmodium falciparum* (strain NF54) or liver sections of *Leishmania donovani* (strain MHOM-ET-67/L82) infected hamster mounted on glass slides. Slides were stored at −80 °C until day of use. For IFA analysis, slides were quickly air-dried at room temperature and fixed with acetone. Sera were diluted in PBS pH 7.2 and applied to the slide-slots. Three control sera were present on each slide; one positive, one equivocal, and one negative control. After 25 min of incubation at 37 °C in a wet chamber, slides were washed with PBS pH 7.2 and air-dried. FITC conjugated F(ab)'2 anti-IgG/A/M (BioRad, #30244) diluted in 0.01% Evans blue in PBS was added, slides were incubated for 25 min at 37 °C, washed, dried, and a cover glass was mounted with buffered glycerol. Slides were examined immediately with a fluorescence microscope. The serodiagnostic test exhibits a sensitivity of 98% for infections with *T.b. rhodesiense* or *T.b. gambiense* and a specificity of >99% for serum samples from healthy blood donors. The IFA exhibits a sensitivity of >99% for *Plasmodium* spp. and a specificity of 98% for healthy blood donor samples. The test has a sensitivity of >96% for visceral leishmaniasis and a specificity of >99% for heathy blood donor sera. Cross reactivity between the mentioned parasites antigens is possible.

2.8. Plasmodium falciparum spp. ELISA

Malaria serology was performed with an in-house screening ELISA for detection of specific *Plasmodium* spp. antibodies. *P. falciparum antigen* (strain NF54) was coated in 0.05 M sodium carbonate buffer, pH 9.6, to Immulon 2HB plates (, Thermo Scientific, Wohlen, Switzerland,). After washing, diluted sera were added to the plates and incubated for 15 min at 37 °C. After additional washing steps, horseradish peroxidase conjugated goat-anti-human-IgG (KPL, 474-1006, BioConcept Ltd, Allschwil, Switzerland) was added. Plates were incubated for 15 min at 37 °C, subsequently washed, and o-Phenylendiamine Dihydrochloride (OPD, Sigma, Buchs, Switzerland) was added. Reaction was stopped with 8 M H_2SO_4, and absorption was read with a Multiscan FC reader (ThermoScientific, Wohlen, Switzerland) at 492 nm. All sera giving positive or equivocal results were additionally tested with an in-house confirmatory Malaria IFA.

2.9. Real-Time PCR

For molecular analysis, 5 mL of whole blood samples were lysed and stored at the hospital site by adding an equal volume of guanidine-HCl 6 M with 0.1 M EDTA pH = 8, according to previous publications [19,20]. These samples were kept at 4 °C until shipment to Switzerland. Upon arrival, samples were immediately processed. For this, samples were heated at 100 °C for 15 min, and 500 μL of the guanidine-HCl-EDTA whole blood was used for extraction using the QIAamp DNA Mini Kit from Qiagen (Hilden, Germany), according to the manufacturer's instructions. DNA was eluted in 100 μL AE buffer (provided by the kit). The PCR targets the 18S rRNA gene of the *Trypanozoon* spp. (including the detection of *T.b. brucei, T.b. gambiense, T.b. rhodesiense, T. evansi,* and *T. equiperdum*) as previously described for a conventional PCR format [21]. Primer and probe sequences were newly designed and adapted to the real-time PCR format (forward primer: 5′-TAGTTTTGTGCCGTGCCAGT-3′, reverse primer: 5′-CGCTCCCGTGTTTCTTGTATC-3′, and TaqMan probe: 5′-FAM-TCGGACGTG-iQ500-TTTTGACCCACGC-BHQ1-3′), resulting in an amplicon of 97 basepairs. The PCR reaction mixture contained 5 μL DNA, 1x GoTaq Probe Master Mix from Promega (Madison, USA), 800 nmol forward and reverse primer, and 200 nmol probe in a total reaction volume of 25 μL. The PCR program started with a step at 50 °C for 2 min and 95 °C for 10 min, followed by 45 cycles of 95 °C for 15 s and 58 °C for 1 min. Plasmid containing the

97 bp amplicon sequence, as well as adjacent base pairs, was used as a positive control. The assay was optimised on *T.b. gambiense* and *T.b. rhodesiense* culture samples and spiked blood samples. Analytical sensitivity of the assay was 1 plasmid copy/µL DNA, and 5–50 parasites/mL spiked whole blood. Specificity was tested against DNA samples from *Babesia divergensis, Cryptosporidium* spp., *Cyclospora cayetanensis, Leishmania aethiopica, L. braziliensis, L. donovani, L. infantum, L. mexicana, Neospora caninum, Plasmodium falciparum, P. vivax, P. knowlesi, P. malariae, P. ovale, Sarcoycstis hominis, Toxoplasma gondii,* and *Trypanosoma cruzi,* and were found to be 100%.

2.10. Statistical Analysis

Categorical characteristics were summarized as counts and proportions, continuous characteristics as means, standard deviations, medians, and interquartile ranges. Paired comparisons were tested using McNemars' exact test or the Wilcoxon signed rank test depending on the nature of the compared factors. SAS version 9.4 (2002–2012, SAS Institute, Cary, NC, USA) was used to perform the statistical analysis. The level of significance was set to an alpha level <0.05.

2.11. Ethics Statement

The study protocol was approved by Ethikkommission Nordwest-und Zentralschweiz (EKNZ) (2017-00471; 12.4.2017) and Comité d'Éthique de l'Université Protestante au Congo (UPC) (CEUPC) (0044; 13.6.2017). Prior to enrolment, all participants gave informed written consent.

3. Results

In the region of Vanga, 96 first stage and 29 second stage HAT patients were recruited into several studies and trials between 2004 and 2005 [12–16]. The recruitment of participants for the present study took place during three visits to the following villages: (i) Kikongo Tango-Milundu, (ii) Nsalu, and (iii) Mayoko-Nkai.

The flowchart of the study, including the number of participants, is shown in Figure 1.

In 69 out of 92 (75%) of the eligible patients, a history and clinical examination could be performed. Fifty-one were previous first stage and 18 were previous second stage HAT patients. Ten out of 92 (11%) were not accessible but, according to oral communication by relatives or friends, were all in good health without any long-term sequelae of HAT. Five out of 92 (5%) died, two of them in the peripartum period of causes unrelated to HAT, and three without a clear diagnosis. Of these three patients, one died due to malnutrition, probably unrelated to HAT, one due to an undefined disease with unspecified swelling but without fever, and the third one due to unknown causes one month after HAT treatment. No information was available for eight out of 92 (9%) of the former patients. There was no history of a confirmed relapse for any of the patients followed up in this study. During the village visits, only clinical investigations, but no specific HAT diagnostic tests, were performed. At this point, no patient was suspected to have HAT; therefore, no blood tests had been planned for this phase of the study.

Table 1 shows the characteristics for patients with previously first (n = 51) and second (n = 18) stage HAT and their matched controls. Tables 2 and 3 show the prevalence of signs and symptoms before treatment and at the long-term follow-up, for first and second stage HAT, respectively. Figures 2 and 3 show the development of these signs and symptoms at the different examined time points.

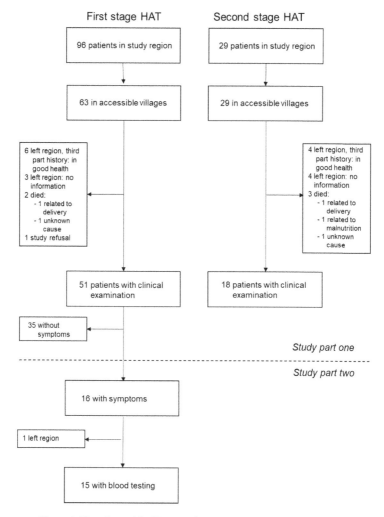

Figure 1. Flow chart of the Human African Trypanosomiasis (HAT) study.

Table 1. Descriptive characteristics for first and second stage HAT patients and their controls.

Characteristic	First Stage HAT		Second Stage HAT	
	Patients (n = 51)	Controls (n = 51)	Patients (n = 18)	Controls (n = 18)
Age * (years):				
Mean ± SD	43.9 ± 12.5	42.7 ± 12.5	52.0 ± 15.8	50.9 ± 14.5
Median (IQR)	41 (35 to 50)	42 (32 to 51)	47.5 (37 to 64)	48 (36 to 64)
Gender: n (%)				
Male	14 (27.5)	14 (27.5)	9 (50.0)	9 (50.0)
Female	37 (72.5)	37 (72.5)	9 (50.0)	9 (50.0)

* Age of controls matched within ±5 years of age of patients; SD = standard deviation; IQR = interquartile range (first to third quartile).

Table 2. First stage HAT: Signs and symptoms for patients before treatment and at 12 year follow-up and for their controls.

Symptom/Sign	Level	Before Treatment n (%)	12 Year Follow-up n (%)	p-Value *	Controls [†] n (%)	p-Value *,[§]
Lymphadenopathy	Absent	1 (2.0)	48 (94.1)	<0.0001	49 (96.1)	0.6547
	Palpable	50 (98.0)	3 (5.9)		2 (3.9)	
Headache	Absent	13 (26.0)	35 (70.0)	<0.0001	43 (86.0)	0.0325
	Present/Unbearable	37 (74.0)	15 [(4)] (30.0)		7 (14.0)	
Pruritus	Absent	37 (72.6)	45 [(4)] (88.2)	0.0005	50 (98.0)	0.0588
	Present/Visible traces of scratching	14 (27.4)	6 [(4)] (11.8)		1 (2.0)	
Daytime sleep	Normal	51 (100.0)	49 (96.1)	-	51 (100.0)	-
	Repeatedly/Continuously	0 (0.0)	2 [(2)] (3.9)		0 (0.0)	
Nighttime sleep	Normal	51 (100.0)	47 (92.2)	-	51 (100.0)	-
	Few hours/Rare	0 (0.0)	4 [(4)] (7.8)		0 (0.0)	
Tremor	Absent	51 (100.0)	48 (94.1)	-	51 (100.0)	-
	Visible/Severe	0 (0.0)	3 [(3)] (5.9)		0 (0.0)	
Speech impairment	Absent	51 (100.0)	50 (98.0)	-	51 (100.0)	-
	Present/Non-interpretable	0 (0.0)	1 [(1)] (2.0)		0 (0.0)	
Abnormal movement	Absent	51 (100.0)	51 (100.0)	-	-	-
Walking disability	Absent	51 (100.0)	51 (100.0)	-	-	-
General motor weakness	Absent	51 (100.0)	51 (100.0)	-	-	-
Unusual behavior	Absent	51 (100.0)	51 (100.0)	-	-	-
Inactivity	Absent	51 (100.0)	51 (100.0)	-	-	-
Aggression	Absent	51 (100.0)	51 (100.0)	-	-	-
Disturbed appetite	Normal	51 (100.0)	51 (100.0)	-	-	-

* McNemar's exact test; [†] Each patient was matched to a control by sex and age (±5 years); [§] For patients at 12 year follow-up and their healthy controls; [(x)] Number of new onsets.

Table 3. Second stage HAT: Signs and symptoms for patients before treatment and at 12 year follow-up and for their controls.

Symptom/Sign	Level	Before Treatment n (%)	12 Year Follow-Up n (%)	p-Value *	Controls [†] n (%)	p-Value *,§
Lymphadenopathy	Absent	1 (5.6)	17(94.4)	0.0020	17 (100.0)	-
	Palpable	17 (94.4)	1 (5.6)		0 (0.0)	
Headache	Absent	8 (44.4)	16 (88.9)	0.0156	17 (94.4)	0.5637
	Present/Unbearable	10 (55.6)	2 [(1)] (11.1)		1 (5.6)	
Pruritus	Absent	9 (50.0)	18 (100.0)	-	18 (100.0)	-
	Present/Visible traces of scratching	9 (50.0)	0 (0.0)		0 (0.0)	
Daytime sleep	Normal	12 (66.7)	18 (100.0)	-	18 (100.0)	-
	Repeatedly/Continuously	6 (33.3)	0 (0.0)		0 (0.0)	
Nighttime sleep	Normal	10 (55.6)	18 (100.0)	-	18 (100.0)	-
	Few hours/Rare	8 (44.4)	0 (0.0)		0 (0.0)	
Tremor	Absent	13 (72.2)	18 (100.0)	-	18 (100.0)	-
	Visible/Severe	5 (27.8)	0 (0.0)		0 (0.0)	
Speech impairment	Absent	16 (88.9)	18 (100.0)	-	18 (100.0)	-
	Present/Non-interpretable	2 (11.1)	0 (0.0)		0 (0.0)	-
Abnormal movement	Absent	18 (100.0)	18 (100.0)	-	18 (100.0)	-
Walking disability	Absent	13 (72.2)	18 (100.0)	-	18 (100.0)	-
	Present/Walking with help/inability to walk	5 (27.8)	0 (0.0)	-	0 (0.0)	
General motor weakness	Absent	14 (77.8)	18 (100.0)	-	18 (100.0)	-
	Ability to stand from chair no hands/No ability to stand	4 (22.0)	0 (0.0)	-	0 (0.0)	
Unusual behavior	Absent	14 (77.8)	18 (100.0)	-	18 (100.0)	-
	Visible/Severe	4 (22.0)	0 (0.0)	-	0 (0.0)	
Inactivity	Absent	11 (61.1)	18 (100.0)	-	18 (100.0)	-
	Reduced workforce/Inability to perform daily tasks	7 (38.9)	0 (0.0)	-	0 (0.0)	
Aggression	Absent	12 (66.7)	18 (100.0)	-	18 (100.0)	-
	Sporadic/Severe, requires observation	6 (33.3)	0 (0.0)	-	0 (0.0)	
Disturbed appetite	Normal	16 (88.9)	18 (100.0)	-	18 (100.0)	-
	Disturbed/Severely	2 (11.1)	0 (0.0)		0 (0.0)	

* McNemar's exact test; [†] Each patient was matched to a control by sex and age (±5 years); [§] For patients at 12 year follow-up and their healthy controls; [(x)] Number of new onsets.

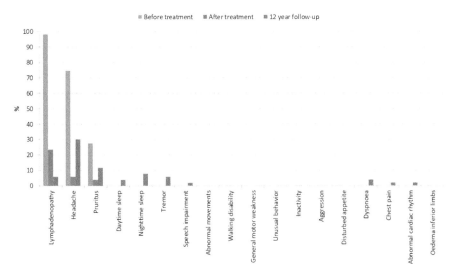

Figure 2. First stage HAT patients: Prevalence of signs and symptoms at different time points. Absence of a bar indicates 0% prevalence at a certain time point, except for dyspnea, chest pain, abnormal cardiac rhythm, and oedema, which were determined only at 12 year follow-up.

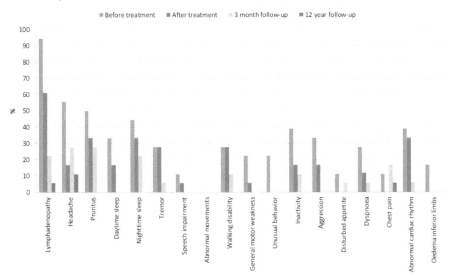

Figure 3. Second stage HAT patients: Prevalence of signs and symptoms at different time points. Absence of a bar indicates 0% prevalence at a certain time point.

3.1. Lymphadenopathy

Lymphadenopathy was the most frequently observed sign before treatment in first stage (98%) and second stage (94.4%) HAT patients. Twelve years after treatment, it was detected only in 5.9% first and in 5.6% second stage patients, which was comparable to the control groups (3.9% and 0%).

3.2. Headache

Headache was the most frequent complaint of HAT patients before treatment and was more frequent in the first stage (74%, including 2% with unbearable headache) than in the second stage (55.6%). In first stage HAT, headaches decreased to 6% at the end of treatment but increased thereafter to 30% (none with unbearable headache) 13 years later, which is significantly higher than in the control group (14%). One patient asked for further examination pertaining to the headache, which revealed the cause of the headache to be posttraumatic after a head injury without association to HAT. In second stage HAT, headaches decreased to 11% 12–13 years after treatment, compared to 5.6% in the control group.

3.3. Pruritus

Pruritus was the second most frequent complaint of HAT patients and was less frequent in the first stage (27.4%, including 6% with scratching marks) than in the second stage (50%) before treatment. It decreased to 4% after treatment and re-increased to 11.8% at the 12 year follow-up (none with scratching marks) in first stage and decreased to none in second stage HAT, comparable to the control group (2%).

3.4. Sleep Disorder

In first stage HAT, sleep disorders were neither observed before nor after treatment, but 3.9% reported daytime sleep and 7.8% reported sleep disorders during the night 12–13 years later. In second stage HAT, daytime sleep decreased from 33% and night time sleep disorders from 44% before treatment stepwise to none 12 years after treatment, equal to the healthy control group.

3.5. Neurological Disorders

In first stage HAT, neurological disorders were not described, before or after treatment, but tremor was reported in 6% and speech disorders in 3% at follow-up. In the second stage, neurological disorders such as speech impairment (11%), walking disability (28%), motor weakness (22%), and unusual behavior (22%) were observed before treatment, decreasing continuously post treatment, and had disappeared completely after 12–13 years.

3.6. Blood Analysis4

Blood analysis was performed only in the second phase of the study for symptomatic follow-up patients from the group with previous first stage HAT. Trypanosomes could not be detected in any of these 15 patients, neither by direct blood examination nor by real time PCR. The CATT was negative for all patients, but IFA using *T. b. brucei* antigen was positive in most patients (see Table 4). None of the 15 patients showed a positive *Leishmania* serology. By contrast, all patients exhibited a positive malaria serology in ELISA and IFA, which can be explained by the region being an endemic area for malaria.

Table 4. Real-time PCR, CATT, *T. brucei*, Malaria, and *Leishmania* serology of 15 follow-up patients.

Serum	Real-time PCR Trypanosoma Result	CATT Test Result	*T. Brucei* Serology IFA (Titre)	*T. Brucei* Serology Result	Malaria Serology ELISA (OD)	Malaria Serology IFA (Titre)	Malaria Serology Result	Leishmania Serology IFA (Titre)	Leishmania Serology Result
P07	negative	negative	1/320	positive	1.59	1/1280	positive	<1/80	negative
P14	negative	negative	1/160	equivocal	1.00	1/1280	positive	<1/80	negative
P28	negative	negative	1/640	positive	1.84	1/1280	positive	<1/80	negative
P29	negative	negative	<1/160	negative	1.62	1/1280	positive	<1/80	negative
P42	negative	negative	1/320	positive	1.95	1/1280	positive	<1/80	negative
P50	negative	negative	1/320	positive	1.82	1/1280	positive	<1/80	negative
P51	negative	negative	1/640	positive	1.76	1/1280	positive	<1/80	negative
P53	negative	negative	1/320	positive	1.65	1/1280	positive	<1/80	negative
P55	negative	negative	1/640	positive	1.71	1/1280	positive	<1/80	negative
P56	negative	negative	1/320	positive	1.73	1/1280	positive	<1/80	negative
P57	negative	negative	1/320	positive	1.30	1/640	positive	<1/80	negative
P58	negative	negative	1/640	positive	1.26	1/1280	positive	<1/80	negative
P62	negative	negative	1/320	positive	1.74	1/1280	positive	<1/80	negative
P63	negative	negative	1/160	equivocal	1.74	1/1280	positive	<1/80	negative
P64	negative	negative	1/320	positive	2.09	1/1280	positive	<1/80	negative

Cutoffs, T. brucei IFA: <1/160 negative, 1/160 equivocal, ≥1/320 positive; Malaria ELISA: <0.15 negative, 0.15–0.29 equivocal, ≥0.30 positive; Malaria IFA: <1/40 negative, 1/40 equivocal, ≥1/80 positive; Leishmania IFA: <1/80 negative, 1/80 equivocal, ≥1/160 positive.

4. Discussion

To the best of our knowledge, this is the first study assessing the long-term sequelae of first and second stage HAT patients more than 10 years after initial treatment, comparing them to healthy controls. The study evaluated the clinical signs and symptoms before treatment, immediately after treatment, and 12–13 years after treatment in 51 first stage and 18 second stage HAT patients. A surprisingly high percentage (75%) of the eligible and accessible patients could be enrolled in the present study, while information on the health condition (including death) of 15% of the patients could be gathered from relatives and friends. In only 10% of the eligible patients was no information available.

Five cases were lost to follow-up because of death. In two of these, HAT could be ruled out as the cause of death, and in the other three, HAT was unlikely as the cause of death according to information from friends and relatives.

In first stage HAT patients, the prevalence of all signs and symptoms (except lymphadenopathy) had decreased 12–13 years after treatment compared to before treatment, but was still higher than immediately after the end of treatment and in the control group. The high prevalence of headaches (31%), pruritus (12%), and even the presence of neuropsychiatric symptoms such as tremor (6%), speech impairment (2%), and sleeping problems (12%) is worrying. All patients with neuropsychiatric symptoms also suffered from headaches. No relapse was clinically suspected in any of the patients or reported by the patients in the time before the long-term follow-up.

In second stage HAT patients treated with melarsoprol, all HAT specific signs and symptoms decreased steadily at the examined time-points towards a range of the healthy control group 12–13 years post-treatment. Only headache was reported in 11%, but this was not significantly different compared to the control group.

The higher prevalence of symptoms in first stage than in second stage HAT patients at follow-up is surprising and contradictory to former studies. In children treated with melarsoprol, signs and symptoms one month to four years after treatment were more frequently reported in second stage patients (22 symptoms in 28 patients) than in their first stage counterparts (25 symptoms in 92 patients) [22]. In contrast to our results, neither headache nor pruritus were the main symptoms, but were primarily neuropsychiatric symptoms: mental confusion (7.5%), changes in character (11.5%), memory problems (11.5%), language problem (3%), and sleeping disorders (5%). Furthermore, changes in growth in young participants, 6–20 years of age, formerly treated for HAT, were more accentuated in second stage HAT compared to first stage HAT [23]. The subjects treated for first and second stage HAT had a smaller body weight (−4.25 kg), were 3 cm shorter, and had a smaller mid-upper-arm circumference (−1.15 cm) than the control group matched for age, sex and residence. These changes were more accentuated in second stage than in first stage patients: body weight from −4.9 to −2.6 kg, height from −4.9 to −2 cm, and mid-upper-arm circumference from −2 to −1 cm [23]. Differences to these studies could eventually be explained by a relatively low number of patients and a different study design (i.e., age of patients, different follow-up period, different context).

In first stage HAT patients, the clear improvement of the signs and symptoms after treatment was expected, but the reappearance of such symptoms 12–13 years post-treatment is surprising. In a follow-up examination of the patients, no trypanosomes could be detected in any of them, neither by direct microscopic examination nor by real time PCR of the blood. The CATT was negative for all 15 former first stage HAT patients with persistent symptoms, but 80% of them were positive in the *Trypanosoma* serology by IFA. In addition, 13% of the 15 participants showed an equivocal result in IFA, and only 7% were negative. The positive *Trypanosoma* serology by IFA could be explained by either long term-persisting anti-trypanosomal antibodies, a boost of immunity without an actual measurable infection due to repetitive infected tsetse bites [24], the presence of subclinical infection, or by cross-reactivity of malaria antibodies to a certain extent.

There are several hypotheses to explain these unexpected results:

First, the patients improved after the treatment and subjectively did not notice remaining minor symptoms at the end of treatment. All these symptoms were generally mild, and the patients did not seek medical help. It could be possible that the symptoms did not really disappear but persisted at a level below immediate perception. This would mean that sequelae persist even more than a decade after treatment and include headaches, pruritus, sleeping disorders, and rare neurological deficits in the absence of persisting parasites. The description of the signs and symptoms described in children [22,23] and case series of adults [10] strengthens the hypothesis of persistence of sequelae.

Secondly, after an initial cure, some patients could have had a relapse or a reinfection with HAT with an oligosymptomatic presentation and trypanosomes below the detection level in the blood. Even if HAT infections are rare events, mainly in the last decade [25], the study design does not allow the exclusion of such reinfection or relapse.

The third hypothesis could be that a few parasites have survived (hiding in other compartments than the blood) and may have caused a persisting oligosymptomatic low-level infection. Treatment with melarsoprol, which reaches nearly all compartments of the body, killed the trypanosomes, but neither pentamidine nor pafuramidine, used against first stage HAT, can penetrate the blood brain barrier and may not have reached all body compartments. Tanowitz described replicating trypanosomes in adipose tissue interacting with adipocytes [26]. Since most drugs used for the treatment of HAT are hydrophilic, their efficacy could be limited in a lipophilic environment, and adipose tissue could represent a safe site for trypanosomes to hide [26]. It has been described that the skin or the CSF could also represent an anatomic reservoir of trypanosomes [21,27]. In addition, the persistence of trypanosomes in the blood below the detection level cannot be ruled out.

Of interest are the results of a study where untreated HAT patients were compared to formerly treated HAT patients [10]. Eleven HAT patients refused treatment, survived, and were evaluated 2–9 years later. Parasites were detected in only one out of 11 patients in the blood (by microscopy and PCR), and HAT specific antibody titres had decreased in only seven out of 10 patients. The study suggests that oligo-or asymptomatic HAT infections may show spontaneous cure over time or persist as low level infection without passage to the CNS [10]. The control group included 18 first stage and 21 second stage HAT patients treated 15 years prior. No parasites could be detected in the blood of any patients, neither by PCR nor by microscopy after mini anion exchange centrifugation technique. A combination of a positive immune trypanolysis test [28] with a negative CATT test was found in 61.5% [10]. In 58% of the treated and in 68% of the untreated patients, non-specific symptoms such as fever and headaches were observed, showing that such symptoms may persist for a long time [10].

The findings lead to the hypothesis that a few surviving trypanosomes in certain compartments could partially be controlled by the immune system, leading to minor persisting symptoms without, however, the development of apparent clinical signs of a relapse of the disease. The persistent survival of trypanosomes could be a source of transmission [10,11] and could explain the reactivity of the serum in the *Trypanosoma* IFA in our study. The negative CATT results could possibly be explained by either a lower sensitivity than the IFA, by the occurrence of trypanosome strains that lack or do not express the LiTat 1.3 gene that has been described for some endemic areas in Nigeria [17], or by the rapid decline of CATT reactivity in treated HAT patients within a few years [29] while other serological tests are still positive. On the other hand, the negative CATT results could also mean that anti-trypanosomal antibodies are no longer present and the positive IFA results are caused by cross-reacting malaria antibodies.

A review of the natural progression of HAT concludes that, in rare cases, an oligosymptomatic chronic carrier stage exists, but duration beyond six to seven years is exceptional [30]. It is also worth paying attention to the broad spectrum of clinical presentations of *T.b. gambiense* HAT, ranging from a chronic oligosymptomatic form to the frequently observed, usually fatal chronic disease in endemic populations to the acute clinical presentation in non-endemic populations [31].

The presented results would be compatible with such a hypothesis, and the presence of antibody titres even 14–15 years after the end of treatment supports this hypothesis, although it needs to be confirmed by more robust data. The study demonstrates a surprisingly high percentage of HAT patients still suffering from symptoms even more than 10 years after treatment. The study was not designed to specify if re-infections, relapses, or parasites surviving in not yet well described body compartments cause the signs and symptoms or if the patients have sequelae without any surviving trypanosomes. These questions should be addressed in further studies.

5. Limitations

The limitations of this study are the subjective character of the symptoms, the difficulties associated with properly assessing third party history, and the relatively low number of patients. Another limitation of the study is that no *Trypanosoma* real time PCR and no *Trypanosoma* and malaria serology was performed for treated asymptomatic patients or control group participants. These data could not be collected due to the study design and the unexpected outcome of the first phase of the study. Finally, cross-reactivity of malaria antibodies against *T. brucei* antigens or vice versa cannot be ruled out.

6. Conclusions

We demonstrated HAT-related signs and symptoms more than 10 years after treatment for the first time in first stage HAT patients without detectable levels of parasites. In first stage HAT patients, the prevalence of all signs and symptoms decreased compared to before treatment, but were still higher than at the end of treatment and in the control group. In second stage HAT patients, all HAT specific findings had continuously decreased to the point where they were in the range of the healthy control group. Persistence of symptoms without detectable levels of parasites in the blood could suggest either parasitaemia below the detection level or the persistence of parasites in some other body compartments. Further studies, including skin or tissue biopsies for detection of trypanosomes by PCR and serologic testing before treatment as well as ten years later, could indicate if there is a reservoir, which could be relevant for subclinical forms and transmission.

Author Contributions: Conceptualization, J.B., C.B., A.B., J.M. and L.G.; methodology, J.B., C.B., A.B., J.M. and L.G.; software, L.G.; validation, J.B. and C.B.; formal analysis, L.G.; investigation, J.B., A.B., J.M., B.N., R.W., M.-T.R. and L.C.; resources, B.N., R.W., M.-T.R., L.C. and J.M.; data curation, L.G., A.B., J.B. and B.N.; writing—original draft preparation, J.B., C.B. and B.N.; writing—review and editing, J.B., C.B., L.G., B.N., M.-T.R., R.W., L.C. and A.B.; visualization, L.G.; supervision, C.B., J.B. and B.N.; project administration, J.B. All authors have read and agreed to the published version of the manuscript.

Funding: This research received no external funding.

Acknowledgments: We thank Monica Cal from the Parasite Chemotherapy Unit, Department of Medical Parasitology and Infection Biology of the Swiss TPH for provision of trypanosomes, Karin Stoll-Rudin from the Diagnostic Center of Swiss TPH, and Patrick Ntumba and Jaques Pombo from the Hôpital Evangélique de Vanga for expert technical assistance. We thank Sven Poppert from the Diagnostic Center of Swiss TPH for his support and critical reading.

Conflicts of Interest: The authors declare no conflict of interest.

References

1. Checchi, F.; Filipe, J.A.; Haydon, D.T.; Chandramohan, D.; Chappuis, F. Estimates of the duration of the early and late stage of gambiense sleeping sickness. *BMC. Infect. Dis.* **2008**, *8*, 16. [CrossRef] [PubMed]
2. WHO. *Interim Guidelines for the Treatment of Gambiense Human African Trypanosomiasis*; World Health Organization: Geneva, Switzerland, 2019.
3. Antoine, P. Neurological and psychological studies of patients with sleeping sickness and their course. *Ann. Soc. Belg. Med. Trop.* **1977**, *57*, 227–248. [PubMed]
4. Ginoux, P.Y.; Frezil, J.L.; Alary, J.C. symptoms of human trypanosomiasis at the first diagnostic phase in the people republic of congo (author's transl). *Med. Trop. (Mars)* **1982**, *42*, 281–287. [PubMed]
5. Kazumba, M.; Kazadi, K.; Mulumba, M.P. characteristics of trypanosomiasis in children. Apropos of 19 case reports at the cnpp (neuro-psycho-pathology center), university hospitals of kinshasa, zaire. *Ann. Soc. Belg. Med. Trop.* **1993**, *73*, 253–259. [PubMed]
6. Blum, J.; Schmid, C.; Burri, C. Clinical aspects of 2541 patients with second stage human african trypanosomiasis. *Acta. Trop.* **2006**, *97*, 55–64. [CrossRef] [PubMed]
7. Brun, R.; Blum, J. Human african trypanosomiasis. *Infect. Dis. Clin. North. Am.* **2012**, *26*, 261–273. [CrossRef]
8. Kazumba, L.M.; Kaka, J.T.; Ngoyi, D.M.; Tshala-Katumbay, D. Mortality trends and risk factors in advanced stage-2 human african trypanosomiasis: A critical appraisal of 23 years of experience in the democratic republic of congo. *PLoS Negl. Trop. Dis.* **2018**, *12*, e0006504. [CrossRef]
9. Buguet, A.; Bourdon, L.; Bisser, S.; Chapotot, F.; Radomski, M.W.; Dumas, M. Sleeping sickness: Major disorders of circadian rhythm. *Med. Trop. (Mars.)* **2001**, *61*, 328–339.
10. Jamonneau, V.; Llboudo, H.; Kaboré, J.; Kaba, D.; Koffi, M.; Solano, P.; Garcia, A.; Courtin, D.; Laveissiere, C.; Lingue, K.; et al. Untreated human infections by trypanosoma brucei gambiense are not 100% fatal. *PLoS Negl. Trop. Dis.* **2012**, *6*, e1691. [CrossRef]
11. Capewell, P.; Atkins, K.; Weir, W.; Jamonneau, V.; Camara, M.; Clucas, C.; Swar, N.K.; Ngoyi, D.M.; Rotureau, B.; Garside, P.; et al. Resolving the apparent transmission paradox of african sleeping sickness. *PLoS Biol.* **2019**, *17*, e3000105. [CrossRef]
12. Blum, J.A.; Burri, C.; Hatz, C.; Kazumba, L.; Mangoni, P.; Zellweger, M.J. Sleeping hearts: The role of the heart in sleeping sickness (human african trypanosomiasis). *Trop. Med. Int. Health* **2007**, *12*, 1422–1432. [CrossRef] [PubMed]
13. Blum, J.A.; Schmid, C.; Hatz, C.; Kazumba, L.; Mangoni, P.; Rutishauser, J.; la Torre, A.; Burri, C. Sleeping glands?—the role of endocrine disorders in sleeping sickness (t.B. Gambiense human african trypanosomiasis). *Acta. Trop.* **2007**, *104*, 16–24. [CrossRef] [PubMed]
14. Blum, J.A.; Schmid, C.; Burri, C.; Hatz, C.; Olson, C.; Fungula, B.; Kazumba, L.; Mangoni, P.; Mbo, F.; Deo, K.; et al. Cardiac alterations in human african trypanosomiasis (t.B. Gambiense) with respect to the disease stage and antiparasitic treatment. *PLoS Negl. Trop. Dis.* **2009**, *3*, e383. [CrossRef] [PubMed]
15. Burri, C.; Yeramian, P.D.; Allen, J.L.; Merolle, A.; Serge, K.K.; Mpanya, A.; Lutumba, P.; Mesu, V.K.; Bilenge, C.M.; Lubaki, J.P.; et al. Efficacy, safety, and dose of pafuramidine, a new oral drug for treatment of first stage sleeping sickness, in a phase 2a clinical study and phase 2b randomized clinical studies. *PLoS Negl. Trop. Dis.* **2016**, *10*, e0004362. [CrossRef] [PubMed]
16. Pohlig, G.; Bernhard, S.C.; Blum, J.; Burri, C.; Mpanya, A.; Lubaki, J.P.; Mpoto, A.M.; Munungu, B.F.; N'Tombe, P.M.; Deo, G.K.; et al. Efficacy and safety of pafuramidine versus pentamidine maleate for treatment of first stage sleeping sickness in a randomized, comparator-controlled, international phase 3 clinical trial. *PLoS Negl. Trop. Dis.* **2016**, *10*, e0004363. [CrossRef]

17. Chappuis, F.; Loutan, L.; Simarro, P.; Lejon, V.; Buscher, P. Options for field diagnosis of human african trypanosomiasis. *Clin. Microbiol Rev.* **2005**, *18*, 133–146. [CrossRef]
18. Bisser, S.; Lumbala, C.; Nguertoum, E.; Kande, V.; Flevaud, L.; Vatunga, G.; Boelaert, M.; Buscher, P.; Josenando, T.; Bessell, P.R.; et al. Sensitivity and specificity of a prototype rapid diagnostic test for the detection of trypanosoma brucei gambiense infection: A multi-centric prospective study. *PLoS Negl. Trop. Dis.* **2016**, *10*, e0004608. [CrossRef]
19. Avila, H.A.; Sigman, D.S.; Cohen, L.M.; Millikan, R.C.; Simpson, L. Polymerase chain reaction amplification of trypanosoma cruzi kinetoplast minicircle DNA isolated from whole blood lysates: Diagnosis of chronic chagas' disease. *Mol. Biochem. Parasitol.* **1991**, *48*, 211–221. [CrossRef]
20. Schijman, A.G.; Bisio, M.; Orellana, L.; Sued, M.; Duffy, T.; Mejia Jaramillo, A.M.; Cura, C.; Auter, F.; Veron, V.; Qvarnstrom, Y.; et al. International study to evaluate pcr methods for detection of trypanosoma cruzi DNA in blood samples from chagas disease patients. *PLoS Negl. Trop. Dis.* **2011**, *5*, e931. [CrossRef]
21. Deborggraeve, S.; Lejon, V.; Ekangu, R.A.; Mumba, N.D.; Pati, P.P.; Ilunga, M.; Mulunda, J.P.; Buscher, P. Diagnostic accuracy of pcr in gambiense sleeping sickness diagnosis, staging and post-treatment follow-up: A 2-year longitudinal study. *PLoS Negl. Trop. Dis.* **2011**, *5*, e972. [CrossRef]
22. Cramet, R. sleeping sickness in children and its long term after-effects. Apropos 110 personal observations at fontem hospital (cameroon). *Med. Trop. (Mars)* **1982**, *42*, 27–31. [PubMed]
23. Aroke, A.H.; Asonganyi, T.; Mbonda, E. Influence of a past history of gambian sleeping sickness on physical growth, sexual maturity and academic performance of children in fontem, cameroon. *Ann. Trop. Med. Parasitol.* **1998**, *92*, 829–835. [CrossRef] [PubMed]
24. Blum, J.; Beck, B.R.; Brun, R.; Hatz, C. Clinical and serologic responses to human 'apathogenic' trypanosomes. *Trans. R. Soc. Trop. Med. Hyg.* **2005**, *99*, 795–797. [CrossRef] [PubMed]
25. Mudji, J.; Benhamou, J.; Mwamba-Miaka, E.; Burri, C.; Blum, J. The Flipside of Eradicating a Disease, Human African Trypanosomiasis in a Woman in Rural Democratic Republic of Congo: A Case Report. *Trop. Med. Infect. Dis.* **2019**, *4*, 142. [CrossRef]
26. Tanowitz, H.B.; Scherer, P.E.; Mota, M.M.; Figueiredo, L.M. Adipose tissue: A safe haven for parasites? *Trends Parasitol.* **2017**, *33*, 276–284. [CrossRef]
27. Capewell, P.; Cren-Travaille, C.; Marchesi, F.; Johnston, P.; Clucas, C.; Benson, R.A.; Gorman, T.A.; Calvo-Alvarez, E.; Crouzols, A.; Jouvion, G.; et al. The skin is a significant but overlooked anatomical reservoir for vector-borne african trypanosomes. *eLife* **2016**, *5*, e17716. [CrossRef]
28. Jamonneau, V.; Bucheton, B.; Kabore, J.; Ilboudo, H.; Camara, O.; Courtin, F.; Solano, P.; Kaba, D.; Kambire, R.; Lingue, K.; et al. Revisiting the immune trypanolysis test to optimise epidemiological surveillance and control of sleeping sickness in west africa. *PLoS Negl. Trop. Dis.* **2010**, *4*, e917. [CrossRef]
29. Paquet, C.; Ancelle, T.; Gastellu-Etchegorry, M.; Castilla, J.; Harndt, I. Persistence of antibodies to trypanosoma brucei gambiense after treatment of human trypanosomiasis in uganda. *Lancet* **1992**, *340*, 250. [CrossRef]
30. Checchi, F.; Filipe, J.A.N.; Barrett, M.P.; Chandramohan, D. The natural progression of gambiense sleeping sickness: What is the evidence? *PLoS Negl. Trop. Dis.* **2008**, *2*, e303. [CrossRef]
31. Blum, J.A.; Neumayr, A.L.; Hatz, C.F. Human african trypanosomiasis in endemic populations and travellers. *Eur. J. Clin. Microbiol. Infect. Dis.* **2012**, *31*, 905–913. [CrossRef]

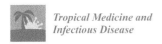

Tropical Medicine and Infectious Disease

Article

Clinical Study on the Melarsoprol-Related Encephalopathic Syndrome: Risk Factors and HLA Association

Jorge Seixas [1,2,*], Jorge Atouguia [1,2], Teófilo Josenando [3], Gedeão Vatunga [4,5], Constantin Miaka Mia Bilenge [6], Pascal Lutumba [7] and Christian Burri [8,9]

[1] Institute of Hygiene and Tropical Medicine, NOVA University, 1349-008 Lisbon, Portugal; j.atouguia@gmail.com
[2] Global Health and Tropical Medicine R&D Center, NOVA University, 1349-008 Lisbon, Portugal
[3] Instituto de Combate e Controlo das Tripanossomíases, Luanda, Angola; josenandot@yahoo.com
[4] Hospital Geral de Luanda, Luanda, Angola; vmlgedeao@live.com
[5] Instituto Superior Politécnico Kalandula de Angola, Luanda, Angola
[6] Programme National de Lutte contre la Trypanosomiase Humaine Africaine, Kinshasa, Democratic Republic of the Congo; tshimbadi@yahoo.fr
[7] Tropical Medicine Department, University of Kinshasa, Kinshasa, Democratic Republic of the Congo; pascal_lutumba@yahoo.fr
[8] Swiss Tropical and Public Health Institute, 4002 Basel, Switzerland; christian.burri@swisstph.ch
[9] University of Basel, 4001 Basel, Switzerland
[*] Correspondence: jseixas@ihmt.unl.pt; Tel.: +351-91-657-97-24

Received: 26 November 2019; Accepted: 25 December 2019; Published: 1 January 2020

Abstract: Melarsoprol administration for the treatment of late-stage human African trypanosomiasis (HAT) is associated with the development of an unpredictable and badly characterized encephalopathic syndrome (ES), probably of immune origin, that kills approximately 50% of those affected. We investigated the characteristics and clinical risk factors for ES, as well as the association between the Human Leukocyte Antigen (HLA) complex and the risk for ES in a case-control study. Late-stage Gambiense HAT patients treated with melarsoprol and developing ES (69 cases) were compared to patients not suffering from the syndrome (207 controls). Patients were enrolled in six HAT treatment centres in Angola and in the Democratic Republic of Congo. Standardized clinical data was obtained from all participants before melarsoprol was initiated. Class I (HLA-A, HLA-B, HLA-Cw) and II (HLA-DR) alleles were determined by PCR-SSOP methods in 62 ES cases and 189 controls. The principal ES pattern consisted in convulsions followed by a coma, whereas ES with exclusively mental changes was not observed. Oedema, bone pain, apathy, and a depressed humour were associated with a higher risk of ES, while abdominal pain, coma, respiratory distress, and a Babinski sign were associated with higher ES-associated mortality. Haplotype C*14/B*15 was associated with an elevated risk for ES (OR: 6.64; *p*-value: 0.008). Haplotypes A*23/C*14, A*23/B*15 and DR*07/B*58 also showed a weaker association with ES. This result supports the hypothesis that a genetically determined peculiar type of immune response confers susceptibility for ES.

Keywords: human African trypanosomiasis; treatment; melarsoprol; adverse event; encephalopathy; human leukocyte antigen; association study

---

1. Introduction

Human African trypanosomiasis (HAT, sleeping sickness) is a neglected tropical disease (NTD) caused by the protozoan parasites *Trypanosoma brucei gambiense* (Gambiense HAT, endemic in West and Central Africa) and *Trypanosoma brucei rhodesiense* (Rhodesiense HAT, endemic in Eastern and Southern

Africa). The disease is transmitted through the bite of infected tsetse flies. HAT caused devastating epidemics at the beginning and the end of the 20th century [1]. As a consequence of intense and sustained control and surveillance activities which developed in endemic countries in the last 25 years, incidence levels were brought down to an all-time historical low (<1000) in 2018. However, HAT cases are still being reported in more than 20 countries in intertropical Africa. Most of the reported cases (98%) are of Gambiense HAT, which usually causes a chronic form of infection and in which humans are the main reservoir of the parasite. Rhodesiense HAT, a zoonotic disease that occasionally affects humans, usually causes a more acute form of disease and accounts for the remaining number of cases. HAT has been targeted by WHO for sustainable elimination by 2030. The essential component of the elimination strategy is the treatment of all diagnosed cases in order to deplete the parasite's reservoir [2,3].

For over 50 years, successful treatment of sleeping sickness depended on correctly evaluating the degree of progression and severity of the disease. Following inoculation, infection remains temporally limited to the hemolymphatic system (hemolymphatic or early stage), but eventually progresses to central nervous system (CNS) invasion (meningo-encephalitic or late-stage). The transition between the early and late stage is insidious, and similar clinical features can exist in both stages [4]. The different penetration into the CNS, the pattern of adverse drug reactions, and the ease of use dictated the selection of the available drugs according to the disease stage until very recently. The early stage was treated with pentamidine or suramin because of the acceptable safety profile but insufficient drug levels in the cerebrospinal fluid (CSF). Late-stage *T.b. gambiense* HAT was typically treated with melarsoprol, and exceptionally with eflornithine. In 2009, the nifurtimox-eflornithine combination therapy (NECT) was added to the WHO essential drug list, replacing the more toxic drug, melarsoprol, as the first line of choice. NECT is, however, unreliable for the treatment of late-stage Rhodesiense HAT, and in this condition, melarsoprol remains the first choice [5]. In 2018, the European Medicines Agency gave a positive scientific opinion on the new oral monotherapy fexinidazole for use against both stages of Gambiense HAT, and subsequently, a marketing authorization was issued in the Democratic Republic of Congo [6]. The WHO updated their treatment guidelines accordingly in August 2019; melarsoprol is now limited to treatment of late-stage *T.b. rhodesiense* and as the last treatment option for relapse cases in *T.b. gambiense* HAT [7]. Clinical research to assess the efficacy of fexinidazole against *T.b. rhodesiense* has recently been initiated (ClinicalTrials.gov Identifier: NCT03974178).

Melarsoprol (Arsobal™), introduced in 1949, was the first drug to efficiently treat both forms of late-stage HAT. Melarsoprol is the combination of melarsen oxide (a trivalent organic arsenical) with dimercaprol (British anti-lewisite, a heavy metal chelator developed as an antidote to arsenical-based nerve gases) [8]. Melarsoprol administration is associated with many adverse drug reactions, but the most severe and feared one is the encephalopathic syndrome (ES). ES is a badly defined, life-threatening neurological complication. ES may occur at any time-point after the first melarsoprol administration and up to 30 days after the last one, with a median and peak occurrence around day nine of treatment [9]. The incidence of ES ranges from 2 to 10% of all melarsoprol treatments, and is associated with a case fatality rate (CFR) of about 50% [10]. In a systematic review on ES, the average frequency appeared to be higher in Rhodesiense HAT (8.0%) than in Gambiense HAT (4.7%), with a CFR of 57% and 44%, respectively [11]. Despite this significant impact and more than 50 years of extensive melarsoprol usage, sound scientific knowledge regarding ES is still scarce.

Melarsoprol-associated ES is mostly described as consisting in the unpredictable and abrupt development of convulsions and intense agitation, followed by coma. However, descriptions of ES characterized only by convulsions or by the sudden onset of coma without previous convulsions also exist [12–15]. Based on restricted clinical–neuropathological correlation data, three independent forms of ES have been suggested, consisting in the separate existence of convulsions, coma, or mental (psychotic) changes. The severe and usually fatal coma type of ES is described as an acute hemorrhagic leukoencephalitis that includes severe abnormalities in the brain stem, with fibrinoid necrosis of small vessels and ring and ball haemorrhages. It is not clear whether these forms correspond to the same etiology or if they are different phenomena. The prognosis of the three hypothetical forms also varies: coma, and to a lesser extent, convulsions are associated with high mortality, whereas the mental form is benign and self-limiting [16]. Furthermore, convulsions, episodes of decreased level of consciousness, and psychotic manifestations are common displays of the severe CNS damage that occurs in late-stage HAT [17].

The cause of ES was generally assumed to be an immune phenomenon occurring mainly in the CNS and involving a complex host–drug–parasite interaction [18–21]. The Human Leukocyte Antigen (HLA) complex is a gene complex encoding the major histocompatibility complex (MHC) proteins in humans [22]. HLA is accepted as the major determinant of the immune response in humans. HLA determines the differentiation between "self" and "non-self", and is involved in auto-immune diseases, as well as in determining susceptibility and resistance to several infectious diseases [23,24].

In order to improve the definition of the syndrome, to identify and quantify clinical risk factors for ES and for the ES case fatality rate, and also to determine whether an association between ES and Class I and II HLA antigens exists, we designed and conducted a case-control study with prospective data collection on the encephalopathic syndrome during treatment of late-stage Gambiense HAT with melarsoprol.

2. Materials and Methods

2.1. Study Design and Conduct

This was a case-control, non-blinded, non-randomized, non-interventive, multi-centre study, with prospective (i.e., before the patients were treated with melarsoprol) clinical data collection. Late-stage Gambiense HAT patients treated with melarsoprol and who developed or did not develop an encephalopathic syndrome were compared. The design of the study was nonparametric and aimed at testing whether or not the alleles of the HLA markers were distributed at random in patients suffering from ES [25]. The study was conducted from June 2002 in Angola and August 2002 in the DRC to November 2003.

Clearances were obtained from the ethical independent ethics committees of both Cantons of Basel (Switzerland) (Protocol approved under number 189/01), and of the Ministries of Health in Luanda (Angola) and Kinshasa (DRC). Informed consent was obtained from all participants or their legal tutors.

2.2. Study Sites

Participants were enrolled in six specialized HAT treatment centres supervised by the Instituto de Combate e Controlo das Tripanossomíases (ICCT) in Angola or by the Programme National de Lutte contre la Trypanosomiase Humaine Africaine (PNLTHA) in the Democratic Republic of Congo. In Angola, these centres were the Centro de Referência e Investigação de Viana (Luanda), N'Dalatando (Kwanza Norte Province), and Uíge (Uíge Province). In the DRC, participating centres were Mbuji Mayi (Kasai Oriental Province), Maluku (Kinshasa), and the Centre Neuro-Psycho-Pathologique (CNPP), Kinshasa.

2.3. Study Population

Inclusion criteria for cases and controls were as follows: (1) the patient had *T. b. gambiense* infection (confirmed either serologically or parasitologically in blood or lymph) and trypanosomes in CSF and/or CSF WBC count > 5 cells/mm^3 and/or clearly defined neurological signs; (2) the patient was treated with melarsoprol; (3) the patient was conscious at admission (Coma Score ≥ 9 in the modified Glasgow Coma Scale) and was not convulsing before the start of melarsoprol treatment; and (4) mental changes of the psychotic type were not reported in the anamnesis or observed before the start of melarsoprol treatment. A patient was considered a case of encephalopathic syndrome when the following criteria were fulfilled: (1) onset of coma; (2) onset of convulsions; and (3) onset of severe mental symptoms, such as psychotic reactions and/or abnormal behaviour (aggressivity, severe confusion or disorientation) requiring a therapeutic intervention.

Exclusion criteria for both cases and controls were as follows: (1) the patient received melarsoprol in association with any other anti-trypanosomal drug; (2) patient follow-up could not be assured for 30 days after discharge.

For each ES case, three controls were enrolled. The controls were selected as the next three HAT patients following an ES case who underwent final discharge examination after having successfully completed treatment with melarsoprol, and did not develop ES during the follow-up period (to cover for the rare possibility of a late-onset ES).

2.4. Study Methodology

Detailed clinical data was obtained from every admitted late-stage HAT patient (and/or from relatives) before melarsoprol was initiated and recorded in a Case Report Form (CRF). When a patient developed an ES, the characteristics of the clinical presentation, of the management and of the final outcome of the syndrome were additionally inserted into the CRF.

Management of HAT patients (i.e., admission, diagnosis, treatment, discharge, and follow-up) and of ES cases in the participating centres followed the guidelines established by the respective national program. A microscopic test for *Plasmodium* was performed if the development of an ES was suspected in a patient. The test result was made available to the clinical staff for adequate management of the patient. No additional changes in routine procedures were introduced.

Blood sample collection for HLA typing was performed once the diagnosis of ES was established (cases) and at discharge for controls. Blood was collected onto filter paper cards (Generation® Sample Collection Cards, Gentra Systems, MN, USA). Dried blood-spotted cards were inserted into sealable plastic bags and stored at room temperature.

2.5. Data Management

Data on CRFs was checked for inclusion and exclusion criteria and for completeness and consistency. Missing data and clarifications were obtained from the local investigators. Data from the CRFs was double-entered into two EpiData (http://epidata.dk/) databases—one for the demographic and clinical information of cases and controls, and the other for the description of ES cases. For analysis, the databases were merged and exported to the SPSS software package (SPSS for Windows, Rel. 15.5.0. 2002. SPSS Inc., Chicago, IL, USA).

2.6. HLA Typization

HLA typing was performed at the Molecular Genetics Laboratory of the Centro de Histocompatibilidade do Norte (North Histocompatibility Centre, CHN), Porto, Portugal, the reference facility for HLA typing for transplantation patients in Northern Portugal. Samples were typed for Class I HLA-A, HLA-B, and HLA-Cw molecules, and for Class II molecules of the HLA-DRB1 category using two different commercially available PCR-based reverse line blot assays that detect specific target DNA sequences by means of multiple immobilized sequence-specific oligonucleotide (SSO) probes [26–29]. The Dynal RELI™ SSO HLA Test (developed by Roche Molecular Systems, Inc. and manufactured by Dynal Biotech Ltd., Wirral, UK) for Class I molecules and the INNO-LiPA HLA-DRB1 Amplification and Hybridization Test (Innogenetics, Ghent, Belgium) for Class II molecules were used.

Hybridization was performed using an AutoLIPA (Innogenetics, Ghent, Belgium) automated assay processor, programmed to fit the Dynal RELI™ SSO HLA or the INNO-LiPA HLA-DRB1 hybridisation tests. To obtain the final HLA type, patterns were interpreted using the Dynal RELI SSO Pattern Matching Program, version 5.11 for Class I molecules (http://imgt.cines.fr) (Lefranc, 2003) or the LiPA interpretation software LiRAS™ for Class II molecules (using the latest available version from Abbott).

2.7. Statistical Analysis

Clinical data of ES cases and controls were compared using Pearson's X^2 or Fisher's test. Risk factors for ES and death from ES were assessed by calculating the corresponding Odds Ratio (OR) and the 95% confidence interval (CI) for binomial variables. The numeric variables' age and white blood cell count (WBC) in CSF were split into quartiles, and the Mann–Whitney test was used to compare medians; standard residual values while applying the X^2 test were checked for values above > [1.96]. For evaluation of the body mass index (BMI) and patient general status on admission, proportions were compared by cross tabulation. Three categories were defined for BMI, corresponding to severe malnutrition (BMI ≤ 18), moderate malnutrition (BMI > 18 and ≤20), and normal nutritional status (BMI > 20). General status was categorized as "Bad", "Fair", or "Good".

For the analysis of the relationship between HLA type and the frequency of ES, allele frequencies were compared among cases and controls by determining the *p* value of the X^2 test applied to a 2 × 2 contingency table. OR and CI were obtained for alleles showing a significant *p* value. Haplotype frequencies were calculated assuming that the two allele loci were in linkage disequilibrium (LD). LD parameter Δ was obtained by constructing a 2 × 2 contingency table and applying the formula originally described by Bodmer and Bodmer in 1970 [30]. LD Δ was then added to the product of allele frequencies. Significant differences in haplotype frequency in cases and controls were subsequently obtained using the X^2 test with Fisher's exact test, with the OR and CI.

3. Results

Case Report Forms of 76 potential cases of encephalopathic syndrome (ES) were received. After checking for inclusion and exclusion criteria, 69 ES cases and 207 control patients were retained and included for analysis. The center of enrolment and outcome of ES patients are described in Table 1.

Table 1. Origin and outcome of enrolled ES patients.

HAT Treatment Centre	Number of ES Patients	Deaths
Mbuji Mayi (DRC)	24 (35%)	10 (41.6%)
Viana (Angola)	21 (30%)	10 (47.6%)
Maluku (DRC)	8 (12%)	4 (50%)
Uíge (Angola)	7 (10%)	4 (57.1%)
N'Dalatando (Angola)	6 (9%)	3 (50%)
CNPP (DRC)	3 (4%)	1 (33.3%)

Thirty (43.3%) patients were female and 39 (56.5%) were male. The age of ES patients ranged from 4 to 67 years, with median and mean values of 26 and 30.6 years, respectively (std. deviation: 14.6 years). Three patients were less than 10 years old, and two patients were above 60 years. Ethnic heterogeneity in the study population was considerable. In Angola, patients belonged to the Kimbondo, Kikongo, Ovimbundo, and Bakongo ethnic groups. The determination of ethnic groups was not available in the DRC, since only the village of birth of the patient was recorded, due to difficulties found in attributing the correct ethnic group to individuals. All but five patients had parasitologically confirmed HAT. These five patients had been previously treated with pentamidine; late-stage HAT diagnosis was established according to a positive card agglutination test for trypanosomiasis (CATT) and more than 5 WBC/mm^3 in CSF. All patients were treated according to the abridged IMPAMEL schedule (2.2 mg/kg/day of melarsoprol for 10 consecutive days).

3.1. Characteristics of the Encephalopathic Syndrome

3.1.1. Clinical Features

ES was mainly characterized by convulsions followed by coma. Variations consisting of isolated convulsions or coma without convulsions occurred with lower frequencies (Table 2). Convulsions were observed in 85.5% of all cases, and 71% of the convulsive episodes were multiple. Convulsions led to coma in 55% of all ES cases, whereas coma not preceded by convulsions was observed in 14.5% of all ES cases. For coma characterization, we used a modified Glasgow Score, where unarousable coma is associated with a score of 7 or less. During the ES episode, the mean minimal score was 4.8, with a median score of 5 (Std. Deviation: 2.6) and the mean maximal score was 6.3, with a median score of 6 (Std. Deviation: 2.5). Additional signs, such as fever and maculopapular cutaneous lesions, were more frequent in the subgroup developing convulsions followed by coma (52% of cases developing fever and maculopapular lesions) than in the coma (20%) and convulsive (5%) sub-groups, respectively. The mental type of ES was not observed in the study.

Table 2. Type of manifestation of ES observed and discriminated according to the outcome. The existence of fever and/or maculopapular cutaneous eruption (urticaria) is also indicated.

Type of Manifestation of ES	Cases N/(%)	Outcome Survival n/%	Additional Signs n	Outcome Death N/%	Additional Signs n
Convulsion and coma	38/(55)	13/(18.8)	Fever in 3 Urticaria in 3 Fever and urticaria in 1	25/(36.2)	Fever in 15 Urticaria in 7 Fever and urticarial in 5
Convulsion without coma	21/(30.5)	19/(27.5)	Fever in 6 Urticaria in 4 Fever and urticaria in 2	2/(2.9)	Fever in 1
Coma without Convulsions	10/(14.5)	5/(7.2)	Fever in 2 Fever and urticaria in 1	5/(7.2)	Fever in 2 Urticaria in 1
Totals	69/(100)	37/(53.6)	Fever in 11 Urticaria in 7 Fever and urticaria in 4	32/(46.4)	Fever in 18 Urticaria in 8 Fever and urticaria in 6

Additional symptoms and signs characterizing ES cases and corresponding degrees are shown in Table 3. Degree 1 was defined as transient, mild, or localized. Degree 2 was defined as durable and needing intervention, intolerable, severe, or diffuse. For fever, Degree 1 was defined as 37.5–38.9 °C, and Degree 2 as more than 39 °C. For tachycardia, Degree 1 was defined as less than 100 bpm, and Degree 2 as more than 100 bpm. For hypotension, Degree 1 was defined as systolic blood pressure less than 80 mmHg, and Degree 2 as shock. Fundoscopic examination was not performed in ES patients.

More than half of the ES patients developed a deep malaise, entered a confusional status, and had fever. Apathy and agitation periods were frequent and could alternate. Two thirds of the patients were tachycardic, but hypotension was present in only 16% of them. Respiratory distress, consisting mainly in irregular respiratory patterns, frequently complicated the advanced phase of ES, preceding death. Nausea and vomiting were present in less than one quarter of the patients. A maculopapular eruption, conjunctival hyperaemia (red eye syndrome), or facial oedema were observed in half, one third, and one fifth of the patients, respectively. Additional signs observed were vertigo in up to one third of the patients and psychotic manifestations (hallucinations, delirium, panic attack, or aggressive behaviour), present in around one tenth of the patients. Damage to the cortical spinal tract, demonstrated by the Babinski sign, was present in one third of the patients. Meningeal irritation, demonstrated by neck rigidity, was observed in only 10% of the patients. Clinical signs of bleeding disorder were not observed.

Table 3. Symptoms and signs characterizing ES, according to the global frequency and discriminated for the degree of severity.

Characterization of ES Symptoms and Signs	Frequency (Global) % (n)	Frequency (Degree 1) %	Frequency (Degree 2) %
Malaise	79.7 (55)	20.3	59.4
Confusional state	78.3 (51)	26.1	52.2
Fever	69.6 (48)	52.2	17.4
Agitation	65.2 (45)	34.8	30.4
Tachycardia	60.9 (42)	39.1	21.7
Respiratory distress	59.4 (41)	36.2	23.2
Headache	56.5 (39)	37.7	18.8
Apathy	56.5 (39)	24.6	31.9
Maculopapular eruption	50.7 (35)	10.1	40.6
Chills	36.2 (25)	24.6	11.6
Red eye syndrome	33.3 (23)	33.3	0
Vertigo	29.0 (20)	20.3	8.7
Oedema (facial)	23.2 (16)	23.2	0
Vomiting	23.2 (16)	14.5	8.7
Babinski sign	20.3 (14)	20.3	0
Panic attack	18.8 (13)	14.5	4.3
Nausea	18.8 (13)	13.0	5.8
Hypotension	15.9 (11)	13.0	2.9
Hallucinations	10.1 (07)	8.7	1.4
Delirium	10.1 (07)	0	10.1
Nucal rigidity	10.1 (07)	10.1	0
Aggressive behaviour	07.2 (05)	4.3	2.9

3.1.2. Laboratory Evaluation of ES

Laboratory evaluation (haemoglobin, leukocyte count in blood and in CSF) within the duration of the ES episode was performed in 15 patients. Neither the leukocyte differential blood count nor the platelet counts were available. ES patients did not show severe anaemia or significant changes in the leukocyte blood count. To check for bacterial meningitis, a Gram-stained smear was performed in 14 CSF samples, always with a negative result. In 11 patients, CSF glucose content was also obtained, but was not simultaneously measured in blood. Half of the patients had glucose levels in CSF close to or below the accepted inferior limit of 50 mg/dL. No increase above the WBC count in CSF on admission was observed during ES. *Plasmodium* smear was negative in all ES cases evaluated for CSF parameters. Additional laboratory parameters for hepatic, renal, respiratory, and metabolic evaluation were not available at the Centres.

3.1.3. Time Point and Outcome for ES

The mean and median numbers of melarsoprol applications associated with the development of ES were 8.5 and 9 doses, respectively (Std. Deviation: 1.9; range: 2 to 10 doses). Melarsoprol was administered on consecutive days in all cases, except in one hypertensive patient due to hypertension peaks, in whom with treatment was interrupted for 2 days; 47.8% of patients developed ES with the 10th dose of melarsoprol. The number of melarsoprol administrations preceding the development of ES was not significantly different whether the initial manifestation of ES consisted of coma or convulsions (p value of the Mann–Whitney test: 0.26; all observed counts not statistically different from to those expected: all std. residuals below 1.96).

The mean time interval between the last application of melarsoprol and start of ES was 35.4 h. This interval is the time between melarsoprol administration and the development of symptoms and signs of an impending encephalopathy, during which subsequent doses of the drug are withheld. Half of the patients developed ES within 23.5 h after the last application, and 75% did so 47.7 h within the last drug application. Figure 1 shows the median time interval distribution for the development of ES after the last melarsoprol application, discriminated according to the outcome of ES. The interval for the occurrence of ES after the last dose of melarsoprol before ES was not significantly different between survivors and fatalities (Mann–Whitney test, *p* value: 0.08).

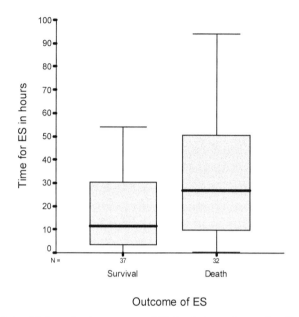

Figure 1. Time interval in hours for the occurrence of ES after the last melarsoprol application according to the final outcome. The inbox line in bold indicates the median. Outliers and extremes are not shown.

Encephalopathic syndromes led to a fatal outcome in 32 patients (46.4%). On average, death occurred 2.5 days after diagnosis of the syndrome (median: 1 day; std. deviation: 2.9 days; range 0–13 days). 80.6% of the patients died within three days after developing ES.

On average, ES manifestations ceased 2.2 days after initiation of the episode in the 37 surviving patients. The majority of surviving patients (73%) did not show any sequelae on discharge. When present, sequelae consisted in tremors (three cases), mental changes (confusion, euphoria, aggressivity) (three cases), paraplegia (two cases, one with urinary retention), speech disturbances (polylalia, dysarthria, aphasia) (three cases), and walking disability (one case).

3.1.4. Patient Management

All centres used corticosteroids (prednisone, hydrocortisone, occasionally combined with promethazine), antimalarials (chloroquine, sulfadoxine-pyrimethamine, or quinine), and anthelminthics (mebendazole, levamisole) and multivitamins for "patient preparation" before melarsoprol administration, aiming at reducing its toxicity.

All ES patients were managed with corticosteroids, except two patients (that survived). Half of the patients under corticosteroid therapy for ES died. Convulsions were managed with standard doses of diazepam and/or phenobarbital, which were frequently used simultaneously with promethazine. The difference in outcome in patients using the three diverse types of antipyretic (paracetamol, acetyl salicylic acid, or dipyrone) was not significant. Antibiotics (mainly ampicillin, in one patient in combination with gentamicin) were used when a severe bacterial infection, usually respiratory, was suspected during ES. The use of quinine, mannitol, furosemide, and adrenaline was associated with high mortality. No evident anomalies in the prescribed dosage of the drugs were detected.

Intravenous fluids (5% glucose in water or Ringer lactate) were used in 61 patients. A urethral catheter was inserted in 40 patients, and a nasogastric tube was used in 13. However, monitoring of fluid and caloric input/output was never recorded. Medical oxygen was not available in the centres.

3.2. Risk Factors for the Encephalopathic Syndrome

3.2.1. Clinical Factors

All variables in the questionnaire were analysed to determine if they constituted risk factors for the development of ES or for death from ES. Table 4 shows the variables obtained on admission that yielded a significant *p* value (<0.05) highlighted in bold. Selected variables with a higher *p* value when the OR indicated a tendency (≥2), even when the lower limit of the 95% CI was below 1, are also indicated. All other variables were below this threshold, and yielded insignificant *p* or OR values.

Table 4. Anamnesis, physical examination, and laboratory variables obtained during admission and corresponding statistical tests for association with the development of ES or death from ES.

Variable	Encephalopathy			Death		
	OR	95% CI	*p*	OR	95% CI	*p*
Anamnesis						
Oedema	**4.0**	**1.0–15.4**	**0.03**	1.8	0.2–11.5	0.09
Bone pain	2.3	1.2–4.3	0.10			
Paralysis	3.0	0.4–22.0	0.20			
Hypoestesia	2.0	0.3–12.2	0.40			
Abdominal pain				**4.5**	**1.5–14.0**	**0.006**
Conjunctivitis				**3.0**	**1.0–8.7**	**0.03**
Pruritus				**3.0**	**1.0–8.7**	**0.04**
Adenomegaly				2.2	0.7–6.1	0.1
Weight loss				2	0.6–6.6	0.2
Weakness/asthenia				2	0.5–7.4	0.3
Diarrhoea				4.9	0.9–25.6	0.4
Physical examination						
Apathy	**1.9**	**1.0–3.8**	**0.04**			
Depression	1.9	0.9–4.2	0.07			
Facial paralysis	3.5	0.6–17.8	0.1			
Incomprehensible Speech	2.2	0.5–7.7	0.2			
Babinski	2.2	0.6–7.7	0.3	3.6	0.4–36.7	0.2
Pale mucosa				2.4	0.2–27.7	0.4
Neck rigidity				2.4	0.2–27.7	0.4
Splenomegaly				2.8	0.2–33.6	0.4
Agitation				2.4	0.2–27.7	0.5

Patients reporting oedema in history or with apathy and/or depressed humour in the physical exam had a significant risk of developing ES. Patients who reported with abdominal pain, conjunctivitis, or pruritus in the anamnesis had a higher risk of dying from ES.

During the ES episode, coma (OR: 2.4, *p* value < 0.001), respiratory distress (OR: 5, *p* value: 0.002) and a Babinski sign (OR: 3.8, *p* value: 0.04) were significantly associated with death. Coma usually developed after convulsions, and respiratory distress often appeared as a terminal event. Respiratory distress was apparently not due to iatrogenic pulmonary oedema (no reference to physical signs of it was found). Tachycardia, hypotension, and, to a lesser extent, agitation were also marginally associated with death.

3.2.2. Laboratory Data

Laboratory evaluation on admission showed that none of the measured biological markers (Haemoglobin, WBC count in blood or in CSF) was clearly associated with the occurrence of ES. CSF WBC count on admission was analysed by dividing the results of the count in quartiles. The limit for the first quartile was found to be 100 WBC/mm^3 in the CSF. Additionally, the more conventional division of WBC count in CSF (less than 20 cells, 21 to 100 cells, and more than 100 cells in CSF) was also used in analysis (data not shown). Trypanosomes were found more frequently in the lymph (*p* value: 0.2, OR: 1.8) and in the CSF (*p* value: 0.2, OR: 2.2) of patients who developed ES, but possibly due to the small numbers, the difference was not statistically significant.

3.2.3. Concomitant Diseases

Of the 58 patients tested for malaria during ES, 13 (22.4%) were positive (thick smear) and 8 (61%) died, while 45 (77.6%) were negative and 23 (51%) died.

Diagnosis of other concomitant diseases on admission included oral candidosis, lymphatic filariasis, pulmonary tuberculosis, and orchitis in one patient each. The patient with oral candidosis did not develop ES, and the three others died from ES. During ES, a clinical diagnosis of respiratory infection was clearly established in two patients, and thereof, one died.

3.2.4. HLA Type

Alleles for every tested HLA category could be clearly determined for 62 ES cases and 189 controls. Samples showing any ambiguity in allele determination were excluded from the analysis. The statistical association between the HLA type and the development of ES is shown in Table 5.

Table 5. Frequency of deducted haplotypes in cases and controls, with OR and CI. (*) indicates Fisher's test was used. LD: linkage disequilibrium.

	Cases	Controls	*p*	OR	CI	LD Cases
C*14/B*15	6/62	3/189	0.008 (*)	6.64	1.35–41.96	0.038
A*23/C*14	3/62	1/189	0.04 (*)	9.56	0.74–50.4	0.01
A*23/B*15	13/62	22/189	0.06	2.0	0.88–4.56	0.04
DR*07/B*58	5/62	5/189	0.07 (*)	3.23	0.71–14.49	0.017

Deducted haplotype C*14/B*15 was associated with a risk more than 6.5 times higher of developing ES. The association is significant (*p* value: 0.008), but the upper limit of the CI is considerably large. Haplotype A*23/C*14 was also found to be potentially associated with ES (*p* value less than 0.05), with a risk nearly 10 times greater of developing ES with this haplotype, but the inferior limit of the CI is below one, suggesting that a greater number of patients is needed for confirmation. A*23/B*15 and DR*07/B*58 showed a tendency for association with ES, but the level of significance for these allele combinations is above a *p* value of 0.05.

4. Discussion

4.1. Characteristics of ES

Until today, this is the largest single study on ES patients that has ever been conducted. So far, the results were only published as a chapter of a PhD thesis [11]. When the study was carried out, melarsoprol was still the only routine option to treat late-stage HAT. Still, the findings have relevance today, since *T.b. rhodesiense* is still treated with this organoarsenic drug, even if we cannot affirm with complete confidence that the risk factors we found in our study will apply to ES associated with this form of sleeping sickness. Nevertheless, our findings are important because they contribute to the understanding of immunological processes in the development of severe adverse drug reactions in the brain.

The results are in line with the majority of publications describing ES. However, they do not support the hypothesis formulated in two publications that three separate forms of the phenomenon exist [9,16], which may rather be the result of observational bias. Our findings, derived from a multi-center prospective study specifically designed to investigate ES and therefore being potentially less bias-prone, suggest that full-blown ES consists in multiple convulsions, where half of the cases are followed by a deep coma. Variations consisting in isolated convulsions or coma without convulsions occurred with lower frequencies around this main pattern. Additional signs, such as fever and maculopapular cutaneous lesions, were more frequent in the subgroup developing convulsions followed by coma than in the coma and convulsive sub-groups. Patients showed profound malaise, mental confusion, and apathy alternating with agitation and tachycardia. Additional signs consisting in conjunctival hyperaemia and facial oedema were present in 1/3 and 1/5 of the patients, respectively.

The exclusively mental type of ES was not observed in the study. Four cases were initially enrolled as belonging to the exclusively mental type of ES. They were, however, excluded from analysis after the presence of severe mental changes in anamnesis in the course of HAT was detected prior to melarsoprol application. This suggests that previous descriptions of this hypothetical type of ES may also suffer from an observational bias, with mental changes already present but not detected in the patient history or under-evaluated in clinical examination. Alternatively, we may speculate that if an exclusively mental type of ES exists, the frequency of the phenomenon is probably very low.

Our patients were all treated with the consecutive 10 day melarsoprol schedule, which has been recommended by the International Scientific Council for Trypanosomiasis Research and Control for late-stage Gambiense HAT in 2003 and by the WHO in 2013 [5], in substitution of older complicated schemes [31]. In accordance with previous data [9], we could confirm that ES occurs preferably after the eighth dose of melarsoprol, and in half of the cases, with the 10th dose. The time-point for occurrence and the prognosis of ES have been the basis for discussions about the etiology and severity of the phenomenon. It has been shown that ES occurs at the same average point in time, independent of whether the abridged 10 consecutive days' constant dosage melarsoprol scheme or an older scheme of progressively increasing intermittent dosage (three series of 4 days with a 7 day interval) is used [31]. A subsequent study showed that both the coma and the convulsive types of ES also tend to occur at the same time-point [9]). In our study, the number of days elapsing before ES developed was similar for both initial manifestations of ES (coma or convulsions) and for the outcome (survival or death). A higher lethality of the hypothetical coma type of ES is described in the literature [9,16]. Our findings indicate that the highest mortality (36.2%) was instead associated with convulsions followed by coma (observed in 55% of the ES cases). Together with our findings on HLA involvement, these results give evidence that ES is an immunological phenomenon and that the different clinical presentations correspond to different severities of the same pathogenetic mechanisms. Further evidence might come from clinical–neuropathological correlation studies, as they would permit confirming the similarities between the neuropathological characteristics of ES and acute hemorrhagic leukoencephalitis (AHLE, Hurst disease), which is considered the most severe form of acute disseminated encephalomyelitis (ADEM). Patients with Hurst disease usually develop a severe CNS condition but, like in ES, different clinical expressions exist [32]). The anatomopathological changes found in AHLE [33] are very similar to the ones described in the coma type of ES by Haller in 1986.

In the literature, the development or intensification of unspecific signs, such as fever, headache, nausea, vomiting, dizziness, tremors, and conjunctival hyperaemia are considered leading signs of ES [34]. The search for distinct heralding signs of ES was an objective of our study protocol, but except for fever, they were generally not reported. However, the fact that clinicians stopped melarsoprol administration in an average of 35.4 h before the inclusion criteria for ES were reached indicates that they suspected the development of the complication.

In 80% of the patients reaching a fatal outcome, death occurred within three days. Surviving patients mostly recovered completely from ES in less than three days. These facts stress the need for careful and adequate patient surveillance while under treatment with melarsoprol so that a prompt diagnosis of ES can be made, and adequate therapeutic measures swiftly initiated. A lethal outcome was the result of ES in nearly half (46.4%) of the cases, with non-significant differences among the participating centres, which is within the range of mortality for ES in Gambiense HAT found in the literature.

None of the limited laboratory variables (haemoglobin and leukocyte count in blood and in CSF) evaluated during ES (rarely reported in the literature) in 15 patients proved useful in the confirmation of an ES diagnosis. We may conclude that there are no useful laboratory markers of ES available for use in the resource-limited rural African health facilities. However, glucose levels in CSF were close to or below the accepted inferior limit of 50 mg/dL in half of the patients, suggesting that low glucose levels in CSF, a potential triggering factor for convulsions, may be frequent in ES. To the best of our knowledge, this original finding could be important for patient management. The CSF Gram stain obtained in 14 ES patients was always negative, showing (with some degree of confidence) that ES patients in the study did not suffer from a confounding and potentially treatable bacterial meningoencephalitis.

4.2. Risk Factors for ES

Haplotype C*14/B*15 was significantly associated with ES. Three additional haplotypes (A*23/B*15, A*23/C*14, and DR*07/B*58) showed lesser degrees of association with ES, but sample size was insufficient for adequate statistical power. Alternatively, we may consider that the genetic component of ES could be polygenic or associated with a single major locus with other loci of small effect. The ethnical diversity observed in the clinical study was considerable, and the low numbers in the different ethnic groups was not sufficient to allow for sufficiently statistically powered ethnic stratification. As usual in genetic association studies, confirmation of these results would be needed in other populations. However, our data does suggest that there is a genetic predisposition for ES. This finding is in line with the described association between acute hemorrhagic leukoencephalitis (AHLE, Hurst disease), and particular, HLA haplotypes [32]. Since the physical map of the HLA complex genes is now available, it would be possible to explore the molecular basis of ES. Linkage of the Class II allele found in the study with Class III genes or non-HLA genes involved in the immune response, especially those related to the synthesis of the cytokines and mediators described in late-stage HAT could be explored to gain further insight into the etiology and pathogenesis of ES.

The following risk factors were consistently identified for ES and for death from ES, respectively: oedema, apathy, and a depressed humour; as well as abdominal pain, pruritus, and conjunctivitis. Additional variables, such as diarrhoea in patient history and facial paralysis and a positive Babinski sign on examination yielded elevated OR values, but their *p* values were below statistical significance. However, the identified symptoms and signs may be transitory and elusive, and may need a careful and detailed evaluation of the patient, which clearly limits their practical value, especially in the African setting. The absence of a clear association between elevated WBC in CSF and presence of trypanosomes in body compartments conflicts with findings from previous studies [9,10,18].

Concomitant infections, particularly malaria, have long been suspected of increasing the risk of ES [9,35]. The issue of concomitant infections and melarsoprol adverse events, including ES, was addressed in a large cohort of patients treated with a concise 10 day schedule [36]. Malaria parasites were found in 22.7% (40/176) of the patients suffering from ES, despite the fact that, as in our study, all patients received a full course of chloroquine or sulfadoxine and pyrimethamine or quinine during the preparation period prior to melarsoprol. In our study, 22.4% (13/58) of the patients showed a positive smear during ES. The role of *Plasmodium* infection in ES is difficult to establish, and its analysis is inherently associated with the quality of the malaria diagnosis, which was frequently low in the participating centres.

Malnutrition is very frequent in patients suffering from HAT. In one report, more than 20% of adults and 56% of the children with Gambiense HAT were affected [37]. A deficient nutritional status and a bad general status are empirically considered as having a significant impact on the risk for ES. However, in our clinical study, neither the general status nor the BMI was correlated with ES or death from ES, which is in accordance with the findings from a large and adequately powered melarsoprol trial (IMPAMEL II) [35].

4.3. Patient Management

Because this was a non-interventive study, and given the multiplicity of the drugs used and the low number of patients enrolled in some centres, we could not evaluate the usefulness of the individual drugs (prednisone, antimalarials, anthelminthics, and multivitamins) used for prevention of ES. Corticosteroids are presently accepted as beneficial in the prevention of ES and widely used for this purpose, but the validity of this intervention is not based on solid evidence [10,11,34].

Management of ES patients in our study with dexamethasone was associated with lower mortality (38.5%) when compared to hydrocortisone (50%), which was the most frequently used corticosteroid. Hydrocortisone has a high sodium retention action when used at the dose needed to reach significant anti-cerebral oedema action, and may contribute to water retention and pulmonary oedema. Dexamethasone, used as in cerebral oedema, offers a more adequate pharmacological profile, and this could explain the tendency for a lower mortality observed with this drug in our study. Limited evidence shows that methylprednisolone, in high (5 to 10 mg/kg/day) or very high (1000 mg/day for an adult) doses, may be useful in critical patients with viral encephalitis, acute disseminated encephalomyelitis (ADEM), and AHLE [38,39]. Such high-dose methylprednisolone schemes could be suitable in ES, given the similarities between these conditions and ES.

Quinine, furosemide, mannitol, and adrenaline can promote or increase cardiovascular arrhythmias, hypoglycaemia, and fluid and electrolyte imbalance, which, in addition to the frequent severe clinical deterioration of ES patients, may explain the high mortality associated with these drugs in our study. Their use in a critically ill ES patient is hazardous (especially without good monitoring equipment and as a combination) and should probably be limited to patients with accurately diagnosed malaria, strong evidence of fluid overload, raised intracranial pressure, shock, or severe bacterial infection.

Human African trypanosomiasis is nowadays considered a rare disease targeted for elimination [40]. Melarsoprol use in HAT is presently limited to rescue therapy of cases refractory to other drug treatments in Gambiense HAT and to Rhodesiense HAT late-stage patients, meaning that melarsoprol-related ES will become a rare event. In our opinion, this also means that patients in need of melarsoprol treatment should preferably be referred to specialized centres where knowledge on the correct management of complications associated with the use of this powerful but dangerous drug persists.

5. Conclusions

In conclusion, our study obtained a more precise definition of ES, which is useful in the correct diagnosis of the condition. The observed clinical risks factors for ES were elusive. A significant statistical association between Class I haplotype C*14/B*15 and ES was found. Patients expressing this haplotype have an almost 6.5 times higher risk of developing ES. Additionally, three other haplotypes were found to be possibly related to ES. This finding corroborates our hypothesis of an immunological involvement in the pathogenesis of ES. This result indicates that a genetically determined individual susceptibility exists that produces a peculiar type of immune response in the central nervous system that, in combination with the presence of trypanosomes and melarsoprol, results in a catastrophic condition in many aspects similar to acute hemorrhagic leukoencephalitis (AHLE, Hurst disease).

Author Contributions: Conceptualization, J.S., J.A. and C.B.; methodology, J.S., C.B.; validation, J.S., C.B., T.J., G.V., C.M.M.B. and P.L.; formal analysis, J.S.; investigation, J.S.; resources, J.S., C.B., T.J., G.V., C.M.M.B. and P.L.; data curation, J.S.; writing—original draft preparation, J.S.; writing—review and editing, J.S., C.B., J.A.,T.J., G.V. and P.L.; visualization, J.S.; supervision, J.S., J.A. and C.B.; project administration, J.S., C.B., T.J., G.V., C.M.M.B. and P.L.; funding acquisition, J.S. and C.B. All authors have read and agreed to the published version of the manuscript.

Trop. Med. Infect. Dis. **2020**, *5*, 5

Funding: The financial support for this study originated mainly from the Swiss Agency for Development and Cooperation (Berne, Switzerland). Additional financial support was also obtained from the Calouste Gulbenkian Foundation (Lisbon, Portugal), the World Health Organization (WHO/CDS, Geneva, Switzerland) and the Fondation Roche de Recherche en Afrique (Abidjan, Ivory Coast).

Acknowledgments: The authors are indebted to the patients and their families, to the clinicians that devoted their time and efforts to their patients in Angola: Amadeo Dala, João Lando, Francisco Manuel, Tito Bage, Francisco António Manuel, Quiala Godi and in the DRC:.Kazadi Kyanza Serge, Wakyhi Ilunga, Kazumba Leon, Kande Victor; to the staff of the North Histocompatibility Center: Helena Alves, Sandra Tafulo, Filomena Mendes and Bruno Lima; to the statistical consultant Luzia Gonçalves; to Cecile Schmid, and Johannes Blum at the Swiss TPH for their scientific advice and support; and to Louis Haller (Fondation Roche de Recherche en Afrique) for all his stimulating efforts to elucidate the nature of the encephalopathic syndromes.

Conflicts of Interest: The authors declare no conflict of interest. The funders had no role in the design of the study; in the collection, analyses, or interpretation of data; in the writing of the manuscript, or in the decision to publish the results.

References

1. Brun, R.; Blum, J.; Chappuis, F.; Burri, C. Human African trypanosomiasis. *Lancet* **2010**, *375*, 148–159. [CrossRef]
2. Franco, J.R.; Cecchi, G.; Priotto, G.; Paone, M.; Diarra, A.; Grout, L.; Simarro, P.P.; Zhao, W.; Argaw, D. Monitoring the elimination of human African trypanosomiasis: Update to 2016. *PLoS Negl. Trop. Dis.* **2018**, *12*, e0006890. [CrossRef] [PubMed]
3. WHO. *Accelerating Work to Overcome the Global Impact of Neglected Tropical Diseases—A Roadmap for Implementation*; WHO/HTM/NTD/2012.1; World Health Organization: Geneva, Switzerland, 2012.
4. Kennedy, P.G.E.; Rodgers, J. Clinical and Neuropathogenetic Aspects of Human African Trypanosomiasis. *Front. Immunol.* **2019**, *10*, 39. [CrossRef] [PubMed]
5. WHO. *Control and Surveillance of Human African Trypanosomiasis*; Technical Report Series No. 984; World Health Organization: Geneva, Switzerland, 2013.
6. Pelfrene, E.; Harvey Allchurch, M.; Ntamabyaliro, N.; Nambasa, V.; Ventura, F.V.; Nagercoil, N.; Cavaleri, M. The European Medicines Agency's. scientific opinion on oral fexinidazole for human African trypanosomiasis. *PLoS Negl. Trop. Dis.* **2019**, *13*, e0007381. [CrossRef] [PubMed]
7. WHO. *WHO Interim Guidelines for the Treatment of Gambiense Human African Trypanosomiasis*; World Health Organization: Geneva, Switzerland, 2019; ISBN 978-92-4-155056-7.
8. Fairlamb, A.H. Chemotherapy of human African trypanosomiasis: Current and future prospects. *Trends Parasitol* **2003**, *19*, 488–494. [CrossRef] [PubMed]
9. Blum, J.; Nkunku, S.; Burri, C. Clinical description of encephalopathic syndromes and risk factors for their occurrence and outcome during melarsoprol treatment of human African trypanosomiasis. *Trop. Med. Int. Health* **2001**, *6*, 390–400. [CrossRef]
10. Pepin, J.; Milord, F.; Khonde, A.N.; Niyonsenga, T.; Loko, L.; Mpia, B.; De Wals, P. Risk factors for encephalopathy and mortality during melarsoprol treatment of Trypanosoma brucei gambiense sleeping sickness. *Trans. R. Soc. Trop. Med. Hyg.* **1995**, *89*, 92–97. [CrossRef]
11. Seixas, J. Investigations on the Encephalopathic Syndrome during Melarsoprol Treatment of Human African Trypanosomiasis. Ph.D. Thesis, Instituto de Higiene e Medicina Tropical, Universidade Nova de Lisboa, Lisboa, Portugal, 2004.
12. Dutertre, J.; Labusquiere, R. La thérapeutique de la trypanosomiase. *Méd. Trop. (Marseille)* **1966**, *26*, 342–356.
13. Bertrand, E.; Serie, F.; Rive, J.; Compaore, P.; Sentilhes, L.; Baudin, L.; Ekra, A.; Philippe, J. La symptomatologie cardio-vasculaire dans la trypanosomiase humaine africaine à Trypanosoma gambiense. *Méd. Afr. Noire* **1973**, *20*, 327–339.
14. Ginoux, P.Y.; Bissadidi, N.; Frezil, J.L. Accidents observes lors du traitement de la trypanosomiase au Congo. *Méd. Trop. (Marseille)* **1984**, *44*, 351–355.
15. Scena, M.R. Melarsoprol toxicity in the treatment of human African trypanosomiasis: Ten cases treated with dimercaprol. *Cent. Afr. J. Med.* **1988**, *34*, 264–268. [PubMed]
16. Haller, L.; Adams, H.; Merouze, F.; Dago, A. Clinical and pathological aspects of human African trypanosomiasis (T. b. gambiense) with particular reference to reactive arsenical encephalopathy. *Am. J. Trop. Med. Hyg.* **1986**, *35*, 94–99. [CrossRef] [PubMed]

17. Atouguia, J.L.M.; Kennedy, P.G.E. Neurological aspects of human African trypanosomiasis. In *Infectious Diseases of the Nervous System*, 1st ed.; Davis, L.E., Kennedy, P.G.E., Eds.; Reed Educational and Professional Publishing Ltd.: Oxford, UK, 2000.

18. Pepin, J.; Milord, F. African trypanosomiasis and drug-induced encephalopathy; risk factors and pathogenesis. *Trans. R. Soc. Trop. Med. Hyg.* **1991**, *85*, 222–224. [CrossRef]

19. Hunter, C.A.; Jennings, F.W.; Adams, J.H.; Murray, M.; Kennedy, P.G.E. Subcurative chemotherapy and fatal post-treatment reactive encephalopathies in African trypanosomiasis. *Lancet* **1992**, *339*, 956–958. [CrossRef]

20. Bouteille, B.; Millet, P.; Enanga, B.; Mezui Me, J.; Keita, M.; Jauberteau, M.O.; Georges, A.; Dumas, M. Human African trypanosomiasis, contributions of experimental models. *Bulletin de la Société de Pathologie Exotique et ses Filiales* **1998**, *91*, 127–132.

21. Keiser, J.; Ericsson, O.; Burri, C. Investigations of the metabolites of the trypanocidal drug melarsoprol. *Clin. Pharmacol. Ther.* **2000**, *67*, 478–488. [CrossRef]

22. Choo, S.Y. The HLA system: Genetics, immunology, clinical testing, and clinical implications. *Yonsei Med. J.* **2007**, *48*, 11–23. [CrossRef]

23. Klein, J.; Sato, A. The HLA system. First of two parts. *N. Engl. J. Med.* **2000**, *343*, 702–709. [CrossRef]

24. Singh, N.; Agrawal, S.; Rastogi, A.K. Infectious diseases and immunity: Special reference to major histocompatibility complex. *Emerg. Infect. Dis.* **1997**, *3*, 41–49. [CrossRef]

25. Abel, L.; Dessein, A.J. Genetic epidemiology of infectious diseases in humans: Design of population-based studies. *Emerg. Infect. Dis.* **1998**, *4*, 593–603. [CrossRef]

26. Saiki, R.K.; Walsh, P.S.; Levenson, C.H.; Erlich, H.A. Genetic analysis of amplified DNA with immobilized sequence-specific oligonucleotide probes. *Proc. Natl. Acad. Sci. USA* **1989**, *86*, 6230–6234. [CrossRef] [PubMed]

27. Buyse, I.; Decorte, R.; Baens, M.; Cuppens, H.; Semana, G.; Emonds, M.P.; Marynen, P.; Cassiman, J.J. Rapid DNA typing of class II HLA antigens using the polymerase chain reaction and reverse dot blot hybridization. *Tissue Antigens* **1993**, *41*, 1–14. [CrossRef] [PubMed]

28. Bugawan, T.L.; Apple, R.; Erlich, H.A. A method for typing polymorphism at the HLA-A locus using PCR amplification and immobilized oligonucleotide probes. *Tissue Antigens* **1994**, *44*, 137–147. [CrossRef] [PubMed]

29. Begovich, A.B.; Erlich, H.A. HLA typing for bone marrow transplantation. New polymerase chain reaction-based methods. *JAMA* **1995**, *273*, 586–591. [CrossRef] [PubMed]

30. Bodmer, J.G.; Bodmer, W.F. Studies on African Pygmies. IV. A comparative study of the HLA polymorphism in the Babinga Pygmies and other African and Caucasian populations. *Am. J. Hum. Genet.* **1970**, *22*, 396–411. [PubMed]

31. Burri, C.; Nkunku, S.; Merolle, A.; Smith, T.; Blum, J.; Brun, R. Efficacy of new, concise schedule for melarsoprol in treatment of sleeping sickness caused by Trypanosoma brucei gambiense: A randomised trial. *Lancet* **2000**, *355*, 1419–1425. [CrossRef]

32. Tenembaum, S.; Chitnis, T.; Ness, J.; Hahn, J.S. Acute disseminated encephalomyelitis. *Neurology* **2007**, *68*, S23–S36. [CrossRef]

33. Lann, M.A.; Lovell, M.A.; Kleinschmidt-DeMasters, B.K. Acute hemorrhagic leukoencephalitis: A critical entity for forensic pathologists to recognize. *Am. J. Forensic. Med. Pathol.* **2010**, *1*, 7–11. [CrossRef]

34. Sina, G.C.; Triolo, N.; Trova, P.; Clabaut, J.M. L'encephalopathie arsenicale lors du traitement de la trypanosomiase humaine africaine a T. gambiense (à propos de 16 cas). *Ann. Société Belg. Méd. Trop.* **1977**, *57*, 67–73.

35. Buyst, H. The treatment of T. rhodesiense sleeping sickness, with special reference to its physio-pathological and epidemiological basis. *Ann. Société Belg. Méd. Trop.* **1975**, *55*, 95–104.

36. Schmid, C.; Richer, M.; Bilenge, C.M.; Josenando, T.; Chappuis, F.; Manthelot, C.R.; Nangouma, A.; Doua, F.; Asumu, P.N.; Simarro, P.P.; et al. Effectiveness of a 10-day melarsoprol schedule for the treatment of late-stage human African trypanosomiasis: Confirmation from a multinational study (IMPAMEL II). *J. Infect. Dis.* **2005**, *191*, 1922–1931. [CrossRef] [PubMed]

37. Blum, J.; Schmid, C.; Burri, C. Clinical aspects of 2541 patients with second stage human African trypanosomiasis. *Acta Trop.* **2006**, *97*, 55–64. [CrossRef] [PubMed]

38. Schwarz, S.; Mohr, A.; Knauth, M.; Wildemann, B.; Storch-Hagenlocher, B. Acute disseminated encephalomyelitis: A follow-up study of 40 adult patients. *Neurology* **2001**, *56*, 1313–1318. [CrossRef] [PubMed]
39. Nakano, A.; Yamasaki, R.; Miyazaki, S.; Horiuchi, N.; Kunishige, M.; Mitsui, T. Beneficial effect of steroid pulse therapy on acute viral encephalitis. *Eur. Neurol.* **2003**, *50*, 225–229. [CrossRef]
40. Büscher, P.; Cecchi, G.; Jamonneau, V.; Priotto, G. Human African trypanosomiasis. *Lancet* **2017**, *390*, 2397–2409. [CrossRef]

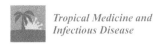

Tropical Medicine and Infectious Disease

Opinion

From Colonial Research Spirit to Global Commitment: Bayer and African Sleeping Sickness in the Mirror of History

Ulrich-Dietmar Madeja * and Ulrike Schroeder

Bayer AG Pharmaceuticals, Müllerstrasse 178, 10785 Berlin, Germany; ulrike.schroeder@bayer.com
* Correspondence: ulrich-dietmar.madeja@bayer.com

Received: 27 January 2020; Accepted: 4 March 2020; Published: 10 March 2020

Abstract: In the early 20th century, a series of epidemics across equatorial Africa brought African sleeping sickness (human African trypanosomiasis, HAT) to the attention of the European colonial administrations. This disease presented an exciting challenge for microbiologists across Europe to study the disease, discover the pathogen and search for an effective treatment. In 1923, the first "remedy for tropical diseases"—Suramin—manufactured by Bayer AG came onto the market under the brand name "Germanin." The development and life cycle of this product—which today is still the medicine of choice for Trypanosoma brucei (T.b), hodesiense infections—reflect medical progress as well as the successes and failures in fighting the disease in the context of historic political changes over the last 100 years.

Keywords: African sleeping sickness; development of treatment; suramin; medical history; political history

---

By the middle of the 19th century, several international health conferences had already set themselves the goal of protecting the colonial countries from tropical diseases such as smallpox, cholera, plague and yellow fever. Then, at the beginning of the 20th century after several epidemics across equatorial Africa, the colonial powers became aware of an additional disease, African sleeping sickness (human African trypanosomiasis, HAT), which posed a threat not only to Europeans travelling to the colonies but also to the local population, as well as to the economic value of the colonies themselves for their ruling countries.

The colonial powers' response was immediate for humanitarian reasons, but humanitarianism reflected the sentiment of the time—"a mixture of benevolent condescension and outright racism" [1] towards the local population—as illustrated by the colonialists' claim that they were "saving hapless Africans from the diseases that plagued them" [1]. However, their intervention was also based on practicalities, such as the need to protect their source of manpower in the thinly populated equatorial zone. Transport at this time relied on human porters or canoes because pack animals were unable to survive in regions infested with tsetse flies. This new epidemic and the resulting deaths among the local population not only caused transport problems, but also aggravated agricultural development, thus threatening to thwart plans to further exploit the colonies [1,2]. However, the turn of the century was also the heyday of microbiology in Europe. Motivated scientists were eager to discover new pathogens, explore life cycles of vectors and develop vaccines and potential new treatments. African sleeping sickness, which posed such a problem for colonial administrations, thus presented a great challenge for microbiologic research [1].

In fact, the challenge was so great as well as worrying that from 1901 to 1913 the colonial administrations sent a total of 15 special research missions to Africa to study the new disease [3,4]. Eight of these missions were from Great Britain, who hosted a major conference on African sleeping sickness in London in 1907–1908 attended mainly by scientists from Britain, France, Germany and Portugal. Recent research findings as well as potential new drugs for treatment and prophylactic measures were discussed. At the same time, Germany and Great Britain were also active on a political level. They implemented steps to stop Africans infected with the disease from crossing borders and then, in 1911, they signed an agreement outlining their plans to jointly fight African sleeping sickness in West Africa.

Bayer, which had been involved in the production and sale of synthetic dyes since its founding in 1863, expanded its activities at the end of the 19th century to include other business areas. In 1891, the chemist and later CEO of Bayer, Carl Duisberg (1861–1935), established a scientific laboratory and efficient research department in Wuppertal-Elberfeld where dyestuffs and their intermediates were developed, as well as pharmaceuticals (e.g., acetylsalicylic acid, Aspirin™). Unlike the first discoveries of medicines which were based on success in the treatment of disease symptoms, research at this time increasingly focused on combating newly discovered pathogens. It was German physician and Nobel prize winner Paul Ehrlich (1854–1915) who defined the term chemotherapy as the "creation of a chemical that would attack a specific pathogen" [1]. He demonstrated that dyes could also be effective against specific pathogens. The so-called trypan dyes were identified as being effective against animal trypanosomes but turned out to be too toxic to be used for treatment of human African trypanosomiasis.

In 1909, Wilhelm Roehl (1881–1929), Ehrlich's former assistant, asked Duisberg to help by providing dyes and money for animal experiments. Heinrich Hoerlein, head of Bayer's Pharmaceutical Department since 1910, realized the importance of Roehl's work and employed him. In 1916, with the help of a small team of chemists, he developed the first effective drug for the treatment of African sleeping sickness: the compound "Bayer 205," a colorless and odorless urea derivative which was later named Suramin.

In 1921, the compound was successfully tested on animals and passed on to the Hamburg Clinic for Tropical Diseases for further testing. There, the English engineer Christopher G. James had been suffering from sleeping sickness for over eight months. James had contracted the infection in Rhodesia and seemed to have little chance of survival. After only a few injections with "Bayer 205," however, Christopher G. James was well again and was able to travel back to Africa [5].

Encouraged by this success, Bayer sent an expedition to South Africa to carry out the necessary field trials on site, despite the difficult conditions after the First World War. The German microbiologist and pharmacologist Friedrich Karl Kleine (1869–1951), an expert in African sleeping sickness research, took the lead. In November 1921, the expedition, equipped with 30 kg of "Bayer 205," set off from Cape Town to Rhodesia (Figures 1–3).

The scientific experiments began in January 1922 and showed that oral applications only had a temporary effect and that injections were much more effective. The results were so convincing that the Governor General of Belgian Congo even invited the expedition to continue its work in the southern Congo region. In 1923, the "remedy for tropical diseases"—Suramin—came onto the market under the patriotic name "Germanin" (Figure 4).

After the First World War, scientific collaborations across Europe slowly resumed. As part of its war reparations and in an attempt to regain possession of its former colonies, Germany expressed its willingness to reveal the secret formula of Suramin. After consultations, France and Great Britain agreed not to accept the offer [1]. A French pharmacologist Ernest Fourneau (1872–1949) succeeded in reverse-engineering the drug based on patents that Bayer had taken out and renamed it "Fourneau 309" [1,6–8]. The pharmaceutical company Rhône-Poulenc marketed it then under the trade name "Moranyl."

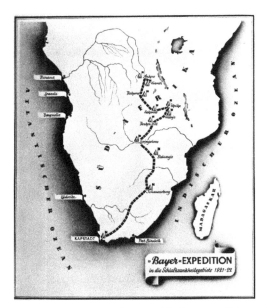

Figure 1. (Bayer Archive. 1921. (Picture 0-19682)) Route of the Bayer expedition starting on 2 November 1921 in Cape Town, travelling to the areas most affected by African sleeping sickness in what is today Tanzania, Burundi, Ruanda, DR Congo as well as a small part of Mozambique, Zimbabwe and Zambia, where the expedition ended in Kiambi in late 1922.

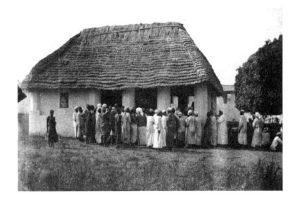

Figure 2. (Bayer Archive. 1921. (Picture 0-34295)) Screening of local population for symptoms of African sleeping sickness in the Urambi camp at Lake Tanganyika in 1921.

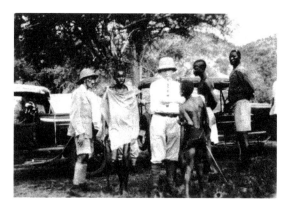

Figure 3. (Bayer Archive. Karl Friedrich Kleine with a Patient (Picture 0-3438301)) Friedrich Karl Kleine demonstrating the palpation of lymph nodes during screening of patients.

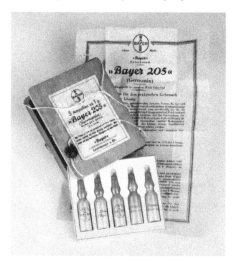

Figure 4. (Bayer Archive. Product "Bayer 205", ca. 1934. (Picture 0-25791)) Pack of ampoules of "Bayer 205" (Germanin), ca. 1934.

Despite being effective in the treatment of the first stage of African sleeping sickness, Suramin was not able to reverse the disease course once the trypanosomes had penetrated the blood-brain barrier. As such, Suramin remained the treatment of choice for acute cases of African sleeping sickness [4].

The availability of Suramin played a significant role in controlling the 1920s epidemic and subsequent outbreaks and in significantly decreasing the number of reported cases until the 1940s. At that time new treatments also became available. Pentamidine, discovered in 1940, started to be used for the treatment of the first stage of T.b. *gambiense* infections. In 1949, Melarsoprol was discovered and used for the treatment of both T.b. *gambiense* and T.b. *rhodesiense* infections. Due to being derived from arsenic, this treatment had many undesirable side effects, some even fatal. Furthermore, increased resistance to Melarsoprol had been observed in certain focal disease areas, particularly in central Africa.

Over the years, the colonial powers introduced extensive screening of populations at risk by mobile teams and implemented early vector control measures [9]. The disease was under control by the mid-1960s with fewer than 5000 cases reported across the African continent (Figure 5) [5].

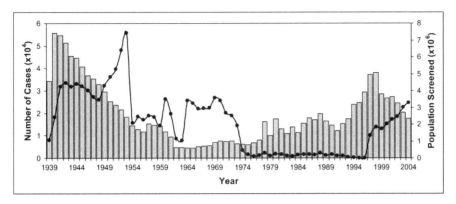

Figure 5. Number of cases of African sleeping sickness reported and population screened [5,10–12]. Graphs show the correlation between population screened (black circles) and number of reported cases (grey columns). Screening and surveillance of endemic disease areas are key to control African sleeping sickness.

By the mid-1960s, most countries affected by African sleeping sickness became independent. Support from the colonial powers ended and most African countries experienced an era of political instability and economic downturn. The effect on health services and on the control and prevention of endemic tropical diseases was disastrous. Consequently, disease control programs were stopped and population screening declined considerably. This situation provoked a new epidemic of African sleeping sickness.

During the 1950s to early 1970s, extensive insecticide spraying was the method of choice for vector control and resulted in a significant reduction in tsetse fly populations, as they are the vector for African sleeping sickness, but concerns about the environmental effect of DDT (Dichlordiphenyltrichlorethan) led to a worldwide ban in the late 1970s.

Since the mid-1970s, decreasing vector control and disease prevention as well as screening and treatment of populations at risk resulted in a steady increase in the number of reported cases of African sleeping sickness. This most recent epidemic lasted until the late 1990s. Around the year 2000, the scale of African sleeping sickness had once again almost reached the levels of the epidemics seen at the beginning of the 20th century (Figure 5) [11,13].

Suramin was added to the "WHO Model List of Essential Medicines" in 1979 and became the medicine of choice for T.b. *rhodesiense* infections, even though the published clinical evidence to support the use of the product remained limited. With no more disease control programs in place in Africa, the demand for medicines to treat African sleeping sickness decreased to a very low level. The only new product, Eflornithine, was registered in 1990. This molecule has shown to be less toxic than Melarsoprol but is only effective against T.b. *gambiense*. Furthermore, the treatment regimen is complex and difficult to apply.

In 1999, pharmaceutical companies started to question whether to continue manufacturing products which were in such low demand. Aventis proposed a substantial increase in price for further supplying Pentamidine, a second-line option to Suramin since 1937. The production of Melarsoprol, used for the treatment of second-stage disease caused by T.b. *rhodesiense* when the central nervous system is involved, became uncertain because of ongoing discussions in Europe over manufacturing the required raw materials containing arsenic. On several occasions, Bayer, which was still producing Suramin on the grounds that no alternative treatments were available, also threatened to halt production [14].

After the colonial-motivated push for research and control of African sleeping sickness in the early 20th century, the increased efforts of WHO, national control programs, bilateral cooperation and nongovernmental organizations (NGOs) have been able to reverse the curve of reported cases after the year 2000, ending the last major epidemic. The availability of novel diagnostic tools such as rapid diagnostic tests (RDTs) and raising awareness in the political will of local countries to fight African sleeping sickness played a crucial role in advancing disease control.

WHO also started public-private partnerships with pharmaceutical companies to secure the supply of the essential medicines to treat African sleeping sickness. In 2001, WHO and the pharmaceutical companies Bayer AG and Aventis (now Sanofi) reached an agreement to provide their medicines to treat African sleeping sickness free of charge for endemic countries. Pharmaceutical companies started to engage beyond donation of medicines and to provide much needed financial contributions for screening of focal disease areas by mobile intervention teals, surveillance and disease mapping, as well as training and public awareness programs. Within the period 2000–2018 the number of reported cases dropped by 95%.

The development of new treatment regimens and products has been part of this success story. In 2009, the new Nifurtimox Eflornithine Combination Therapy (NECT) was introduced for the treatment of T.b. *gambiense* infections. It simplified the use of eflornithine by reducing the duration of treatment and the number of intravenous infusions. In the same year, the combination of Nifurtimox (produced by Bayer) and originally registered for the treatment of American trypanosomiasis, with Eflornithine (produced by Sanofi) was included in the "WHO List of Essential Medicines" and is currently recommended as first-line treatment for the T.b. *gambiense* form. Since 2009, both pharmaceutical companies have been providing these products free of charge to WHO for endemic countries. The products are packed in a patient treatment kit containing all the material needed for their administration in remote rural areas [15].

In 2005, the development of Fexinidazole as the first-all oral treatment for T.b. *gambiense* infected patients started. On 10 July 2019, the WHO added the product to the "WHO List of Essential Medicines." Fexinidazole is indicated for first stage and non-severe second stage and it can simplify and facilitate case management of human African trypanosomiasis caused by T.b. *gambiense* [16].

Under the lead of WHO and the implementation of efficient disease control programs, the number of reported cases of African sleeping sickness dropped below 10,000 (9878) in 2009 for the first time in 50 years and continued to decline with only 997 new cases reported in 2018, the lowest level since the start of systematic global data-collection 80 years ago [15].

One hundred years ago, Suramin was discovered as the first effective treatment of African sleeping sickness. The history of this product and the motivation for fighting African sleeping sickness have changed significantly over time and reflect the historic medical and political changes. In 2012, the "WHO Roadmap on Neglected Tropical Diseases (NTDs)" set the goal to achieve the sustainable elimination of African sleeping sickness as a public health problem by 2020. This goal was reached by WHO and partners a concerted high-impact approach.

New clinical developments are essential to overcome the development of cross-resistance of currently used substances and to advance treatment options. Surely, one of these "will finally put suramin to rest and ease this esteemed great-grandfather of chemotherapy into a well-deserved retirement" [17]. Along with other interventions, the next goal of achieving disruption of transmission of African sleeping sickness, as outlined in the "WHO NTD Roadmap 2030," seems now to be very feasible.

Author Contributions: Both authors equally contributed. All authors have read and agreed to the published version of the manuscript.

Funding: This research received no external funding.

Conflicts of Interest: The authors declare no conflict of interest.

Trop. Med. Infect. Dis. **2020**, *5*, 42

References

1. Headrick, D.R.; Büscher, P.H. Sleeping Sickness Epidemics and Colonial Responses in East and Central Africa, 1900–1940. *PLoS Negl. Trop. Dis.* **2014**, *8*, 4. [CrossRef] [PubMed]
2. Neill, D.J. *Networks in Tropical Medicine: Internationalism, Colonialism, and the Rise of a Medical Specialty, 1890–1930*; Stanford University Press: Stanford, CA, USA, 2012; pp. 104, 105, 111–133, 158–175.
3. Tilley, H. Ecologies of complexity: Tropical environments, African trypanosomiasis, and the science of disease control in British colonial Africa, 1900–1940. *Osiris* **2004**, *19*, 21–38. [CrossRef] [PubMed]
4. Tilley, H. *Africa as a Living Laboratory*; University of Chicago Press: Chicago, IL, USA, 2011; pp. 176–191.
5. Steverding, D. The history of African trypanosomiasis. *Parasit. Vectors* **2008**, *1*, 3. [CrossRef] [PubMed]
6. Ehlers, S. *Europa und die Schlafkrankheit: Koloniale Seuchenbekämpfung, Europäische Identitäten und Moderne Medizin 1890–1950*; Vandenhoeck & Ruprecht: Göttingen, Germany, 2019.
7. Fourneau, E.; Théfouël, J.; Vallée, J. Sur une nouvelle série de médicaments trypanocides. *C. R. Séances L'acad. Sci.* **1924**, *178*, 675.
8. Pope, W.J. Synthetic therapeutic agents. *BMJ* **1924**, *1*, 413–414. [CrossRef] [PubMed]
9. Fourneau, E.; Tréfouël, J.; Tréfouël, T.B.; Vallée, J. Recherches de chimiothérapie dans la série du 205 Bayer: Urées des acides aminobenzoylaminonaphtaléniques. *Ann. L'inst. Pasteur* **1924**, *38*, 81–114.
10. De Raadt, P. The History of Sleeping Sickness. WHO. 2005. Available online: http://www.who.int/trypanosomiasis_african/country/history/en (accessed on 9 March 2020).
11. WHO/CDS/CSR/ISR/2000.1. *WHO Report on Global Surveillance of Epidemic-Prone Infectious Diseases*; Chapter 8—African Trypanosomiasis; World Health Organization: Geneva, Switzerland, 2000; pp. 95–106.
12. WHO. Human African Trypanosomiasis (sleeping sickness): Epidemiological update. *Wkly. Epidemiol. Rec.* **2006**, *81*, 71–80.
13. Stich, A.; Steverding, D. Trypanosomen—Die Rückkehr einer Seuche. *Biol. Unserer Zeit* **2002**, *32*, 294–302. [CrossRef]
14. Etchegorry, M.G.; Helenport, J.P.; Pecoul, B.; Jannin, J.; Legros, D. Availability and Affordability of treatment for Human African Trypanosomiasis. *Trop. Med. Int. Health* **2002**, *6*, 957–959. [CrossRef] [PubMed]
15. WHO/HAT. Available online: https://www.who.int/trypanosomiasis_african/en/ (accessed on 20 January 2020).
16. DNDi/HAT/Fexinidazole. Available online: https://www.dndi.org/diseases-projects/portfolio/fexinidazole/ (accessed on 1 March 2020).
17. De Koning, H.P. The Drugs of Sleeping Sickness: Their Mechanisms of Action and Resistance, and a Brief History. *Trop. Med. Infect. Dis.* **2020**, *5*, 14. [CrossRef] [PubMed]

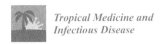 *Tropical Medicine and Infectious Disease*

Review

The Drugs of Sleeping Sickness: Their Mechanisms of Action and Resistance, and a Brief History

Harry P. De Koning

Institute of Infection, Immunity and Inflammation, University of Glasgow, Glasgow G12 8TA, UK; Harry.de-Koning@glasgow.ac.uk; Tel.: +44-141-3303753

Received: 19 December 2019; Accepted: 16 January 2020; Published: 19 January 2020

Abstract: With the incidence of sleeping sickness in decline and genuine progress being made towards the WHO goal of eliminating sleeping sickness as a major public health concern, this is a good moment to evaluate the drugs that 'got the job done': their development, their limitations and the resistance that the parasites developed against them. This retrospective looks back on the remarkable story of chemotherapy against trypanosomiasis, a story that goes back to the very origins and conception of chemotherapy in the first years of the 20 century and is still not finished today.

Keywords: sleeping sickness; human African trypanosomiasis; trypanosoma brucei; drugs; drug resistance; history

1. Introduction

The first clue towards understanding drug sensitivity and, conversely, resistance, in human African trypanosomiasis (HAT) is that most drugs are very old and quite simply toxic to any cell—if they can enter it. That places the mechanisms of uptake at the centre of selectivity, toxicity and resistance issues for all the older trypanocides such as diamidines (e.g., pentamidine, pafuramidine, diminazene), suramin and the melaminophenyl arsenicals. Significantly, none of these drug classes, dating from the 1910s to the 1940s, were designed for a specific intracellular target and even today identification of their targets has defied all attempts with advanced postgenomic, proteomic and metabolomic techniques—in short, they are examples of polypharmacology, where the active agent acts on multiple cellular targets. One might say they are non-specifically toxic. As such, resistance is unlikely to occur from mutations that change the binding site of a particular intracellular protein. Rather, the resistance mechanisms have been associated with mechanisms of cellular uptake and/or distribution. Some of the newer drugs have a more defined mode of action, and are selective at target level, but resistance to eflornithine, at least, is still associated with the loss of the *T. brucei* transporter that internalises it, rather than with the target enzyme. In the sections below I will examine these issues for each drug separately and show how resistance and treatment failure have changed clinical treatment of sleeping sickness and stimulated the development of the newer generations of drugs, culminating in the latest additions to the arsenal (fexinidazole, acoziborole) [1–4].

2. Diamidines

The development of the diamidines arose from the observations that advanced (animal) trypanosomiasis is often associated with hypoglycaemia [5,6] and trypanosomes metabolise glucose at a phenomenal rate. This suggested that the chemical induction of hypoglycaemia might be deleterious to trypanosomes in the bloodstream. Several groups tested insulin and other hypoglycaemia-inducing therapies against trypanosomiasis but with at best mild and variable success [7,8]. However, the synthetic insulin substitute synthalin (**1**; for structures see Figure 1) did have remarkable, curative trypanocidal activity [8,9] and, importantly, was not cross-resistant with the aromatic arsenicals used at the time, nor with suramin ("Bayer 205") [10]. Although it was not immediately clear to what extent this could be attributed to effects on blood sugar levels, that question was rapidly settled by the trypanocidal effects of synthalin on ex vivo trypanosomes [11]. By 1939, Lourie and Yorke, in collaboration with A. J. Ewins of May & Baker Ltd, reported on a large series of new diamidine compounds, among them 4,4'-diamidinostilbene (stilbamidine, **2**) and 4,4'-diamidino,1,5-diphenoxy pentane (pentamidine, **3**) [12]. Stilbamidine was the most active compound—curative with 25–50 µg per 20 g mouse (1.25–2.5 mg/kg b.w.) and a therapeutic index of 30—closely followed by propamidine (**4**) and pentamidine, which displayed a slightly lower therapeutic index of 15. To appreciate the enormous advance this signified, these numbers need to be compared to the dramatically higher minimum curative doses for the aromatic arsenicals then in use: 1000 mg/kg for tryparsamidine (**5**) or 250 mg/kg for atoxyl (**6**), each with a therapeutic index of just two [12]! As stilbamidine appeared to induce adverse neurological sequelae in early clinical trials [13], it was abandoned and pentamidine became the drug of choice for early stage HAT, especially of the *gambiense* variety. The now exclusively veterinary analogue diminazene aceturate ("Berenil", **7**) has also been used initially (and later sporadically) against HAT [14,15], but this practice has long been discontinued.

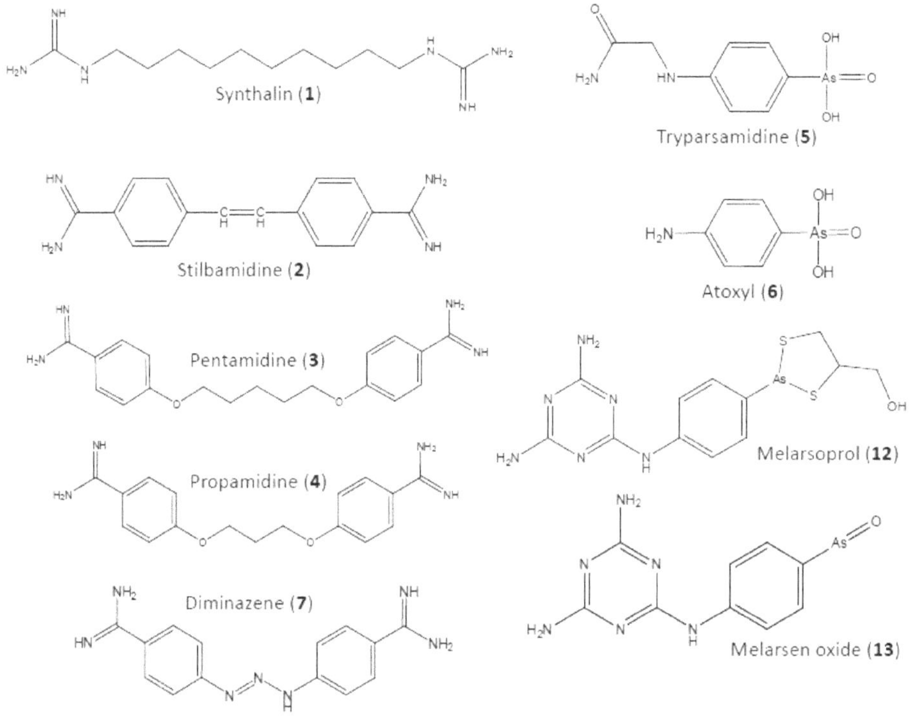

Figure 1. *Cont.*

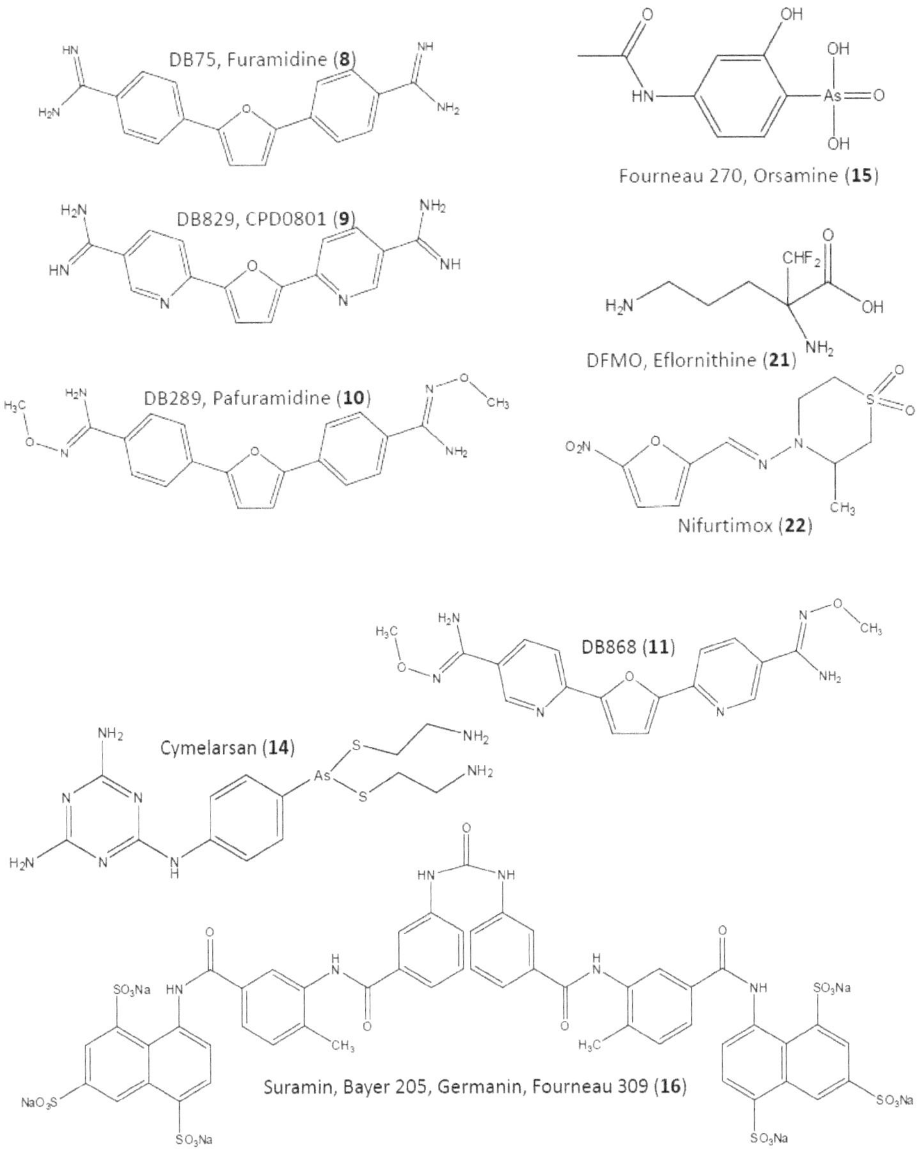

Figure 1. *Cont.*

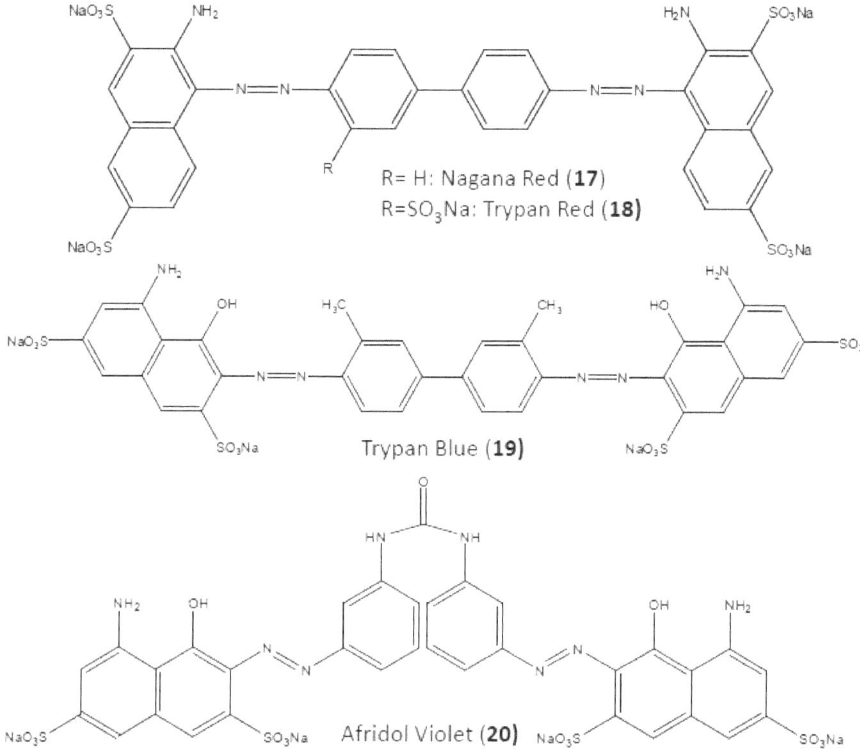

Figure 1. Structural formulas of trypanocides.

Diamidines are believed to be minor groove binders and as such bind to the DNA double helix, particularly targeting AT-rich sequences [16–19], impeding replication and transcription processes in the kinetoplast and/or nucleus. Usually, they accumulate strongly in the trypanosome's single mitochondrion (and mitochondria of cancer cells [20]), the compartmentalisation of these dications being driven by the mitochondrial membrane potential and binding to the kinetoplast DNA (kDNA) (for a schematic of the trypanosome structure, see Figure 2). Indeed, fluorescent diamidines light up the kinetoplast within 1 minute of administration, a process that is much delayed in resistant parasites [21]. Thus, pentamidine is known to accumulate up to mM levels inside trypanosomes [22] and does not exit the cell when the extracellular drug is removed [23]. Furamidine (8) and its analogues reportedly accumulate to > 10 mM, associating strongly with kinetoplast and nuclear DNA [17,24]. Similar processes drive mitochondrial accumulation of other cationic trypanocidal agents including isometamidium [25], symmetrical compounds with choline-like head groups [26], furamidines [21,27,28], shielded bis-phosphonium compounds [29] and inhibitors of Trypanosome Alternative Oxidase (TAO) linked to a lipophilic cation [30,31]. Resistance to minor groove binders cannot occur via mutations in the target and the binding affinity does not need to be very high if the accumulation of the drug is to the high local concentrations reported. Thus, resistance is associated with the inability of the diamidine to reach its target, either by preventing its uptake into the cell altogether, or at least preventing its accumulation in the mitochondrion. The latter mechanism was demonstrated in pentamidine-resistant *Leishmania mexicana* parasites [32].

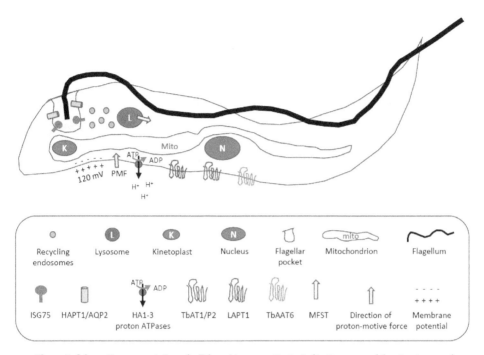

Figure 2. Schematic representation of a *T. brucei* trypomastigote, indicating some of the structures and proteins involved in the uptake or mechanism of action of trypanocides.

While pentamidine is used exclusively for the treatment of stage I (haemolymphatic) HAT, there have been reports of successes with 'early late stage' infections, where the parasite has crossed the blood-brain barrier (BBB) but not yet fully penetrated the brain parenchyma [33]. In particular, a study from 1996 reported a cure rate of 94% of early-late stage HAT patients with pentamidine [34]. Thus, pentamidine must be aided across the BBB by a transporter, and Sekhar et al. identified the Organic Cation Transporter 1 (OCT1) as responsible for the process [35], as previously reported in experiments with cell lines expressing all three human OCT isoforms [36]. The reason that pentamidine is not active against cerebral trypanosomiasis, then, is because it is actively extruded again from the CNS to the blood, by P-glycoproteins (P-gp), Multidrug Resistance-Associated Proteins (MRPs) or other extrusion transporters [37]; Yang et al (2014) later reported that pentamidine and the furamidines are not substrates for P-gps [38]. Other diamidines such as diminazene and furamidine are equally ineffective against cerebral trypanosomiasis [39–41], and the distribution of DB75, although readily detectable in-whole brain extracts, was limited to the cells lining the BBB and blood–cerebrospinal fluid (CSF) barriers as it did not penetrate the brain parenchyma [36].

However, DB829 (2,5-bis(5-amidino-2-pyridyl)furan; (**9**)), a close analogue of furamidine, did display remarkable efficacy against cerebral trypanosomiasis in mice and in vervet monkeys [42,43]. This was taken as evidence that DB829 is either recognized more efficiently than furamidine by a BBB transporter importing it into the CSF, or less efficiently extruded from the CSF by a P-gp-type transporter; both compounds have a similar pK_a and are dications at physiological pH, precluding any notion that they could simply diffuse across the barrier. However, the late failure of the clinical trials with pafuramidine (**10**), as a result of delayed nephrotoxicity in a small number of patients [40], also impeded clinical development of the all too similar DB829 and its prodrug DB868 (**11**).

The first resistance mechanism identified for the diamidines pentamidine and diminazene (the most-used drugs for early-stage HAT and for AAT, respectively) was loss of the P2 aminopurine transporter [44–46], which is encoded by the gene *TbAT1* [47]. Deletion of this gene did result in

Trop. Med. Infect. Dis. **2020**, *5*, 14

modest loss of in vitro pentamidine sensitivity in *T. b. brucei* bloodstream forms (and high-level resistance to diminazene [48]) but not to the extent that it would lead to clinical treatment failure. Indeed, Graf et al. [49] established that field isolates of *T. b. gambiense* from HAT patients that carry the *TbAT1* resistance allele were highly resistant to diminazene but only marginally less sensitive to pentamidine, compared to strains carrying the reference *TbAT1* allele. The *TbAT1^R* allele contained several amino acid changes and a 1-codon deletion, compared to the reference. These mutations were systematically evaluated, separately and in groups, by expressing the various mutant forms in a *tbat1*-null strain of *T. b. brucei* [50]. Surprisingly, none of the single amino acid mutations changed pentamidine transport or sensitivity much, but the introduction of two and particularly three such changes at the same time all but disabled the transporter's capacity for pentamidine uptake. The mutational studies were combined with homology modelling of the TbAT1 protein and produced a strong model of substrate binding, in which both aminopurines and pentamidine are bound via dual H-bonds with Asp140 and aromatic interactions with phenylalanines 19 and 316 [50]. This binding mode confirmed earlier binding models based on substrate binding energies with a large set of adenosine and diamidine analogues [51,52].

However, the transport of [3H]-pentamidine by *T. b. brucei* is inhibited only partially by P2/TbAT1 substrates adenine and adenosine, leading to the unambiguous conclusion that (an)other transporter(s) must also be involved [45,53]. Two additional transporters were identified, with K_m values of 36 ± 6 nM and 56 ± 8 µM (compare 0.43 ± 0.02 µM for TbAT1) and were accordingly designated the High Affinity Pentamidine Transporter (HAPT1) and the Low Affinity Pentamidine Transporter (LAPT1) [53]. Adaptation of the *tbat1*-null cell line to higher levels of pentamidine in vitro produced a strain, B48, that had lost HAPT1 activity and was 130-fold resistant to pentamidine in vitro (and was also highly resistant to melaminophenyl arsenicals, vide infra) [54]. This clonal strain had lost the HAPT1 transporter but retained normal LAPT function [54]; efforts to induce even higher levels of pentamidine and induce mutations in LAPT1 were unsuccessful [55]. The conclusion from this work was that the HAPT1 transporter was the most important contributor to pentamidine sensitivity in *T. brucei*, with LAPT playing only a minor role at therapeutically relevant drug concentrations.

A genome-wide screen for genes conferring pentamidine sensitivity with an RNAi library identified two loci, encoding for the plasma membrane proton ATPases HA1, HA2 and HA3, and for the aquaglyceroporins TbAQP2 and TbAQP3, respectively [56]. The involvement of the proton pumps indicates that pentamidine uptake is dependent on the proton-motive force or plasma membrane potential (as previously reported for procyclic *T. b. brucei* [53]), which the ATPases help maintain, but the latter RNAi 'hit' was harder to explain, as aquaporins are not known to engage in the uptake of relatively large molecules such as pentamidine, and certainly no cations. However, deletion of TbAQP2, but not of TbAQP3, resulted in a high-level of pentamidine resistance [57], and expression of TbAQP2 in *Leishmania mexicana* promastigotes, which are normally not very sensitive to pentamidine, increased their sensitivity ~40-fold and introduced a high affinity transport function that was indistinguishable from HAPT1 of *T. b. brucei* by K_m and inhibitor profile [55].

One possible explanation for the implausible uptake of dicationic pentamidine by an aquaporin is that pentamidine simply binds to the extracellular face of TbAQP2 and is internalised through endocytosis when the protein is internalised for turnover [58]. However, the rate of high affinity pentamidine transport in *T. brucei* procyclic cells is > 10-fold higher than in bloodstream forms [53,59], despite a much lower rate of endocytosis [60]. Moreover, although TbAQP2 is solely localised to the flagellar pocket in bloodstream forms [57], it is located all over the plasma membrane of procyclic forms, and the flagellar pocket is the sole site of endocytosis in trypanosomes [61]. For the same reasons, the high rate of pentamidine uptake in *L. mexicana* promastigotes expressing *TbAQP2* [55] seems incompatible with the endocytosis model. The alternative explanation is that pentamidine does in fact traverse the TbAQP2 channel, and this is explained by the unique changes to the selectivity filter motifs characteristic of aquaporins; these changes have the combined effect of making the pore much wider and removing the cation-excluding arginine residue [57,62]. This allowed docking of the stretched-out pentamidine in a low-energy conformation inside the pore of a model of TbAQP2 [62]. Much work has subsequently been done to supply definitive proof of either model, and this has definitively come down on the side of uptake through the TbAQP2 pore [63].

In summary, pentamidine resistance is principally associated with changes in *TbAQP2* through mutations, deletions and chimeric rearrangements with the adjacent *TbAQP3* gene. Interestingly, resistance can be bypassed with a nanotechnology formulation of pentamidine in chitosan nanoparticles coated with single domain nanobodies that specifically target trypanosomal surface proteins [64].

3. Melaminophenyl Arsenicals

Arsenic-based drugs were the very first treatments against sleeping sickness, starting with the use of inorganic sodium arsenite to treat animal trypanosomiasis or 'nagana' by David Livingstone in 1847 or 1848 [65] and David Bruce in 1895 [66]. Although neither of these pioneers achieved a full cure with this treatment (the animals eventually relapsed), it led to the development of the first organo-arsenic compound for sleeping sickness, atoxyl (**6**) as early as 1905, at the time of the major sleeping sickness epidemic in Central and East Africa [67]. However, atoxyl, meaning 'non-toxic' had severe side effects and was only active against early stage HAT, and was followed by tryparsamide (**5**) in 1919 [68]. Tryparsamidine was the first drug to be active against the late stage; however, it was only used against *gambiense* HAT and was considered of little use to either the early or late stage of the Rhodesian form [7,69,70]. A very similar compound, acetyl-*p*-amino-O-oxophenylarsenic acid, known as Fourneau 270 or Orsanine (**15**), was synthesised by Ernest Fourneau at the Institut Pasteur in Paris [71] and had very similar properties as tryparsamide [72,73]; indeed, it was claimed to have twice the selectivity index of tryparsamidine [74] and was in use for approximately 15 years [75].

The melaminophenyl arsenicals (MPA) replaced these earlier arsenicals, particularly tryparsamide, partly because melarsoprol (**12**) had better penetration into the central nervous system ('rendered trypanocidal the cerebrospinal fluid of rabbits' [76]) and tryparsamidine was poorly active against the early stage of the disease [14]. In fact, the MPAs were the first cure for late stage Rhodesian sleeping sickness, which had been considered incurable up to then [72]. More importantly yet, resistance to tryparsamide had developed and had become widespread throughout the early 1940s, to the point that the drug had become ineffective in most cases, particularly in French West Africa and Belgian Congo [77]; in 1947, 80% of new cases in Congo were reportedly resistant to what was then the only treatment for late stage HAT [7,14]. Moreover, resistance to both atoxyl and tryparsamide had been shown to be highly stable over prolonged periods, with Yorke and Murgatroyd concluding that it 'persists indefinitely', even when passed repeatedly through tsetse flies [78]. The MPAs were introduced in the late 1940s [14,69], despite reservations about their toxicity [79], largely driven by concerns about tryparsamide resistance. Extensive experience with MPAs in French West Africa was contained in a 1953 report by the Service Général d'Hygiène Mobile et de Prophylaxie de l'Afrique Occidentale Française [80] and concluded that the proposed "detoxified melarsen oxide", Mel B (melarsoprol, "Arsobal") was at least as toxic as melarsen oxide (**13**) itself but less active, and strongly recommended a return to melarsen oxide. However, the report also acknowledged that the MPAs as a class were a step forward and active against strains resistant to the older arsenicals. Ian Apted, in his comprehensive 1970 review of HAT treatments, states that melarsoprol, developed from melarsen oxide by reaction with Dimercaprol, also called British anti-Lewisite (BAL; antidote for arsenic poisoning) was less toxic than the original melarsen and melarsen oxide [72]. However, even after melarsoprol became the standard treatment for late stage sleeping sickness, the high level of severe adverse effects, with an estimated 10% of patients suffering from reactive encephalitis, half fatal [81,82] remained acceptable only for lack of alternatives. The introduction of an optimised 10-day administration schedule in 2005 [83] reduced the total amount administered and saved money but did not reduce the adverse effects significantly. A further and highly promising development was the proposal of melarsoprol cyclodextrin complexes as the first oral treatment of HAT [84]. In mouse models, this protocol appeared to be much safer, and it negated the need for intravenous administration of melarsoprol, as a caustic solution in propylene glycol. The melarsoprol cyclodextrin complex was awarded orphan drug status by the European Medicines Agency (EMA) in October 2012 [85] and by the U.S. Food and Drug Administration (FDA) in 2013. A protocol for phase 2 clinical trials of oral complexed melarsoprol in late stage *T. b. rhodesiense* HAT in Uganda was subsequently approved by the EMA (Peter Kennedy, personal communication). However, this has not yet been implemented for lack of funding, presumably because new human trials with arsenicals would be hard to get funding for, and NECT and fexinidazole came along as timely alternatives, at least for *gambiense* HAT (see below).

The discovery of the resistance mechanisms for the MPA melarsoprol (and its veterinary analogue cymelarsan (**14**)) is very similar, and parallel to that of the diamidines. Indeed, the phenomenon of pentamidine-melarsoprol cross-resistance (MPXR) was first reported almost 70 years ago [86,87], and at the time hypothesised to be due to the presence of similar motifs in the melamine-phenyl group and benzamidine moieties and thus 'loss of permeability to, or adsorption affinity of, the melamine grouping in the melarsen-resistant strain may possibly prevent initial uptake of the amidine-type drugs' as well [86]. This insight, based solely on cross-resistance patterns and a faint structural similarity, has now been well validated [88].

The association of MPAs with uptake via P2/TbAT1 was first discovered by Carter and Fairlamb in 1993, who found that out of a large number of biochemicals only adenine, adenosine and the transport inhibitor dipyridamole partly blocked the trypanocidal activity of melarsen oxide, and that an MPA-resistant strain had lost the function of one purine transporter, which they termed P2 [89]. This was later confirmed by other researchers [90], and the joint recognition motif for adenosine, diamidines and MPAs formally established [51,52,91]. As related in the previous section, the P2-encoding gene, *TbAT1*, was identified in 1999 and an allele bearing multiple polymorphisms was found to confer resistance [47]. A similar resistance allele was reported from Uganda in 2001 and was found more frequently in melarsoprol relapse patients than in those cured [92,93]. This was followed by experimental evidence that the deletion of *TbAT1* led to a loss in in vitro MPA sensitivity [48].

As reviewed elsewhere [94], concerns of melarsoprol treatment failure had been rising throughout the 1990s and early 2000s [95–98]. The confirmation of *TbAT1* resistance alleles, as well as the well-documented toxicity of melarsoprol [81] and the confirmation that the treatment failures could not be attributed to individual patients' differences in melarsoprol pharmacokinetics and distribution [99], shifted first-line treatment in many centres, including Omugo in Uganda, to eflornithine monotherapy. Resampling of clinical isolates 4 years later no longer detected the *TbAT1^R* allele in Omugo; in contrast, the mutant allele was readily amplified from patients, including five relapse cases, in the Moyo treatment centre, also in Northern Uganda, that had continued to use melarsoprol as the first-line drug [100]. Similarly, no *TbAT1^R* alleles and no MPA-resistant isolates were found in a 2007 clinical study in South Sudan—an area that had also switched to eflornithine in 2001 after high melarsoprol relapse rates [101]. However, in the latter study it remained unproven whether the *TbAT1* mutations had disappeared after melarsoprol treatment had been largely discontinued or that, alternatively, the treatment failures had not been due to *TbAT1* mutations in the first place, as no sampling had been done before the switch to eflornithine. Conversely, the Ugandan study had not tested the *TbAT1^R*-bearing isolates MPA for sensitivity in vitro or in a controlled animal model, and thus the link of clinical melarsoprol failure and *TbAT1* mutations has remained formally unproven, although highly plausible. Specifically, it could not be ruled out that additional factors (whether patient- or trypanosome-related) also played a role.

Meanwhile, Bridges et al. [54] showed that MPA resistance was much higher in laboratory strains that had functionally lost both the TbAT1/P2 transporter and the HAPT1 transport functions. As related in the previous section, HAPT1 was found to be encoded by *TbAQP2* [57] and the MPA resistance was due to a chimeric rearrangement in the *TbAQP2-TbAQP3* locus [55]. Several studies subsequently found such TbAQP2-3 chimeras, or outright TbAQP2 deletions, in clinical isolates from South Sudan and the DRC, demonstrating a clear link between *AQP2* mutations and MPXR [49,62,101]. The definitive word on this was the demonstration that the introduction of a wild-type *AQP2* gene in the resistant

T. b. gambiense isolates restored sensitivity, whereas the expression of two different chimeric AQP2/3 genes, from an MPXR *T. b. gambiense* isolate and from the MPXR *T. b. brucei* clone B48, into an *aqp2/aqp3* null cell line of *T. b. brucei*, did not [55,102]. *TbAQP2* deletions were also found in two *T. b. rhodesiense* strains adapted in vitro to pentamidine and melarsoprol, respectively [103], and as such there is little remaining doubt, if any, that mutations in the *TbAQP2* gene are the principal determinant of MPXR, and that its unique pore architecture is what made *T. brucei* spp. highly sensitive to them in the first place. Interestingly, the veterinary trypanosome *T. congolense*, which lacks paralogues of both *TbAT1* [104] and *TbAQP2*, is orders of magnitude less sensitive to pentamidine than the *brucei* species.

4. Suramin

While melarsoprol and pentamidine were developed in the 1930s or 1940s, suramin (**16**) is by some distance the oldest trypanocide still in routine clinical use. It was developed out of a series of trypanocidal dyes tested by Paul Ehrlich, starting with Nagana Red (**17**), which displayed only weak trypanocidal properties, followed by the more water-soluble form Trypan Red (**18**) in 1904 [105], which turned out to be both curative and prophylactic for *T. equinum* infections in mice [105–107]. As Jim Williamson [7] put it: "This was the classic first cure of an experimentally produced disease by administration of a single dose of a synthetic organic substance of known chemical composition", and it has had enormous impact on the pursuit of chemotherapy. The 7-amino derivative of Trypan Red was used in a trial in Africa by Robert Koch, but unsuccessfully [107]. Further experimentation with Nagana Red also led to the concepts of acquired drug resistance ('serum-fast') in infectious agents and the whole concept of specific targets for different drugs ('chemo-receptors') to explain cross-resistance patterns observed [7,108]. However, Nagana Red and its successors, such as Trypan Blue (**19**), all displayed unacceptable side effects at curative doses. Only Trypan Blue was effective in animal models of trypanosomiasis [109,110] and was taken into use as a veterinary drug (against babesiosis), but it stained the meat and skin blue, which did not serve to make it popular and precluded its use on human patients [107]. Further development to an active (and colourless!) trypanocide was undertaken by Maurice Nicolle and Felix Mesnil at the Institut Pasteur [111] in collaboration with by Wilhelm Röhl and Bernhard Heymann at Bayer [7], who via Afridol Violet (**20**), the first of the symmetrical ureas of the series, and after synthesis of >1000 of related structures, found 'Bayer 205' in 1916 [112]. This was introduced clinically under the name Germanin, and the formula was kept secret and supplied only to German clinicians, i.e., in German colonial territories [113,114]. As related by Dietmar Steverding [107], the German authorities offered the formula of Bayer 205 to the British Government in return for their lost colonies after World War I, but this was declined. The formula of Germanin was elucidated by Fourneau in 1924 [115,116], and promptly reissued under the name Fourneau 309 [114]. Bayer confirmed the structure 4 years later [107].

For decades now, suramin has only been used for early stage *T. b. rhodesiense* infections, with pentamidine preferred against the *gambiense* disease. There have been few reports of treatment failure with suramin, and it is generally assumed that most of these could have been related to misdiagnosis of cerebral stage HAT. Apted also proposed that in some cases suramin may simply not attain the curative concentration in blood [117], which would constitute treatment failure rather than resistance. However, Pépin and Milord, in their authoritative 1994 review [118], discuss several reports of significant relapse rates in East Africa, and suramin resistance can also be induced experimentally [119], but it is reportedly less stable than tryparsamide resistance, with experimental *T. b. rhodesiense* strains gradually regaining full sensitivity [78].

Suramin has six negative charges at physiological pH and this ensures of course that it will not cross biological membranes unless aided by an active process. One consequence is that suramin must be administered parenterally (i.v. because i.m. and s.c. causes inflammation and necrosis at the injection site [118]) and has no activity against cerebral trypanosomiasis as it is unable to cross the BBB. Another is that this large (MW = 1296 for the free acid, 1429 for the sodium salt), clumsy, un-drug-like molecule that breaks all the Lipinski rules [120], must enter the trypanosomal cell body in order to impact its viability, via an active mechanism. The size and charge of the molecule all but precludes uptake via a nutrient transporter, channel or suchlike. It was proposed that suramin, which binds strongly to Low Density Lipoprotein (LDL) was taken up together with this serum protein by *T. brucei*, via receptor-mediated endocytosis [121,122], but later work, while consistent with uptake via endocytosis, found no correlation between LDL internalization rates and suramin sensitivity [123].

As for several other trypanocides, genome-wide screening for loss-of function with an RNAi library in bloodstream form *T. b. brucei* revealed new details of the suramin mode of action and resistance [56]. Most of the hits from this screen concerned its mechanism of uptake, confirming endocytosis, whereas it gave few clues about its mechanism of action, strengthening the view that suramin exhibits polypharmacology. Indeed, suramin has been shown to inhibit many trypanosomal enzymes including dihydrofolate reductase [124], thymidine kinase [125], all the glycolytic enzymes [126] and many others [118,127]. The RNAi screen revealed the suramin receptor to be an Invariant Surface Glycoprotein, ISG75, and also highlighted the involvement of a number of endosomal proteins, lysosomal proteases (Cathepsin L) and a lysosome-based member of the Major Facilitator Superfamily, designated MFST [56]. This has resulted in the current model of suramin uptake, via binding (either free or in complex with a serum protein) to ISG75, delivery to the lysosome by the endosomal system, degradation of the proteinous receptor and finally exit from the lysosome via MFST in to the cytoplasm [127,128].

5. Eflornithine

Eflornithine (DL-α-difluoromethylornithine; DFMO; **21**) is chemically a close analogue of the amino acid ornithine and pharmacologically a suicide inhibitor of Ornithine Decarboxylase (ODC), i.e., it binds the protein active site irreversibly, via a chemical reaction with a cysteine residue (Cys360 in mouse ODC [129]). ODC is the key enzyme in the cellular production of polyamines (spermine, spermidine, putrescine), which are essential for cell division and as such eflornithine was developed to inhibit cancer cell proliferation [130]. While this was insufficiently effective, due to the very rapid turnover/replacement rate of mammalian ODC ($t_{1/2}$ ~20 min), the drug is currently being investigated by cancer researchers as a chemoprevention agent [131,132].

Eflornithine started being tested, with both oral and i.v. formulations, against *gambiense* sleeping sickness from the mid-1980s, with promising results even against late-stage disease [133–136]. Because it was able to cure melarsoprol-refractory cases and patients already too frail to survive the arsenic-based treatment, it became known as the 'resurrection drug' [137]. By the early 2000s, the consensus treatment regimen was established as 100 mg/kg b.w. every 6 h for 14 days, by infusions [138]. However, the treatment was much less successful against *rhodesiense* sleeping sickness than against the *T. b. gambiense* infection [139,140]. The relative refractoriness of *T. b. rhodesiense* was also seen in a test with clinical isolates in mice [141], and Iten et al. [142] concluded that *T. b. rhodesiense* are innately tolerant to eflornithine.

Probably the most important reason that eflornithine worked better against trypanosomiasis than against cancer is that the *T. b. gambiense* ODC is very stable, with a half-life time in excess of 18 h. Thus, the irreversible inhibition of the enzyme by eflornithine ensures that the cell is deprived of polyamines, which it cannot obtain any other way, for a long time (African trypanosomes do not have polyamine transporters, as there are no polyamines in the blood). This seems also to be a main difference with *T. b. rhodesiense* (ODC $t_{1/2}$ ~4.3 h), although the total ODC activity in this species is also higher than in *T. b. gambiense* [141,143]. There was no difference in DFMO uptake between *T. b. rhodesiense* and *T. b. gambiense* [143]. However, several early studies showed reduced eflornithine uptake in resistant cells, which were readily produced in the laboratory [144,145].

One debate [146] with respect to the eflornithine mechanism of action was whether its uptake might be transporter-mediated [145], or by simple diffusion [143,144,147]. This debate has been definitively settled in favour of mediated uptake, as should be expected of a highly soluble, zwitterionic compound with an experimental LogP of −2.7. Vincent et al. [148] induced eflornithine resistance in *T. b. brucei* bloodstream forms and found no mutations in *ODC* but again saw a strongly diminished rate of eflornithine uptake. However, a systematic amplification and sequencing of amino acid transporter genes identified deletions of the gene encoding amino acid transporter 6 (*TbAAT6*) in two independently generated resistant lines. Specific ablation of this transporter by RNAi in a sensitive line resulted in eflornithine resistance, whereas the (re)-introduction of a wild-type *TbAAT6* allele into a resistant strain restored sensitivity [148]. This paper was almost immediately followed by the publication of two other, independent studies using RNAi library screens, which each also identified *TbAAT6* as the main determinant of eflornithine resistance [56,149].

While clinical reports about eflornithine resistance in the field are scarce, the fact remains that it is easily induced in the laboratory and that a single point mutation in a non-essential gene (*TbAAT6*) will cause a high level of resistance. Considering that the dosage regimen of eflornithine monotherapy is already severe as well as expensive, and cannot easily be increased in amount or duration, this placed serious question marks over the longevity of the drug, and was a major driver, along with both the cost, duration and logistics of administration, and the adverse effects of 14-day i.v. eflornithine [150], in the development of combination therapies. This included a trial, reported in 2002, of a short treatment with eflornithine followed by three daily injections with melarsoprol, giving a probability of cure of 93% [151]. In 2006, a trial with 54 patients was reported, testing three combinations: melarsoprol-nifurtimox, melarsoprol-eflornithine and eflornithine-nifurtimox [152]. The trial was halted because of the toxicity of the melarsoprol-plus-nifurtimox combination (which also gave only a 44% cure rate), but the eflornithine-nifurtimox performed significantly better than the eflornithine-melarsoprol combination (94.1 versus 78.4%; $P < 0.05$) and resulted in fewer adverse effects. In 2007, two studies, in Uganda [153] and the Republic of Congo [154], described further trials with eflornithine-nifurtimox combination therapy (NECT), which were subsequently extended to a full multi-centre non-inferiority trial [155]. The overall conclusions were that the combination is non-inferior to eflornithine monotherapy and has considerable advantages such as protection against resistance, lower cost, easier and shorter administration as well as a reduction in adverse effects by 50% [155,156].

NECT was added to the WHO Essential Medicines list in April 2009 and was adopted as the new first-line treatment for late stage *gambiense* sleeping sickness [156]. At this point, the phasing-out of melarsoprol was considered to be one of the main remaining challenges, as it was still used for ~50% of cases in the Democratic Republic of Congo (DRC), for instance [156]. In 2012, a pharmacovigilance evaluation of 1735 patient outcomes from 9 different countries found that although adverse effects were quite common (60.1%) serious adverse effects were rarely observed (1.1%) and the case fatality rate was 0.5% [157]. This of course compared very well with melarsoprol, the use of which by then had dropped to 12% of all second stage *gambiense* HAT cases [150]. Two further clinical reports, describing NECT outcomes in 684 second stage patients in the DRC [158] and 109 patients in Uganda [159] provided a further evidence base for the selection of NECT as the first-line treatment for cerebral stage infection with *T. b. gambiense*. Based on the low efficacy of eflornithine against *T. b. rhodesiense*, no clinical trials with either eflornithine monotherapy or NECT were initiated against late stage *rhodesiense* sleeping sickness, and to date melarsoprol remains the only approved treatment for that condition.

6. Nifurtimox

Nifurtimox (**22**) has been used since 1969 against *Trypanosoma cruzi* (i.e., Chagas Disease) [160,161] and, given the urgent need to replace melarsoprol for late-stage HAT, has been investigated as a possible treatment for African trypanosomiasis as well [69]. As related by Janssens and De Muynck [162], the first tests with nifurtimox against African trypanosomiasis were conducted by Marc Wéry who found, apparently to everybody's great surprise, 'a definite activity on the chronic infection' in rats, justifying a first trial in humans. That first trial, of just four patients, used 3×120 mg or 3×150 mg daily for 60 or 120 days or however long the drug was tolerated. The trial results were mixed, and it was concluded that nifurtimox was not the sought-after, reliable and low-toxicity replacement of melarsoprol that was hoped for, but that it might serve as a drug of last resort for melarsoprol-refractory patients that were thus untreatable at the time [162]. A subsequent trial in Zaire with 12.5–15.0 mg/kg b.w. daily (in three doses) for 2 months reported cures of 7-out-of-8 melarsoprol-refractory cases and 5-out-of-7 new late-stage cases [163]. In contrast, using essentially the same treatment schedule, Pépin and co-workers reported a relapse rate of 63% in 1989 and concluded that a higher dose would be necessary for cure in most patients [164]. However, after a trial with 30 mg/kg b.w./day for 30 days they concluded that this regimen was 'significantly toxic' and that the (only slight) improvement in efficacy did not outweigh the increase in toxicity [165]. Their overall conclusion was that nifurtimox is inferior to eflornithine, then becoming available, as a mono-therapy treatment for arseno-tolerant HAT. Van Nieuwenhove, summarizing the emerging evidence on eflornithine and nifurtimox monotherapy in 1992, strongly advocated trials of combinations of the three available treatments of late-stage HAT [166]. While a treatment regimen starting with melarsoprol alone 2 doses) followed by 10 days of nifurtimox-plus-melarsoprol gave superior cure rates to melarsoprol or nifurtimox alone [167], the combination of eflornithine with nifurtimox (NECT) was eventually adopted, as related in the previous section.

With the trialling and implementation of NECT, the question of nifurtimox' mode of action and potential resistance mechanism became one of acute importance. It had long been known that nitro-heterocyclic trypanocides can generate free radicals such as superoxide [168], although direct evidence of this being the principal mechanism of action for nifurtimox and related nitro compounds was lacking. However, the deletion of a gene encoding a glycosomal and cytosolic superoxide dismutase, *TbSODB1*, significantly increased sensitivity to nifurtimox and benznidazole, which was restored to wild-type levels upon re-introduction of the gene; this was specific to *TbSODB1* as deletion of the related glycosomal *TbSODB2* had no effect [169]. Further confirmation of the mechanism of action came with the identification of a mitochondrial NADPH-dependent nitroreductase, NTR, that proved to be essential for the efficacy of a nitro-heterocyclic drug in *T. brucei* and *T. cruzi* [170]. Both species have one copy of this type 1 nitroreductase in their genome. A *T. cruzi* cell line induced for nifurtimox resistance was highly cross-resistant to a variety of nitro-heterocyclic compounds and purified NTR was shown to efficiently reduce all of them. Worryingly, deletion of just one *TbNTR* allele created a heterozygous $NTR^{+/-}$ *T. brucei* that displayed no growth phenotype but was three-fold resistance to the nitro-heterocyclic drugs; the double deletion (*ntr*-null) *T. brucei* cell line was even more resistant but also displayed significant growth impairment, leading to the conclusion that the gene is essential [170]. The same gene was subsequently identified in genome-wide RNAi library screens with nifurtimox and benznidazole [171]. As overexpression of *NTR1* resulted in hypersensitivity to the nitro drugs [170] it is clear that *NTR1* is the main determinant of nitro-heterocyclic sensitivity in trypanosomes, and that a single mutation in one allele could eliminate their small therapeutic window, as the main biochemical difference with host cells, as pertains to nifurtimox' mode of action, is cancelled.

This conclusion was put to the test by Alan Fairlamb, who induced two nifurtimox-resistant *T. brucei* lines in vitro, which both showed cross-resistance to other nitro-heterocyclic drugs including fexinidazole [172]. The resistant strain displayed unimpeded virulence in mice and, most worryingly, nifurtimox had little effect on the in vivo progression of the infection with this strain [172].

The accumulation of nifurtimox across the BBB was investigated by Sarah Thomas using both a murine perfusion system and an in vitro model based on immortalised human BBB cells [173,174]. Nifurtimox readily crossed the BBB and blood–CSF barriers and this was not significantly different in healthy mice or infected mice where the barrier integrity had been compromised [173]. This almost certainly means that the uptake of nifurtimox at the BBB is trans-cellular rather than paracellular (i.e., between cells). Nor was there any difference between the standard model and mice deficient in the BBB efflux transporter P-gp. This was consistent with an earlier study in rats, which found that ^{35}S-nifurtimox is rapidly distributed throughout the host, and that both the blood-brain or placental barriers were permeable to the drug [175]. This could be the result of its lipophilicity (octanol-saline partition coefficient = 5.46 [173]), which might allow a simple diffusion across membranes. Certainly, no transporter for nifurtimox uptake has, to date, been identified, either in the host or in trypanosomes, including with RNAi library screens [171]. Yet, nifurtimox, bearing a polar nitro group, is not *very* lipophilic, the trans-cellular uptake at the BBB is consistent with a transporter, and it has been argued that almost all drugs require a transport mechanism [176] and that absence of proof for the involvement of a transporter simply means we haven't looked well enough [177]. Moreover, Jeganathan et al. reported a higher concentration of ^{3}H-nifurtimox in the CNS compared with plasma [173], which would be hard to explain without active import, especially since there is also a component of extrusion across the barrier (see below). Of potential importance for NECT, eflornithine reduced CNS accumulation of ^{3}H-nifurtimox by > 50%, presumably by interfering at the level of a transporter at the barrier [173], although that result could not be reproduced in the later study with cultured human BBB cells [174]. If nifurtimox uptake is indeed transporter-mediated, the failure to identify transporter genes with the genome-wide RNAi library could reflect uptake by multiple transporters (non-dependence on a single gene) or the gene being essential (knockdown being lethal).

Although the existence of a plasma membrane transporter importing nifurtimox has not (yet) been established, Thomas's studies with the BBB did provide evidence for extrusion across the BBB, despite the non-involvement of P-gp [173,174]. For instance, coadministration with pentamidine enhanced CNS accumulation in the mouse perfusion system, likely indicating an interaction with the ^{3}H-nifurtimox efflux transporter at the barrier [173], as also observed with ^{3}H-pentamidine distribution [37]. In the follow-on study using immortalised human BBB cells, it was found that accumulation across the barrier was strongly increased by inhibitors of the breast cancer resistance protein (BCRP) but not of P-gp; BCRP is an ATP-dependent efflux transporter of the ABC super family and depletion of ATP in the cell line had the same effect as inhibitors of BCRF [174].

Nifurtimox appears to be similarly effective against *T. b. rhodesiense* and *T. b. gambiense*, at least in vitro [178,179]. However, if nifurtimox has been tested clinically on *rhodesiense* HAT, I have been unable to find any reference to it. Certainly, no systematic trials have been held and, considering that NECT is unlikely to work on that infection because of the eflornithine component (see above), the effort would seem almost redundant, and the ethics might be debatable. As such, melarsoprol is still the only approved option for late-stage *rhodesiense* sleeping sickness, although the Drugs for Neglected Diseases initiative (DNDi) started a programme in September 2018 to develop fexinidazole, the newly approved oral drug for late stage *gambiense* disease [180] that does not require co-treatment with eflornithine [181], for the equivalent condition with *T. b. rhodesiense* (https://www.dndi.org/diseases-projects/portfolio/fexinidazole-tb-rhodesiense/).

As regards fexinidazole, the EMA issued a positive opinion in November of 2018, based on the DNDiFEX004-6 trials, clearing the way for its implementation [182]. However, fexinidazole monotherapy was somewhat less effective than NECT (91.2% vs. 97.6% cure) [181], within the predetermined acceptability margin. However, as pointed out by François Chappuis, this is compensated for by the ease of administration and approved access to medicine that this oral formulation brings to the HAT treatment options [181,183]. Moreover, fexinidazole, was reportedly > 98% curative for early and early-late stage *gambiense* HAT (trial NCT03025789) and can thus be used without having to perform the invasive lumber punctures still required for determination of HAT stage [183]. The most important limitation of fexinidazole, however, seems to be a relatively low curative rate of 86.9% for the patients with the most severe meningoencephalitic HAT (defined as > 100 white blood cells/ml CSF) [1,182]. Thus, for these patients NECT remains the best option [182,184].

7. A Perspective on Drug Resistance in African Trypanosomiasis

It is a dogma in the pharmacology of infectious diseases that resistance will (eventually) occur for any drug. Certainly, the infectious agents have many tricks up their proverbial sleeves, often not anticipated [185]. Yet, there is no proof of suramin resistance in African trypanosomes, despite approximately 100 years of usage in East Africa. Additionally, there is no clear proof of pentamidine resistance either, despite intensive use against *gambiense* HAT since the 1940s, including highly successful mass treatments, particularly by the French and Belgian colonial authorities [33]. This even though resistance to either drug can be induced in the laboratory without apparent loss of viability. Thus, there has been relatively little incentive to develop new treatments for the early stage disease and the target product profile of the DNDi has, since its inception, been for late-stage disease. While there was a significant element in this of the need for new treatments with reduced toxicity and cost, leading to optimisation of use of melarsoprol with a shorter 10-day protocol, for instance [83,186], most of the new drug development was driven by resistance to the then-standard treatment. It is questionable whether melarsoprol would have ever been taken into clinical use if not for the catastrophically high levels of resistance with tryparsamide. Similarly, a major factor in the introduction of eflornithine, in addition to melarsoprol's dangerous toxicity, was the rapid rise in cases refractory to melarsoprol in Central Africa. The well-founded fear of resistance to eflornithine monotherapy (and the anecdotal reports of increasing failures with the drug) helped drive urgent trials with eflornithine and nifurtimox combinations. Every time, we were on our last or only drug against late stage sleeping sickness and the introduction of replacements was sheer necessity.

So, where are we now, in 2020? The number of patients, particularly with *gambiense* HAT, is in steep decline, human-to-human transmission is low, possibly at an all-time low, and we have in hand first-stage treatments that have stood the no-resistance test of time (pentamidine, suramin), and a combination therapy for late stage that is safer than we ever had. The introduction of fexinidazole [181–184] and potentially acoziborole [2,3], safe oral drugs that are active against both stages of the disease, is finally eliminating the need for risky lumbar punctures for determining the disease stage. The fact that there are finally multiple treatment options would allow clinicians to rotate treatments, should the need arise, but as long as continued vigilance keeps transmission very low, resistance is much less likely to develop. Does this mean sleeping sickness is 'done'? We have thought this once before, when cases were few, in the 1960s, and have hopefully learned that we must continue the vigilance, awareness and training of medical personnel. More work is also still needed on early detection/diagnosis, detection of asymptomatic cases, animal reservoirs. As far as resistance is concerned, the cross-resistance between fexinidazole and nifurtimox is of potential concern as any strains surviving fexinidazole monotherapy would likely also cause failure with NECT. Thus, the completion of the clinical development and registration of acoziborole and/or melarsoprol-cyclodextrin complex is still of great importance, as is the trial of fexinidazole for late stage *rhodesiense* HAT. Currently Rhodesian HAT is the most neglected disease, still treated with suramin from ~1920 and the awful i.v. melarsoprol in propylene glycol for the late stage. Hopefully one of these new options will finally put suramin to rest and ease this esteemed great-grandfather of chemotherapy into a well-deserved retirement—and i.v. melarsoprol as well.

Conflicts of Interest: The author declares no conflict of interest.

References

1. Fairlamb, A.H. Fexinidazole for the treatment of human African trypanosomiasis. *Drugs Today* **2019**, *55*, 705–712. [CrossRef] [PubMed]
2. Eperon, G.; Balasegaram, M.; Potet, J.; Mowbray, C.; Valverde, O.; Chappuis, F. Treatment options for second-stage gambiense human African trypanosomiasis. *Expert Rev. Anti-Infect. Ther.* **2014**, *12*, 1407–1417. [CrossRef] [PubMed]
3. R&D Portfolio Update February 2019: DNDi Sleeping Sickness Programme. Available online: www.dndi.org/2019/media-centre/news-views-stories/news/sleepingsickness_rnd_status_2019/ (accessed on 15 December 2019).
4. Jacobs, R.T.; Nare, B.; Wring, S.A.; Orr, M.D.; Chen, D.; Sligar, J.M.; Jenks, M.X.; Noe, R.A.; Bowling, T.S.; Mercer, L.T.; et al. SCYX-7158, an orally-active benzoxaborole for the treatment of stage 2 human African trypanosomiasis. *PLoS Negl. Trop. Dis.* **2011**, *5*, e1151. [CrossRef] [PubMed]
5. Dubois, A. Mort par hypoglycémie dans les trypanosomiases aiguës. *CR Soc. Biol.* **1928**, *99*, 656–657.
6. Nieman, R.E.; Kelly, J.J.; Waskin, H.A. Severe African trypanosomiasis with spurious hypoglycemia. *J. Infect. Dis.* **1989**, *159*, 360–362. [CrossRef]

7. Williamson, J. Review of chemotherapeutic and chemoprophylactic drugs. In *The African Trypanosomiases*; Mulligan, H.W., Ed.; George Allen/Unwin Ltd.: London, UK, 1970; pp. 125–221.

8. Schern, K.; Artagaveytia-Allende, R. Zur glykopriven Therapie und Prophylaxe mit sowohl toxische als auch atoxische wirkende Substanzen bei der experimentellen Trypanosomen-und Treponemen-Infektion. *Z Immun. Exp. Ther.* **1936**, *89*, 21–64.

9. Von Janscó, N.; Von Janscó, H. Chemotherapeutische Wirkung und Kohlehydratstoffwechsel: Die Heilwirkung von Guanidinderivaten auf die Trypanosomeninfektion. *Z Immun. Exp. Ther.* **1935**, *86*, 1–30.

10. King, H.; Lourie, E.M.; Yorke, W. New trypanocidal substances. *Lancet* **1937**, *223*, 1360–1363. [CrossRef]

11. Lourie, E.M.; Yorke, W. Studies in Chemotherapy XVI: The trypanocidal action of synthalin. *Ann. Trop. Med. Parasitol.* **1937**, *31*, 435–445. [CrossRef]

12. Lourie, E.M.; Yorke, W. Studies in Chemotherapy XVI: The trypanocidal action of certain aromatic diamidines. *Ann. Trop. Med. Parasitol.* **1939**, *33*, 289–304. [CrossRef]

13. Napier, L.E.; Sen Gupta, P.C. A peculiar neurological sequel to administration of 4:400-diamidino-diphenyl-ethylene (M&B 744). *Indian Med. Gaz.* **1942**, *77*, 71–74.

14. Friedheim, E.A.H. MelB in the treatment of human trypanosomiasis. *Am. J. Trop. Med.* **1949**, *29*, 173–180. [CrossRef]

15. Temu, S. Summary of cases of human early trypanosomiasis treated with Berenil at EATRO. *Trans. R. Soc. Trop. Med. Hyg.* **1975**, *69*, 277.

16. Lansiaux, A.; Tanious, F.; Mishal, Z.; Dassonneville, L.; Kumar, A.; Stephens, C.E.; Hu, Q.; Wilson, W.D.; Boykin, D.W.; Bailly, C. Distribution of furamidine analogues in tumor cells: Targeting of the nucleus or mitochondria depending on the amidine substitution. *Cancer Res.* **2002**, *62*, 7219–7229. [PubMed]

17. Mathis, A.M.; Bridges, A.S.; Ismail, M.A.; Kumar, A.; Francesconi, I.; Anbazhagan, M.; Hu, Q.; Tanious, F.A.; Wenzler, T.; Saulter, J.; et al. Diphenyl furans and aza analogs: Effects of structural modification on in vitro activity, DNA binding, and accumulation and distribution in trypanosomes. *Antimicrob. Agents Chemother.* **2007**, *51*, 2801–2810. [CrossRef] [PubMed]

18. Nguyen, B.; Lee, M.P.H.; Hamelberg, D.; Joubert, A.; Bailly, C.; Brun, R.; Neidle, S.; Wilson, W.D. Strong binding in the DNA minor groove by an aromatic diamidine with a shape that does not match the curvature of the groove. *J. Am. Chem. Soc.* **2002**, *124*, 13680–13681. [CrossRef] [PubMed]

19. Wilson, W.D.; Tanious, F.A.; Mathis, A.; Tevis, D.; Hall, J.E.; Boykin, D.W. Antiparasitic compounds that target DNA. *Biochimie* **2008**, *90*, 999–1014. [CrossRef] [PubMed]

20. Liu, L.; Wang, F.; Tong, Y.; Li, L.-F.; Liu, Y.; Gao, W.-Q. Pentamidine inhibits prostate cancer progression via selectively inducing mitochondrial DNA depletion and dysfunction. *Cell Prolif.* **2019**, e12718. [CrossRef] [PubMed]

21. Stewart, M.L.; Krishna, S.; Burchmore, R.J.S.; Brun, R.; De Koning, H.P.; Boykin, D.W.; Tidwell, R.R.; Hall, J.E.; Barrett, M.P. Detection of arsenical drug resistance in *Trypanosoma brucei* using a simple fluorescence test. *Lancet* **2005**, *366*, 486–487. [CrossRef]

22. Damper, D.; Patton, C.L. Pentamidine transport and sensitivity in *brucei*-group trypanosomes. *J Protozool* **1976**, *23*, 39–356. [CrossRef]

23. Damper, D.; Patton, C.L. Pentamidine transport in *Trypanosoma brucei*—Kinetics and specificity. *Biochem. Pharmacol.* **1976**, *25*, 271–276. [CrossRef]

24. Mathis, A.M.; Holman, J.L.; Sturk, L.M.; Ismail, M.A.; Boykin, D.W.; Tidwell, R.R.; Hall, J.E. Accumulation and intracellular distribution of antitrypanosomal diamidine compounds DB75 and DB820 in African trypanosomes. *Antimicrob. Agents Chemother.* **2006**, *50*, 2185–2191. [CrossRef] [PubMed]

25. Eze, A.A.; Gould, M.K.; Munday, J.C.; Tagoe, D.N.A.; Stelmanis, V.; Schnaufer, A.; De Koning, H.P. Loss of mitochondrial membrane potential is a late adaptation of *Trypanosoma brucei brucei* to isometamidium preceded by mutations in the γ subunit of the F_1F_0-ATPase. *PLoS Negl. Trop. Dis.* **2016**, *10*, e0004791. [CrossRef] [PubMed]

26. Ibrahim, H.M.; Al-Salabi, M.I.; El Sabbagh, N.; Quashie, N.B.; Alkhaldi, A.A.; Escale, R.; Smith, T.K.; Vial, H.J.; De Koning, H.P. Symmetrical choline-derived dications display strong anti-kinetoplastid activity. *J. Antimicrob. Chemother.* **2011**, *66*, 111–125. [CrossRef]

27. Ward, C.P.; Wong, P.E.; Burchmore, R.J.; De Koning, H.P.; Barrett, M.P. Trypanocidal furamidine analogues: Influence of pyridine nitrogens on trypanocidal activity, transport kinetics and resistance patterns. *Antimicrob. Agents Chemother.* **2011**, *55*, 2352–2361. [CrossRef] [PubMed]

28. Lanteri, C.A.; Tidwell, R.R.; Meshnick, S.R. The mitochondrion is a site of trypanocidal action of the aromatic diamidine DB75 in bloodstream forms of *Trypanosoma brucei*. *Antimicrob. Agents Chemother.* **2008**, *52*, 875–882. [CrossRef] [PubMed]

29. Alkhaldi, A.A.M.; Martinek, J.; Panicucci, B.; Dardonville, C.; Ziková, A.; De Koning, H.P. Trypanocidal action of bisphosphonium salts through a mitochondrial target in bloodstream form *Trypanosoma brucei*. *Int. J. Parasitol. Drugs Drug. Res.* **2016**, *6*, 23–34. [CrossRef]

30. Ebiloma, G.U.; Balogun, E.O.; Cueto Díaz, E.J.; De Koning, H.P.; Dardonville, C. Alternative Oxidase inhibitors: Development and efficient mitochondrion-targeting as a strategy for new drugs against pathogenic parasites and fungi. *Med. Res. Rev.* **2019**, *39*, 1553–1602. [CrossRef]

31. Fueyo González, F.J.; Ebiloma, G.U.; Izquierdo García, C.; Bruggeman, V.; Sánchez Villamañán, J.M.; Donachie, A.; Balogun, E.O.; Inaoka, D.K.; Shiba, T.; Harada, S.; et al. Conjugates of 2,4-dihydroxybenzoate and salicylhydroxamate and lipocations display potent anti-parasite effects by efficiently targeting the *Trypanosoma brucei* and *Trypanosoma congolense* mitochondrion. *J. Med. Chem.* **2017**, *60*, 1509–1522. [CrossRef]

32. Basselin, M.; Denise, H.; Coombs, G.H.; Barrett, M.P. Resistance to pentamidine in *Leishmania mexicana* involves exclusion of the drug from the mitochondrion. *Antimicrob. Agents Chemother.* **2002**, *46*, 3731–3738. [CrossRef]

33. Bray, P.G.; Barrett, M.P.; Ward, S.A.; De Koning, H.P. Pentamidine uptake and resistance in pathogenic protozoa. *Trends Parasitol.* **2003**, *19*, 232–239. [CrossRef]

34. Doua, F.; Miezan, T.W.; Sanon Singaro, J.R.; Boa Yapo, F.; Baltz, T. The efficacy of pentamidine in the treatment of early-late stage *Trypanosoma brucei gambiense* trypanosomiasis. *Am. J. Trop. Med. Hyg.* **1996**, *55*, 586–588. [CrossRef] [PubMed]

35. Sekhar, G.N.; Georgian, A.R.; Sanderson, L.; Vizcay-Barrena, G.; Brown, R.C.; Muresan, P.; Fleck, R.A.; Thomas, S.A. Organic cation transporter 1 (OCT1) is involved in pentamidine transport at the human and mouse blood-brain barrier (BBB). *PLoS ONE* **2017**, *12*, e0173474. [CrossRef] [PubMed]

36. Sturk, L.M.; Brock, J.L.; Bagnell, C.R.; Hall, J.E.; Tidwell, R.R. Distribution and quantitation of the anti-trypanosomal diamidine 2,5-bis (4-amidinophenyl) furan (DB75) and its N-methoxy prodrug DB289 in murine brain tissue. *Acta Trop.* **2004**, *91*, 131–143. [CrossRef]

37. Sanderson, L.; Dogruel, M.; Rodgers, J.; De Koning, H.P.; Thomas, S.A. Pentamidine movement across the murine blood-brain and blood-CSF barriers; effect of trypanosome infection, combination therapy, P-glycoprotein and MRP. *J. Pharmacol. Exp. Ther.* **2009**, *329*, 967–977. [CrossRef]

38. Yang, S.; Wenzler, T.; Miller, P.N.; Wu, H.; Boykin, D.W.; Brun, R.; Wang, M.Z. Pharmacokinetic comparison to determine the mechanisms underlying the differential efficacies of cationic diamidines against first- and second-stage human African trypanosomiasis. *Antimicrob. Agents Chemother.* **2014**, *58*, 4064–4074. [CrossRef]

39. Myburgh, E.; Coles, J.A.; Ritchie, R.; Kennedy, P.G.; McLatchie, A.P.; Rodgers, J.; Taylor, M.C.; Barrett, M.P.; Brewer, J.M.; Mottram, J.C. In vivo imaging of trypanosome-brain interactions and development of a rapid screening test for drugs against CNS stage trypanosomiasis. *PLoS Negl. Trop. Dis.* **2013**, *7*, e2384. [CrossRef]

40. Paine, M.; Wang, M.; Boykin, D.; Wilson, W.D.; De Koning, H.P.; Olson, C.; Polig, G.; Burri, C.; Brun, R.; Murilla, G.A.; et al. Diamidines for human African trypanosomiasis. *Curr. Opin. Investig. Drugs* **2010**, *11*, 876–883.

41. Pohlig, G.; Bernhard, S.C.; Blum, J.; Burri, C.; Mpanya, A.; Lubaki, J.P.; Mpoto, A.M.; Munungu, B.F.; N'tombe, P.M.; Deo, G.K.; et al. Efficacy and safety of pafuramidine versus pentamidine maleate for treatment of first stage sleeping sickness in a randomized, comparator-controlled, international phase 3 clinical trial. *PLoS Negl. Trop. Dis.* **2016**, *10*, e0004363. [CrossRef]

42. Wenzler, T.; Boykin, D.W.; Ismail, M.A.; Hall, J.E.; Tidwell, R.R.; Brun, R. New treatment option for second-stage African sleeping sickness: In vitro and in vivo efficacy of aza analogs of DB289. *Antimicrob. Agents Chemother.* **2009**, *53*, 4185–4192. [CrossRef]

43. Thuita, J.K.; Wolf, K.K.; Murilla, G.A.; Bridges, A.S.; Boykin, D.W.; Mutuku, J.N.; Liu, Q.; Jones, S.K.; Gem, C.O.; Ching, S.; et al. Chemotherapy of second stage human African trypanosomiasis: Comparison between the parenteral diamidine DB829 and its oral prodrug DB868 in vervet monkeys. *PLoS Negl. Trop. Dis.* **2015**, *9*, e0003409. [CrossRef] [PubMed]

44. Carter, N.S.; Berger, B.J.; Fairlamb, A.H. Uptake of diamidine drugs by the P2 nucleoside transporter in melarsen-sensitive and -resistant *Trypanosoma brucei brucei*. *J. Biol. Chem.* **1995**, *270*, 28153–28157. [PubMed]
45. De Koning, H.P.; Jarvis, S.M. Uptake of pentamidine in *Trypanosoma brucei brucei* is mediated by the P2 adenosine transporter and at least one novel, unrelated transporter. *Acta Trop.* **2001**, *80*, 245–250. [CrossRef]
46. De Koning, H.P.; Anderson, L.F.; Stewart, M.; Burchmore, R.J.S.; Wallace, L.J.M.; Barrett, M.P. The trypanocide diminazene aceturate is accumulated predominantly through the TbAT1 purine transporter; additional insights in diamidine resistance in African trypanosomes. *Antimicrob. Agents Chemother.* **2004**, *48*, 1515–1519. [CrossRef] [PubMed]
47. Mäser, P.; Sütterlin, C.; Kralli, A.; Kaminsky, R. A nucleoside transporter from *Trypanosoma brucei* involved in drug resistance. *Science* **1999**, *285*, 242–244.
48. Matovu, E.; Stewart, M.; Geiser, F.; Brun, R.; Mäser, P.; Wallace, L.J.M.; Burchmore, R.J.; Enyaru, J.C.K.; Barrett, M.P.; Kaminsky, R.; et al. The mechanisms of arsenical and diamidine uptake and resistance in *Trypanosoma brucei*. *Eukaryot. Cell* **2003**, *2*, 1003–1008. [CrossRef]
49. Graf, F.E.; Ludin, P.; Wenzler, T.; Kaiser, M.; Pyana, P.; Büscher, P.; De Koning, H.P.; Horn, D.; Mäser, P. Aquaporin 2 mutations in *Trypanosoma b. gambiense* field isolates correlate with decreased susceptibility to pentamidine and melarsoprol. *PLoS Negl. Trop. Dis.* **2013**, *7*, e2475. [CrossRef]
50. Munday, J.C.; Tagoe, D.N.A.; Eze, A.A.; Krezdorn, J.A.; Rojas López, K.E.; Alkhaldi, A.A.M.; McDonald, F.; Still, J.; Alzahrani, K.J.; Settimo, L.; et al. Functional analysis of drug resistance-associated mutations in the *Trypanosoma brucei* adenosine transporter 1 (TbAT1) and the proposal of a structural model for the protein. *Mol. Microbiol.* **2015**, *96*, 887–900. [CrossRef]
51. De Koning, H.P.; Jarvis, S.M. Adenosine transporters in bloodstream forms of *T. b. brucei*: Substrate recognition motifs and affinity for trypanocidal drugs. *Mol. Pharmacol.* **1999**, *56*, 1162–1170. [CrossRef]
52. Collar, C.J.; Al-Salabi, M.I.; Stewart, M.L.; Barrett, M.P.; Wilson, W.D.; De Koning, H.P. Predictive computational models of substrate binding by a nucleoside transporter. *J. Biol. Chem.* **2009**, *284*, 34028–34035. [CrossRef]
53. De Koning, H.P. Uptake of pentamidine in *Trypanosoma brucei brucei* is mediated by three distinct transporters. Implications for crossresistance with arsenicals. *Mol. Pharmacol.* **2001**, *59*, 586–592. [CrossRef] [PubMed]
54. Bridges, D.; Gould, M.K.; Nerima, B.; Mäser, P.; Burchmore, R.J.S.; De Koning, H.P. Loss of the High Affinity Pentamidine Transporter is responsible for high levels of cross-resistance between arsenical and diamidine drugs in African trypanosomes. *Mol. Pharmacol.* **2007**, *71*, 1098–1108. [CrossRef] [PubMed]
55. Munday, J.C.; Eze, A.A.; Baker, N.; Glover, L.; Clucas, C.; Aguinaga Andrés, D.; Natto, M.J.; Teka, I.A.; McDonald, J.; Lee, R.S.; et al. *Trypanosoma brucei* Aquaglyceroporin 2 is a high affinity transporter for pentamidine and melaminophenyl arsenic drugs and is the main genetic determinant of resistance to these drugs. *J. Antimicrob. Chemother.* **2014**, *69*, 651–663. [CrossRef] [PubMed]
56. Alsford, S.; Eckert, S.; Baker, N.; Glover, L.; Sanchez-Flores, A.; Leung, K.F.; Turner, D.J.; Field, M.C.; Berriman, M.; Horn, D. High-throughput decoding of antitrypanosomal drug efficacy and resistance. *Nature* **2012**, *482*, 232–236. [CrossRef]
57. Baker, N.; Glover, L.; Munday, J.C.; Aguinaga Andrés, D.; Barrett, M.P.; De Koning, H.P.; Horn, D. Aquaglyceroporin 2 controls susceptibility to melarsoprol and pentamidine in African trypanosomes. *Proc. Natl. Acad. Sci. USA* **2012**, *109*, 10996–11001. [CrossRef]
58. Song, J.; Baker, N.; Rothert, M.; Henke, B.; Jeacock, L.; Horn, D.; Beitz, E. Pentamidine is not a permeant but a nanomolar inhibitor of the *Trypanosoma brucei* Aquaglyceroporin-2. *PLoS Pathog.* **2016**, *2*, e1005436. [CrossRef]
59. Teka, I.A.; Kazibwe, A.; El-Sabbagh, N.; Al-Salabi, M.I.; Ward, C.P.; Eze, A.A.; Munday, J.C.; Mäser, P.; Matovu, E.; Barrett, M.P.; et al. The diamidine diminazene aceturate is a substrate for the High Affinity Pentamidine Transporter: Implications for the development of high resistance levels. *Mol. Pharmacol.* **2011**, *80*, 110–116. [CrossRef]
60. Langreth, S.G.; Balber, A.E. Protein uptake and digestion in bloodstream and culture forms of *Trypanosoma brucei*. *J. Protozool.* **1975**, *22*, 40–55. [CrossRef]
61. Field, M.C.; Carrington, M. The trypanosome flagellar pocket. *Nat. Rev. Microbiol.* **2009**, *7*, 775–786. [CrossRef]
62. Munday, J.C.; Settimo, L.; De Koning, H.P. Transport proteins determine drug sensitivity and resistance in a protozoan parasite, *Trypanosoma brucei*. *Front. Pharmacol.* **2015**, *6*, 32. [CrossRef]

63. Alghamdi, A.; Munday, J.C.; Campagnaro, G.; Eze, A.A.; Svensson, F.; Martin Abril, E.; Milic, P.; Dimitriou, A.; Wielinska, J.; Smart, G.; et al. Pentamidine enters *Trypanosoma brucei* by passing through the pore of the aquaglyceroporin TbAQP2. 2020; (submitted).

64. Unciti-Broceta, J.D.; Arias, J.L.; Maceira, J.; Soriano, M.; Ortiz-González, M.; Hernández-Quero, J.; Muñóz-Torres, M.; De Koning, H.P.; Magez, S.; Garcia-Salcedo, J.A. Specific cell targeting therapy bypasses drug resistance mechanisms in African trypanosomiasis. *PloS Pathog.* **2015**, *11*, e1004942. [CrossRef] [PubMed]

65. Livingstone D (1858) Arsenic as a remedy for the tsetse bite. *Brit. Med. J.* **1858**, *1*, 360–361.

66. Bruce, D. *Preliminary Report on the Tsetse Fly Disease or Nagana*; Zululand: Harrison and Sons, London, 1895.

67. *The African Trypanosomiases*; Mulligan, H.W. (Ed.) George Allen and Unwin Ltd.: London, UK, 1970; pp. 41–88.

68. Jacobs, W.A.; Heidelberger, M. Aromatic arsenic compounds v. N-substituted glycylarsanilic acids. *J. Am. Chem. Soc.* **1919**, *41*, 1809–1821. [CrossRef]

69. Van Nieuwenhove, S. Present strategies in the treatment of human African trypanosomiasis. In *Progress in Human African Trypanosomiasis, Sleeping Sickness*; Dumas, M., Bouteille, B., Buguet, A., Eds.; Springer: Paris, France, 1999; pp. 253–281.

70. Dukes, P. Arsenic and old taxa: Subspeciation and drug sensitivity in *Trypanosoma brucei*. *Trans. R. Soc. Trop. Med. Hyg.* **1984**, *78*, 711–725. [CrossRef]

71. Fourneau, E.; Tréfouël, J.; Tréfouël, T.; Benoit, G. Sur les isomères de l'acide para-oxy-3-amino-phényl-arsinique et de son dérivé acétylé (stovarsol). *Bull. Soc. Chim. Fr.* **1927**, *41*, 499–514.

72. Apted, F.I.C. Treatment of human trypanosomiasis. In *The African Trypanosomiases*; Mulligan, H.W., Ed.; George Allen and Unwin Ltd.: London, UK, 1970; pp. 684–710.

73. Ledentu, G.; Daude, J. Essai du traitement de la trypanosomiase humaine par le 270 Fourneau. *Ann. Inst. Pasteur* **1926**, *40*, 830–845.

74. Laveissière, C.; Penchenier, L. *Manuel De Lutte Contre La Maladie Du Sommeil*; éditions de l'Institut de recherche pour le développement, coll. Didactiques. IRD Editions: Marseille, France, 2005; Volume 4, p. 273.

75. Ollivier, G.; Legros, D. Trypanosomiase humaine africaine: Historique de la thérapeutique et de ses échecs. *Trop. Med. Int. Health* **2001**, *6*, 855–863. [CrossRef]

76. Rollo, I.M.; Williamson, J.; Lourie, E.M. Studies on the chemotherapy of melaminyl arsenicals and antimonials in laboratory trypanosome infections. *Ann. Trop. Med. Parasitol.* **1949**, *43*, 194–208. [CrossRef]

77. Van Hoof, L.; Henrard, C.; Peel, E. Pentamidine is the prevention and treatment of trypanosomiasis. *Trans. R. Soc. Trop. Med. Hyg.* **1944**, *37*, 271–280. [CrossRef]

78. Murgatroyd, F.; Yorke, W. Studies in chemotherapy XIV—The stability of drug-resistance in trypanosomes. *Ann. Trop. Med. Parsitol.* **1937**, *31*, 165–172. [CrossRef]

79. Wery, M. therapy for African trypanosomiasis. *Curr. Opin. Infect. Dis.* **1991**, *4*, 838–843. [CrossRef]

80. Jonchere, H.; Gomer, J.; Reynaud, R. Contribution à l'étude de produits a radical mélaminyl dans le traitement de la trypanosmiase humaine à Tr gambiense. *Bull. Soc. Pathol. Exot.* **1953**, *3*, 386–396.

81. Blum, J.; Nkunku, S.; Burri, C. Clinical description of encephalopathic syndromes and risk factors for their occurrence and outcome during melarsoprol treatment of human African trypanosomiasis. *Trop. Med. Int. Health* **2001**, *6*, 390–400. [CrossRef] [PubMed]

82. Pépin, J.; Milord, F.; Khonde, A.; Niyonsenga, T.; Loko, L.; Mpia, B. Gambiense trypanosomiasis: Frequency of, and risk factors for, failure of melarsoprol therapy. *Trans. R. Soc. Trop. Med. Hyg.* **1994**, *88*, 447–452. [CrossRef]

83. Schmid, C.; Richer, M.; Bilenge, C.M.; Josenando, T.; Chappuis, F.; Manthelot, C.R.; Nangouma, A.; Doua, F.; Asumu, P.N.; Simarro, P.P.; et al. Effectiveness of a 10-day melarsoprol schedule for the treatment of late-stage human African trypanosomiasis: Confirmation from a multinational study (IMPAMEL II). *J. Infect. Dis.* **2005**, *191*, 1922–1931. [CrossRef]

84. Rodgers, J.; Jones, A.; Gibaud, S.; Bradley, B.; McCabe, C.; Barrett, M.P.; Gettinby, G.; Kennedy, P.G.E. Melarsoprol Cyclodextrin Inclusion Complexes as Promising Oral Candidates for the Treatment of Human African Trypanosomiasis. *PLOS Negl. Trop. Dis.* **2011**, *5*, e1308. [CrossRef]

85. Committee for Orphan Medicinal Products (COMP) Meeting Report on the Review of Applications for Orphan Designation. 8 October 2012. Available online: https://www.ema.europa.eu/en/documents/committee-

report/comp-meeting-report-review-applications-orphan-designation-october-2012_en.pdf (accessed on 17 January 2020).

86. Rollo, I.M.; Williamson, J. Acquired resistance to 'Melarsan', tryparsamidine and amidines in pathogenic trypanosomes. *Nature* **1951**, *167*, 147–148. [CrossRef]
87. Baker, N.; De Koning, H.P.; Mäser, P.; Horn, D. Drug resistance in African trypanosomiasis: The melarsoprol and pentamidine story. *Trends Parasitol.* **2013**, *29*, 110–118. [CrossRef]
88. De Koning, H.P. The ever-increasing complexities of arsenical-diamidine cross-resistance in African trypanosomes. *Trends Parasitol.* **2008**, *24*, 345–349. [CrossRef]
89. Carter, N.S.; Fairlamb, A.H. Arsenical-resistant trypanosomes lack an unusual adenosine transporter. *Nature* **1993**, *361*, 173–176. [CrossRef] [PubMed]
90. De Koning, H.P.; MacLeod, A.; Barrett, M.P.; Cover, B.; Jarvis, S.M. Further evidence for a link between melarsoprol resistance and P2 transporter function in African trypanosomes. *Mol. Biochem. Parasitol.* **2000**, *106*, 181–185. [CrossRef]
91. Carter, N.S.; Barrett, M.P.; De Koning, H.P. A drug resistance determinant from *Trypanosoma brucei*. *Trends Microbiol.* **1999**, *7*, 469–471. [CrossRef]
92. Nerima, B.; Matovu, E.; Lubega, G.W.; Enyaru, J.C. Detection of mutant P2 adenosine transporter (TbAT1) gene in *Trypanosoma brucei gambiense* isolates from northwest Uganda using allele-specific polymerase chain reaction. *Trop. Med. Int. Health* **2007**, *12*, 1361–1368. [CrossRef] [PubMed]
93. Matovu, E.; Geiser, F.; Schneider, V.; Mäser, P.; Enyaru, J.C.; Kaminsky, R.; Gallati, S.; Seebeck, T. Genetic variants of the TbAT1 adenosine transporter from African trypanosomes in relapse infections following melarsoprol therapy. *Mol. Biochem. Parasitol.* **2001**, *117*, 73–81. [CrossRef]
94. Barrett, M.P.; Vincent, I.M.; Burchmore, R.J.S.; Kazibwe, A.J.N.; Matovu, E. Drug resistance in human African trypanosomiasis. *Future Microbiol.* **2011**, *6*, 1037–1047. [CrossRef]
95. Brun, R.; Schumacher, R.; Schmid, C.; Kunz, C.; Burri, C. The phenomenon of treatment failures in Human African Trypanosomiasis. *Trop. Med. Int. Health* **2011**, *6*, 906–914. [CrossRef]
96. Legros, D.; Fournier, C.; Gastellu Etchegorry, M.; Maiso, F.; Szumilin, E. Therapeutic failure of melarsoprol among patients treated for late stage *T.b. gambiense* human African trypanosomiasis in Uganda. *Bull. Soc. Pathol. Exot.* **1999**, *92*, 171–172.
97. Moore, A.; Richer, M. Re-emergence of epidemic sleeping sickness in southern Sudan. *Trop. Med. Int. Health* **2001**, *6*, 342–347. [CrossRef]
98. Robays, J.; Nyamowala, G.; Sese, C.; Betu Ku Mesu Kande, V.; Lutumba, P.; Van der Veken, W.; Boelaert, M. High failure rates of melarsoprol for sleeping sickness, Democratic Republic of Congo. *Emerg. Infect. Dis.* **2008**, *14*, 966–967. [CrossRef]
99. Burri, C.; Keiser, J. Pharmacokinetic investigations in patients from northern Angola refractory to melarsoprol treatment. *Trop. Med. Int. Health* **2001**, *6*, 412–420. [CrossRef]
100. Kazibwe, A.J.N.; Nerima, B.; De Koning, H.P.; Mäser, P.; Barrett, M.P.; Matovu, E. Genotypic status of the TbAT1/P2 adenosine transporter of *Trypanosoma brucei gambiense* isolates from North western Uganda following melarsoprol withdrawal. *PLoS Negl. Trop. Dis.* **2009**, *3*, e523. [CrossRef] [PubMed]
101. Pyana Pati, P.; Van Reet, N.; Mumba Ngoyi, D.; Ngay Lukusa, I.; Karhemere Bin Shamamba, S.; Büscher, P. Melarsoprol sensitivity profile of *Trypanosoma brucei gambiense* isolates from cured and relapsed sleeping sickness patients from the Democratic Republic of the Congo. *PLoS Negl. Trop. Dis.* **2014**, *8*, e3212. [CrossRef]
102. Graf, F.E.; Baker, N.; Munday, J.C.; De Koning, H.P.; Horn, D.; Mäser, P. Chimerization at the *AQP2-AQP3* locus is the genetic basis of melarsoprol-pentamidine cross-resistance in clinical *Trypanosoma brucei gambiense* isolates. *Int. J. Parasitol. Drugs Drug Res.* **2015**, *5*, 65–68. [CrossRef] [PubMed]
103. Graf, F.E.; Ludin, P.; Arquint, C.; Schmidt, R.S.; Schaub, N.; Kunz-Renggli, C.; Munday, J.C.; Krezdorn, J.; Baker, N.; Horn, D.; et al. Comparative genomics of drug resistance of the sleeping sickness parasite *Trypanosoma brucei rhodesiense*. *Cell. Mol. Life Sci.* **2016**, *73*, 3387–3400. [CrossRef] [PubMed]
104. Munday, J.C.; Rojas López, K.E.; Eze, A.A.; Delespaux, V.; Van Den Abbeele, J.; Rowan, T.; Barrett, M.P.; Morrison, L.J.; De Koning, H.P. Functional expression of TcoAT1 reveals it to be a P1-type nucleoside transporter with no capacity for diminazene uptake. *Int. J. Parasitol. Drugs Drug Resist.* **2013**, *3*, 69–76. [CrossRef] [PubMed]
105. Ehrlich, P.; Shiga, K. Farben therapeutische Versuche bei Trypanosomerkrankung. *Berl. Klin. Wochenschr.* **1904**, *14*, 362–365.

106. Ehrlich, P.; Shiga, K. Farbentherapeutische Versuche bei Trypanosomenerkrankung. *Berl. Klin. Wochenschr.* **1904**, *41*, 329–332.

107. Steverding, D. The development of drugs for treatment of sleeping sickness: A historical review. *Parasit. Vectors* **2010**, *3*, 15. [CrossRef]

108. Ehrlich, P. Aus Theorie und Praxis der Chemotherapie. *Folia Serol.* **1911**, *7*, 697–714.

109. Nicolle, M.; Mesnil, F. Traitement des trypanosomiases par les couleurs de benzidine. Première partie—Étude chemique. *Ann. Inst. Pasteur.* **1906**, *20*, 417–448.

110. Mesnil, F.; Nicolle, M. Traitement des trypanosomiases par les couleurs de benzidine. Second partie—Étude expérimentale. *Ann. Inst. Pasteur.* **1906**, *20*, 513–538.

111. Tréfouël, J. Le rôle de Maurice Nicolle en chimiothérapie anti-trypanosome. *Bull. Soc. Pathol. Exotique.* **1962**, *55*, 200–207.

112. Travis, A.S. Paul Ehrlich: A hundred years of chemotherapy 1891-1991. *Biochemist* **1991**, *13*, 9–12.

113. Schlitzer, M. Wirkstoffe zur Behandlung der Afrikanischer Schlafkrankheit. *Pharm. Unsere Zeit.* **2009**, *6*, 552–558. [CrossRef] [PubMed]

114. Pope, W.J. Synthetic therapeutic agents. *Br. Med. J.* **1924**, *1*, 413–414. [CrossRef]

115. Fourneau, E.; Tréfouël, J.; Vallée, J. Sur une nouvelle série de médicaments trypanocides. *Comptes Rendus des Séances de l'Académie des Sciences* **1924**, *178*, 675.

116. Fourneau, E.; Tréfouël, J.; Vallée, J. Recherches de chimiothérapie dans la série du 205 Bayer. Urées des acides aminobenzoylaminonaphtaléniques. *Ann. Inst. Pasteur.* **1924**, *38*, 81–114.

117. Apted, F.I.C. Present status of chemotherapy and chemoprophylaxis of human trypanosomiasis in the Eastern hemisphere. *Pharmac. Ther.* **1980**, *11*, 391–413. [CrossRef]

118. Pépin, J.; Milord, F. The treatment of human African trypanosomiasis. *Adv. Parasitol.* **1994**, *33*, 1–47.

119. Scott, A.G.; Tait, A.; Turner, C.M. Characterisation of cloned lines of *Trypanosoma brucei* expressing stable resistance to MelCy and suramin. *Acta Trop.* **1996**, *60*, 251–262. [CrossRef]

120. Lipinski, C.A.; Lombardo, F.; Dominy, B.W. Experimental and computational approaches to estimate solubility and permeability in drug discovery and development settings. *Adv. Drug Deliv. Rev.* **2001**, *46*, 3–26. [CrossRef]

121. Coppens, I.; Opperdoes, F.R.; Courtoy, P.J.; Baudhuin, P. Receptor-mediated endocytosis in the blood-stream form of *Trypanosoma brucei. J. Protozool.* **1987**, *34*, 465–473. [CrossRef] [PubMed]

122. Vansterkenburg, E.L.M.; Coppens, I.; Wilting, J.; Bos, O.J.M.; Fischer, M.J.E.; Janssen, L.H.M.; Opperdoes, F.R. The uptake of the trypanocidal drug Suramin in combination with low-density lipoproteins by *Trypanosoma brucei* and its possible mode of action. *Acta Trop.* **1993**, *54*, 237–250. [CrossRef]

123. Pal, A.; Hall, B.S.; Field, M.C. Evidence for a non-LDL-mediated entry route for the trypanocidal drug suramin in *Trypanosoma brucei. Mol. Biochem. Parasitol.* **2002**, *122*, 217–221. [CrossRef]

124. Jaffe, J.J.; McCormack, J.J.; Meymariam, E. Comparative properties of schistosomal and filarial dihydrofolate reductase. *Biochem. Pharmacol.* **1972**, *21*, 719–731. [CrossRef]

125. Chello, P.L.; Jaffe, J.J. Comparative properties of trypanosomal and mammalian thymidine kinases. *Comp. Biochem. Physiol. B* **1972**, *43*, 543–562. [CrossRef]

126. Willson, M.; Callens, M.; Kuntz, D.A.; Perié, J.; Opperdoes, F.R. Synthesis and activity of inhibitors highly specific for the glycolytic enzymes from *Trypanosoma brucei. Mol. Biochem. Parasitol.* **1993**, *59*, 201–210. [CrossRef]

127. Zoltner, M.; Horn, D.; De Koning, H.P.; Field, M.C. Exploiting the Achilles' heel of membrane trafficking in trypanosomes. *Curr. Opin. Microbiol.* **2016**, *34*, 97–103. [CrossRef]

128. Alsford, S.; Field, M.C.; Horn, D. Receptor-mediated endocytosis for drug delivery in African trypanosomes: Fulfilling Paul Ehrlich's vision of chemotherapy. *Trends. Parasitol.* **2013**, *29*, 207–212. [CrossRef]

129. Poulin, R.; Lu, L.; Ackermann, B.; Bey, P.; Pegg, A.E. Mechanism of the irreversible inactivation of mouse ornithine decarboxylase by alpha-difluoromethylornithine. Characterization of sequences at the inhibitor and coenzyme binding sites. *J. Biol. Chem.* **1992**, *267*, 150–158.

130. Weeks, C.E.; Herrmann, A.L.; Nelson, F.R.; Slaga, T.J. α-Difluoromethylornithine, an irreversible inhibitor of ornithine decarboxylase, inhibits tumor promoter-induced polyamine accumulation and carcinogenesis in mouse skin. *Proc. Natl. Acad. Sci. USA* **1982**, *79*, 6028–6032. [CrossRef]

131. Meyskens, F.L., Jr.; Gerner, E.W. Development of difluoromethylornithine (DFMO) as a chemoprevention agent. *Clin. Cancer Res.* **1999**, *5*, 945–951. [PubMed]

132. Gerner, E.W.; Meyskens, F.L., Jr. Polyamines and cancer: Old molecules, new understanding. *Nat. Rev. Cancer* **2004**, *4*, 781–792. [CrossRef]

133. Milord, F.; Pépin, J.; Loko, L.; Ethier, L.; Mpia, B. Efficacy and toxicity of eflornithine for treatment of *Trypanosoma brucei gambiense* sleeping sickness. *Lancet* **1992**, *340*, 652–655. [CrossRef]

134. Van Nieuwenhove, S.; Schechter, P.J.; Declercq, J.; Bone, G.; Burke, J.; Sjoerdsma, A. Treatment of gambiense sleeping sickness in Sudan with oral DFMO (DL-alpha-difluoromethylornithine), an inhibitor of ornithine decarboxylase: First field trial. *Trans. R. Soc. Trop. Med. Hyg.* **1985**, *79*, 692–698. [CrossRef]

135. Taelman, H.; Schechter, P.J.; Marcelis, L.; Sonnet, J.; Kazyumba, G.; Dasnoy, J.; Haegele, K.D.; Sjoerdsma, A.; Wery, M. Difluoromethylornithine, an effective new treatment of Gambian trypanosomiasis. Results in five patients. *Am. J. Med.* **1987**, *82*, 607–614. [CrossRef]

136. Eozenou, P.; Jannin, J.; Ngampo, S.; Carme, B.; Tell, G.P.; Schechter, P.J. Essai de traitement de la trypanosomiase a *Trypanosoma brucei gambiense* par l'eflornithine en Republique Populaire du Congo. *Med. Trop.* **1989**, *49*, 149–154.

137. Ebikeme, C. The death and life of the resurrection drug. *PLoS Negl. Trop. Dis.* **2014**, *8*, e2910. [CrossRef]

138. Burri, C.; Brun, R. Eflornithine for the treatment of human African trypanosomiasis. *Parasitol. Res.* **2003**, *90*, S49–S52. [CrossRef]

139. Kennedy, P.G. Clinical features, diagnosis, and treatment of human African trypanosomiasis (sleeping sickness). *Lancet Neurol.* **2013**, *12*, 186–194. [CrossRef]

140. Bales, J.D.; Harison, S.M.; Mbwabi, D.L.; Schechter, P.J. Treatment of arsenical refractory Rhodesian sleeping sickness in Kenya. *Ann. Trop. Med. Parasitol.* **1989**, *83* (Suppl. S1), 111–114. [CrossRef] [PubMed]

141. Bacchi, C.J.; Nathan, H.C.; Livingston, T.; Valladares, G.; Saric, M.; Sayer, P.D.; Njogu, A.R.; Clarkson, A.B., Jr. Differential susceptibility to DL-alpha-difluoromethylornithine in clinical isolates of *Trypanosoma brucei rhodesiense*. *Antimicrob. Agents Chemother.* **1990**, *34*, 1183–1188. [CrossRef] [PubMed]

142. Iten, M.; Matovu, E.; Brun, R.; Kaminsky, R. Innate lack of susceptibility of Ugandan *Trypanosoma brucei rhodesiense* to DL-alpha-difluoromethylornithine (DFMO). *Trop. Med. Parasitol.* **1995**, *46*, 190–194. [PubMed]

143. Iten, M.; Mett, H.; Evans, A.; Enyaru, J.C.; Brun, R.; Kaminsky, R. Alterations in ornithine decarboxylase characteristics account for tolerance of *Trypanosoma brucei rhodesiense* to D,L-alpha-difluoromethylornithine. *Antimicrob. Agents Chemother.* **1997**, *41*, 1922–1925. [CrossRef]

144. Bellofatto, V.; Fairlamb, A.H.; Henderson, G.B.; Cross, G.A.M. Biochemical changes associated with alpha-difluoromethylornithine uptake and resistance in *Trypanosoma brucei*. *Mol. Biochem. Parasitol.* **1987**, *25*, 227–238. [CrossRef]

145. Phillips, M.A.; Wang, C.C. A *Trypanosoma brucei* mutant resistant to alpha-difluoromethylornithine. *Mol. Biochem. Parasitol.* **1987**, *22*, 9–17. [CrossRef]

146. Delespaux, V.; De Koning, H.P. Drugs and drug resistance in African trypanosomiasis. *Drug Resist. Updat.* **2007**, *10*, 30–50. [CrossRef]

147. Bitonti, A.J.; Bacchi, C.J.; McCann, P.P.; Sjoerdsma, A. Uptake of alpha-difluoromethylornithine by *Trypanosoma brucei brucei*. *Biochem. Pharmacol.* **1986**, *35*, 351–354. [CrossRef]

148. Vincent, I.M.; Creek, D.; Watson, D.G.; Kamleh, M.A.; Woods, D.J.; Wong, P.E.; Burchmore, R.J.; Barrett, M.P. A molecular mechanism for eflornithine resistance in African trypanosomes. *PLoS Pathog.* **2010**, *6*, e1001204. [CrossRef]

149. Schumann Burkard, G.; Jutzi, P.; Roditi, I. Genome-wide RNAi screens in bloodstream form trypanosomes identify drug transporters. *Mol. Biochem. Parasitol.* **2011**, *175*, 91–94. [CrossRef]

150. Simarro, P.P.; Franco, J.; Diarra, A.; Postigo, J.A.; Jannin, J. Update on field use of the available drugs for the chemotherapy of human African trypanosomiasis. *Parasitology* **2012**, *139*, 842–846. [CrossRef] [PubMed]

151. Mpia, B.; Pépin, J. Combination of eflornithine and melarsoprol for melarsoprol-resistant Gambian trypanosomiasis. *Trop. Med. Int. Health* **2002**, *7*, 775–779. [CrossRef] [PubMed]

152. Priotto, G.; Fogg, C.; Balasegaram, M.; Erphas, O.; Louga, A.; Checchi, F.; Ghabri, S.; Piola, P. Three drug combinations for late-stage *Trypanosoma brucei gambiense* sleeping sickness: A randomized clinical trial in Uganda. *PLoS Clin. Trials.* **2006**, *1*, e39. [CrossRef] [PubMed]

153. Checchi, F.; Piola, P.; Ayikoru, H.; Thomas, F.; Legros, D.; Priotto, G. Nifurtimox plus Eflornithine for late-stage sleeping sickness in Uganda: A case series. *PLoS Negl. Trop. Dis.* **2007**, *1*, e64. [CrossRef] [PubMed]

154. Priotto, G.; Kasparian, S.; Ngouama, D.; Ghorashian, S.; Arnold, U.; Ghabri, S.; Karunakara, U. Nifurtimox-eflornithine combination therapy for second-stage *Trypanosoma brucei gambiense* sleeping sickness: A randomized clinical trial in Congo. *Clin. Infect. Dis.* **2007**, *45*, 1435–1442. [CrossRef]

155. Priotto, G.; Kasparian, S.; Mutombo, W.; Ngouama, D.; Ghorashian, S.; Arnold, U.; Ghabri, S.; Baudin, E.; Buard, V.; Kazadi-Kyanza, S.; et al. Nifurtimox-eflornithine combination therapy for second-stage African *Trypanosoma brucei gambiense* trypanosomiasis: A multicentre, randomised, phase III, non-inferiority trial. *Lancet* **2009**, *374*, 56–64. [CrossRef]

156. Yun, O.; Priotto, G.; Tong, J.; Flevaud, L.; Chappuis, F. NECT is next: Implementing the new drug combination therapy for *Trypanosoma brucei gambiense* sleeping sickness. *PLoS Negl. Trop. Dis.* **2010**, *4*, e720. [CrossRef]

157. Franco, J.R.; Simarro, P.P.; Diarra, A.; Ruiz-Postigo, J.A.; Samo, M.; Jannin, J.G. Monitoring the use of nifurtimox-eflornithine combination therapy (NECT) in the treatment of second stage gambiense human African trypanosomiasis. *Res. Rep. Trop. Med.* **2012**, *3*, 93–101. [CrossRef]

158. Alirol, E.; Schrumpf, D.; Amici Heradi, J.; Riedel, A.; de Patoul, C.; Quere, M.; Chappuis, F. Nifurtimox-eflornithine combination therapy for second-stage gambiense human African trypanosomiasis: Médecins Sans Frontières experience in the Democratic Republic of the Congo. *Clin. Infect. Dis.* **2013**, *56*, 195–203. [CrossRef]

159. Kansiime, F.; Adibaku, S.; Wamboga, C.; Idi, F.; Kato, C.D.; Yamuah, L.; Vaillant, M.; Kioy, D.; Olliaro, P.; Matovu, E. A multicentre, randomised, non-inferiority clinical trial comparing a nifurtimox-eflornithine combination to standard eflornithine monotherapy for late stage *Trypanosoma brucei gambiense* human African trypanosomiasis in Uganda. *Parasit. Vectors* **2018**, *11*, 105. [CrossRef]

160. Wegner, D.H.G.; Rohwedder, R.W. The effect of nifurtimox on acute Chagas' infection. *Arzneim. Forsch.* **1972**, *22*, 1624–1635.

161. Ribeiro, V.; Dias, N.; Paiva, T.; Hagström-Bex, L.; Nitz, N.; Pratesi, R.; Hecht, M. Current trends in the pharmacological management of Chagas disease. *Int. J. Parasitol. Drugs Drug Resist.* **2019**, *12*, 7–17. [CrossRef] [PubMed]

162. Janssens, P.G.; De Muynck, A. Clinical trials with "nifurtimox" in African trypanosomiasis. *Ann. Soc. Belg. Med. Trop.* **1977**, *57*, 475–479. [PubMed]

163. Moens, F.; De Wilde, M.; Ngato, K. Essai de traitement au nifurtimox de la trypanosomiase humaine Africaine. *Ann. Soc. Belg. Med. Trop.* **1984**, *64*, 37–43.

164. Pepin, J.; Milord, F.; Mpia, B.; Meurice, F.; Ethier, L.; DeGroof, D.; Bruneel, H. An open clinical trial of nifurtimox for arseno-resistant *Trypanosoma brucei gambiense* sleeping sickness in central Zaire. *Trans. R. Soc. Trop. Med. Hyg.* **1989**, *83*, 514–517. [CrossRef]

165. Pépin, J.; Milord, F.; Meurice, F.; Ethier, L.; Loko, L.; Mpia, B. High-dose nifurtimox for arseno-resistant *Trypanosoma brucei gambiense* sleeping sickness: An open trial in central Zaire. *Trans. R. Soc. Trop. Med. Hyg.* **1992**, *86*, 254–256. [CrossRef]

166. Van Nieuwenhove, S. Advances in sleeping sickness therapy. *Ann. Soc. Belg. Med. Trop.* **1992**, *72* (Suppl. S1), 39–51.

167. Bisser, S.; N'Siesi, F.X.; Lejon, V.; Preux, P.M.; Van Nieuwenhove, S.; Miaka Mia Bilenge, C.; Büscher, P. Equivalence trial of melarsoprol and nifurtimox monotherapy and combination therapy for the treatment of second-stage *Trypanosoma brucei gambiense* sleeping sickness. *J. Infect. Dis.* **2007**, *195*, 322–329. [CrossRef]

168. Docampo, R.; Stoppani, A.O. generation of superoxide anion and hydrogen peroxide induced by nifurtimox in *Trypanosoma cruzi*. *Arch. Biochem. Biophys.* **1979**, *197*, 317–321. [CrossRef]

169. Prathalingham, S.R.; Wilkinson, S.R.; Horn, D.; Kelly, J.M. Deletion of the *Trypanosoma brucei* superoxide dismutase gene sodb1 increases sensitivity to nifurtimox and benznidazole. *Antimicrob. Agents Chemother.* **2007**, *51*, 755–758. [CrossRef]

170. Wilkinson, S.R.; Taylor, M.C.; Horn, D.; Kelly, J.M.; Cheeseman, I. A mechanism for cross-resistance to nifurtimox and benznidazole in trypanosomes. *Proc. Natl. Acad. Sci. USA* **2008**, *105*, 5022–5027. [CrossRef] [PubMed]

171. Baker, N.; Alsford, S.; Horn, D. Genome-wide RNAi screens in African trypanosomes identify the nifurtimox activator NTR and the eflornithine transporter AAT6. *Mol. Biochem. Parasitol.* **2011**, *176*, 55–57. [CrossRef] [PubMed]

172. Sokolova, A.Y.; Wyllie, S.; Patterson, S.; Oza, S.L.; Read, K.D.; Fairlamb, A.H. Cross-resistance to nitro drugs and implications for treatment of human African trypanosomiasis. *Antimicrob. Agents Chemother.* **2010**, *54*, 2893–2900. [CrossRef] [PubMed]

173. Jeganathan, S.; Sanderson, L.; Dogruel, M.; Rodgers, J.; Croft, S.; Thomas, S.A. The distribution of nifurtimox across the healthy and trypanosome-infected murine blood–brain and blood-CSF barriers. *J. Pharmacol. Exp. Ther.* **2010**, *336*, 506–515. [CrossRef] [PubMed]

174. Watson, C.P.; Dogruel, M.; Mihoreanu, L.; Begley, D.J.; Weksler, B.B.; Couraud, P.O.; Romero, I.A.; Thomas, S.A. The transport of nifurtimox, an anti-trypanosomal drug, in an in vitro model of the human blood-brain barrier: Evidence for involvement of breast cancer resistance protein. *Brain Res.* **2012**, *1436*, 111–121. [CrossRef] [PubMed]

175. Duhm, B.; Maul, W.; Medenwald, H.; Patzschke, K.; Wegner, L.A. Investigations on the pharmacokinetics of nifurtimox-^{35}S in the rat and dog. *Arzneimittelforschung* **1972**, *22*, 1617–1624. [PubMed]

176. Kell, D.B.; Oliver, S.G. How drugs get into cells: Tested and testable predictions to help discriminate between transporter-mediated uptake and lipoidal bilayer diffusion. *Front. Pharmacol.* **2014**, *5*, 231. [CrossRef]

177. Kell, D.B.; Dobson, P.D.; Oliver, S.G. Pharmaceutical drug transport: The issues and the implications that it is essentially carrier-mediated only. *Drug Discov. Today* **2011**, *16*, 704–714. [CrossRef]

178. Baliani, A.; Bueno, G.J.; Stewart, M.L.; Yardley, V.; Brun, R.; Barrett, M.P.; Gilbert, I.H. Design and synthesis of a series of melamine-based nitroheterocycles with activity against Trypanosomatid parasites. *J. Med. Chem.* **2005**, *48*, 5570–5579. [CrossRef]

179. Maina, N.; Maina, K.J.; Mäser, P.; Brun, R. Genotypic and phenotypic characterization of *Trypanosoma brucei gambiense* isolates from Ibba, South Sudan, an area of high melarsoprol treatment failure rate. *Acta Trop.* **2007**, *104*, 84–90. [CrossRef]

180. Deeks, E.D. Fexinidazole: First global approval. *Drugs* **2019**, *79*, 215–220. [CrossRef]

181. Mesu, V.K.B.K.; Kalonji, W.M.; Bardonneau, C.; Mordt, O.V.; Blesson, S.; Simon, F.; Delhomme, S.; Bernhard, S.; Kuziena, W.; Lubaki, J.F.; et al. Oral fexinidazole for late-stage African *Trypanosoma brucei gambiense* trypanosomiasis: A pivotal multicentre, randomised, non-inferiority trial. *Lancet* **2018**, *391*, 144–154. [CrossRef]

182. Pelfrene, E.; Harvey Allchurch, M.; Ntamabyaliro, N.; Nambasa, V.; Ventura, F.V.; Nagercoil, N.; Cavaleri, M. The European Medicines Agency's scientific opinion on oral fexinidazole for human African trypanosomiasis. *PLoS Negl. Trop. Dis.* **2019**, *13*, e0007381.

183. Chappuis, F. Oral fexinidazole for human African trypanosomiasis. *Lancet* **2018**, *391*, 100–102. [CrossRef]

184. Lindner, A.K.; Lejon, V.; Chappuis, F.; Seixas, J.; Kazumba, L.; Barrett, M.P.; Mwamba, E.; Erphas, O.; Akl, E.A.; Villanueva, G.; et al. New WHO guidelines for treatment of gambiense human African trypanosomiasis including fexinidazole: Substantial changes for clinical practice. *Lancet Infect. Dis.* **2019**. [CrossRef]

185. De Koning, H.P. Drug resistance in protozoan parasites. *Emerg. Top. Life Sci.* **2017**, *1*, 627–632.

186. Blum, J.; Burri, C. Treatment of late stage sleeping sickness caused by T. b. gambiense: A new approach to the use of an old drug. *Swiss. Med. Wkly.* **2002**, *132*, 51–56. [PubMed]

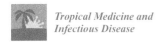

Review

New Drugs for Human African Trypanosomiasis: A Twenty First Century Success Story

Emily A. Dickie [1], Federica Giordani [1], Matthew K. Gould [1], Pascal Mäser [2], Christian Burri [2,3], Jeremy C. Mottram [4], Srinivasa P. S. Rao [5] and Michael P. Barrett [1,*]

[1] Wellcome Centre for Integrative Parasitology, Institute of Infection, Immunity and Inflammation, University of Glasgow, Glasgow G12 8TA, UK; emily.dickie@glasgow.ac.uk (E.A.D.); federica.giordani@glasgow.ac.uk (F.G.); matthew.gould@glasgow.ac.uk (M.K.G.)

[2] Swiss Tropical and Public Health Institute, Socinstrasse 57, 4002 Basel, Switzerland; pascal.maeser@swisstph.ch (P.M.); christian.burri@swisstph.ch (C.B.)

[3] University of Basel, Petersplatz 1, 4000 Basel, Switzerland

[4] York Biomedical Research Institute, Department of Biology, University of York, Wentworth Way, Heslington, York YO10 5DD, UK; jeremy.mottram@york.ac.uk

[5] Novartis Institute for Tropical Diseases, 5300 Chiron Way, Emeryville, CA 94608, USA; srinivasa.rao@novartis.com

* Correspondence: michael.barrett@glasgow.ac.uk

Received: 16 January 2020; Accepted: 14 February 2020; Published: 19 February 2020

Abstract: The twentieth century ended with human African trypanosomiasis (HAT) epidemics raging across many parts of Africa. Resistance to existing drugs was emerging, and many programs aiming to contain the disease had ground to a halt, given previous success against HAT and the competing priorities associated with other medical crises ravaging the continent. A series of dedicated interventions and the introduction of innovative routes to develop drugs, involving Product Development Partnerships, has led to a dramatic turnaround in the fight against HAT caused by *Trypanosoma brucei gambiense*. The World Health Organization have been able to optimize the use of existing tools to monitor and intervene in the disease. A promising new oral medication for stage 1 HAT, pafuramidine maleate, ultimately failed due to unforeseen toxicity issues. However, the clinical trials for this compound demonstrated the possibility of conducting such trials in the resource-poor settings of rural Africa. The Drugs for Neglected Disease initiative (DNDi), founded in 2003, has developed the first all oral therapy for both stage 1 and stage 2 HAT in fexinidazole. DNDi has also brought forward another oral therapy, acoziborole, potentially capable of curing both stage 1 and stage 2 disease in a single dosing. In this review article, we describe the remarkable successes in combating HAT through the twenty first century, bringing the prospect of the elimination of this disease into sight.

Keywords: human African trypanosomiasis; sleeping sickness; elimination; chemotherapy; fexinidazole; pafuramidine; acoziborole

1. Introduction

The current drugs used for human African trypanosomiasis (HAT) (Figure 1) have served their purpose for many years. The incidence of HAT is now at a historic low (fewer than 1000 cases reported in 2018 [1]). Two forms of the disease occur. The one found in West and Central Africa is caused by *Trypanosoma brucei gambiense*, and the other, found in East and Southern Africa, is caused by *Trypanosoma brucei rhodesiense*. The former causes a chronic disease, taking years between infection and death, while the latter may kill within weeks to months. Parasites injected into the bloodstream cause a stage 1 infection, where replication is primarily associated with blood and lymph. However, the parasites then invade other organs, including the central nervous system (CNS). Once replicating in the CNS, the disease progresses to stage 2, where many of the symptoms of sleeping sickness become manifest. The current drugs suffer many drawbacks [2]. For stage 1 disease, either suramin or pentamidine is used for HAT caused by *T. b. rhodesiense* and *T. b. gambiense*, respectively. Both drugs must be given by injection for a prolonged period, and both carry a risk of adverse events. For stage 2 disease, the highly toxic melarsoprol is still the treatment of choice for rhodesiense HAT. Melarsoprol causes an encephalopathic syndrome that is fatal in up to one in twenty people taking the drug [3]. For gambiense HAT, the past decade has seen the introduction of a combination therapy. Intravenous eflornithine is given for 10 days alongside oral nifurtimox for 14 days [4].

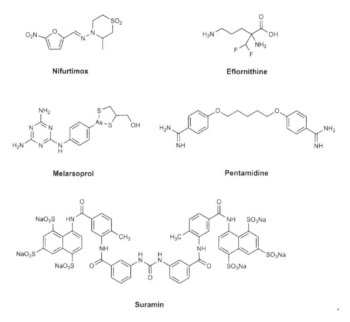

Figure 1. Different drugs have been used to treat HAT depending on the trypanosome subspecies causing the disease, and whether progression is at stage 1 or 2. For the past decade nifurtimox and eflornithine combination therapy has been the treatment of choice for stage 2 *T. b. gambiense* disease, and pentamidine for stage 1. For rhodesiense HAT, stage 2 is treated with melarsoprol and stage 1 with suramin.

The combination is relatively safe and efficacious. However, the delivery of kilogram quantities of eflornithine and many liters of sterile saline brings substantial logistical difficulty. For melarsoprol, resistance was a growing problem in the early 2000s [5], and for eflornithine [6] and nifurtimox [7] independently, resistance can be readily selected in the laboratory. There is no doubt that better drugs for use against HAT are required [8].

The first two decades of the twenty first century can be seen as a major success story in regards to intervention against this neglected tropical disease. HAT was running out of control in the late twentieth century, with an estimated 300,000 people infected [9]. In response, the international community launched several key initiatives, which can be seen as having converged to turn the tide. Consequently, the twenty first century has witnessed a dramatic change in the trajectory of HAT.

In 1999, Médecins Sans Frontières (MSF) initiated their "Access" campaign to encourage a re-engagement of the pharmaceutical industry with neglected diseases, including HAT [10]. A key study [11] revisited the administration regimen of melarsoprol based on pharmacokinetic data.

An effective 10-day administration protocol, which diminished hospitalization time for patients [12], albeit without increasing safety, was introduced to great effect [13]. This IMPAMEL program ("improved application of melarsoprol") was crucial in implementing the first modern clinical trials on HAT, and also in demonstrating the feasibility of conducting trials in extremely resource-limited conditions according to Good Clinical Practice, laying the foundation for future developments.

Eflornithine had been shown to be far safer than melarsoprol as treatment for stage 2 disease [14]. Yet, by the late 1990s, no pharmaceutical company was prepared to make this compound for HAT treatment. However, when it was discovered that the same compound could prevent the growth of unwanted facial hair in women, a number of drug companies saw an opportunity to market the compound for this purpose [15]. MSF, already campaigning for access to essential medicines, were able to make a compelling case that society needed to rethink drug discovery paradigms for neglected diseases [16]. Aventis (now Sanofi) were persuaded to develop the drug and donate it at no cost to the World Health Organization (WHO) for distribution in Africa. Millions of dollars were also provided by Aventis/Sanofi to WHO, who could now develop new screening and intervention programs. The Bill and Melinda Gates Foundation selected HAT to be one of the first diseases they targeted through the Consortium of Parasitic Drug Development (CPDD) [17], and the Drugs for Neglected Diseases initiative (DNDi) was founded through MSF [18] to seek new drugs for diseases including HAT. In diagnostics, the Foundation for Innovative New Diagnostics (FIND) sought novel ways of improving our ability to detect HAT patients [19], and new ways of combating the tsetse fly were rolled out too [20]. A number of pharmaceutical companies also regained an interest in HAT, including GlaxoSmithKline (GSK) through their Tres Cantos Open Lab foundation [21] and the Novartis Institute for Tropical Diseases (NITD) [22]. Small companies too, such as Immtech Pharmaceuticals Inc., Scynexis and Anacor Pharmaceuticals Inc. in the USA, also raised investment to develop new drugs against HAT. The first twenty years of the twenty first century have now seen the clinical trials and ultimate failure of a new orally available diamidine prodrug [23], the registration of the first all-orally available therapy against stage 2 disease [24], and the entry into clinical trials of a compound that may cure stage 2 HAT with a single oral administration [25]. This article outlines the successes seen in the development of new drugs for HAT in the twenty first century.

2. Pafuramidine—A New Paradigm in Anti-Trypanosomal Drug Development

Among the currently used drugs for HAT is pentamidine, a diamidine that was introduced in the 1940s, and has been the mainstay in the treatment of stage 1 gambiense HAT for nearly 80 years [26]. Another diamidine, diminazene, is used in treating veterinary trypanosomiasis [27]. The diamidines are di-cations, with positive charges at either end, which renders them highly polar, precluding bioavailability if taken orally [28]. Pentamidine is typically given by intramuscular injection for seven days. Das and Boykin showed in the 1970s that methoxy-derivatives of other diamidines acted as orally available prodrugs, and the methoxy group metabolized back to the amidine systemically [29].

The Bill and Melinda Gates Foundation was founded in 2000, a time when the resurgence of HAT was at its pinnacle. Among the Foundation's earliest supported projects was the development of the diamidine methoxy-prodrug approach towards new drugs for HAT through the CPDD.

DB289 (Figure 2) (pafuramidine maleate; 2,5-bis(4-amidinophenyl)-furan-bis-*O*-methylamidoxime), the methoxy product of furamidine (2,5-bis(4-amidinophenyl)-furan), in which the benzamidine moieties are separated by a furan ring, emerged as the lead compound for progression.

Furamidine is highly polar and unable to traverse lipid bilayers without the assistance of transporters (see later). Pafuramidine, however, has much greater capacity to diffuse across membranes [30], including the intestinal epithelium, giving it considerable oral bioavailability. Once systemic, it is metabolized via various cytochrome P450 enzymes and cytochrome b5 reductase [31–36] to furamidine. Preclinical safety and efficacy results [37,38] were sufficient to enable the passage to clinical trials.

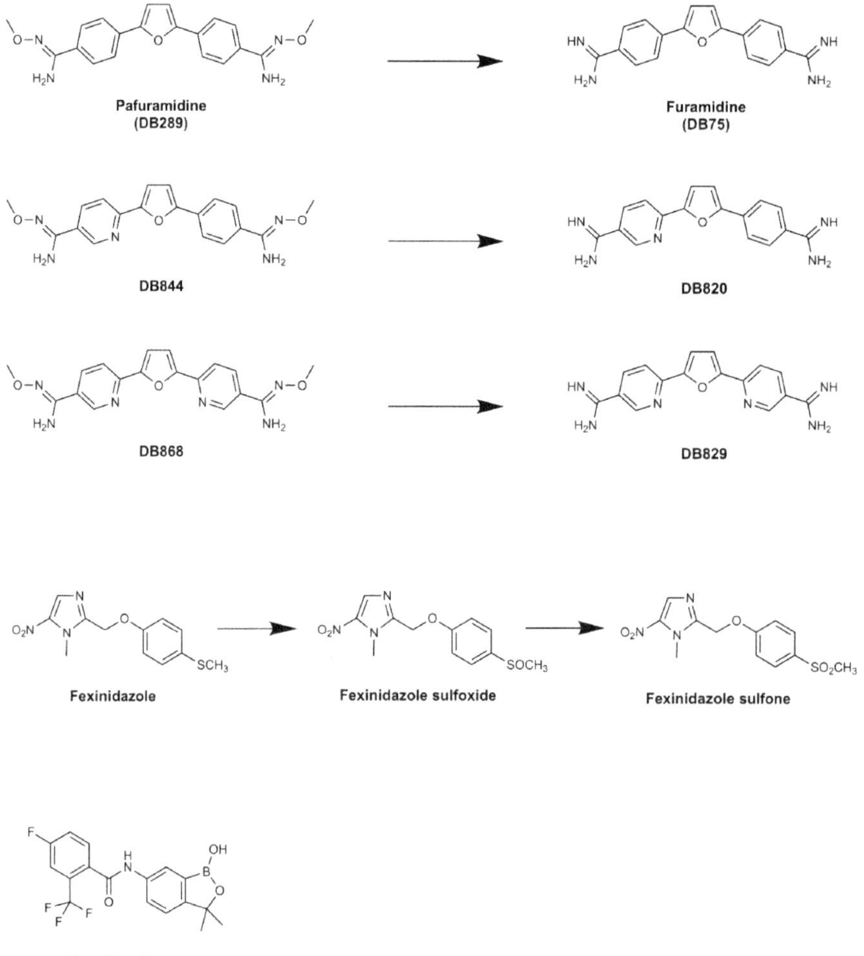

Figure 2. Clinical trials with pafuramidine (DB289), which is the prodrug of furamidine (DB75), failed due to the appearance of renal toxicity during extended phase I safety profiling. The aza-derivatives including DB868—a prodrug of DB829, and DB844—a prodrug of DB820, also showed activity against stage 2 disease, but development was halted following identification of the toxicity associated with pafuramidine. Fexinidazole has been approved for use by the European Medicines Agency in 2018. The compound is converted to sulfoxide then sulfone derivatives after administration. Acoziborole is a benzoxaborole in clinical trials, where the efficacy of a single dosing of the drug as an oral medication against stage 2 disease is being assessed.

2.1. Clinical Trials of Pafuramidine

Ultimately pafuramidine failed in clinical trials [23,39]. However, those trials were of great importance, not only in testing the efficacy of this promising lead compound, but also in informing on any criteria required to conduct clinical trials for regulatory purposes in a cohort of patients in difficult places to work. These trials also helped to establish protocols for patient seeking, screening, drug administration, record keeping and patient follow-up post-treatment. The very fact that over 350,000 individuals were screened in the quest for patients to include in the trials had a major impact on the incidence of the disease. Patients testing positive but failing inclusion criteria (i.e., not clearly in stage 1 disease), were treated with other drugs appropriate to their stage.

An original phase I safety study (unpublished), carried out in healthy Caucasian volunteers in Germany in 2001 showed the drug to be well tolerated in single and multi-dose testing (100 mg twice per day (b.i.d.)) and up to 600 mg in a single dose.

A phase IIa study [39] in Viana, Angola and the CDTC Maluku, Democratic Republic of the Congo (DRC) with 32 patients showed that 100 mg of pafuramidine orally twice a day for 5 days yielded loss of all visible trypanosomes in blood 24 h after treatment cessation in 93% of cases, compared to 100% efficacy with 7-day pentamidine treatment. However, prolonged follow up began to pick up enhanced relapse rates from this five-day dosing (by 24 months, only 67% of pafuramidine-treated patients were considered cured). 81 patients had entered a phase IIb trial, at the same 5-day dosing (40 for pafuramidine and 41 for pentamidine) [39] by this time. However, the high relapse rate after prolonged follow up in the phase IIa-1 trial prompted a decision to use a 10-day dosing of 100 mg pafuramidine b.i.d. instead, and 30 more patients were enrolled for this phase IIa-2 trial. The dose was well tolerated over 10 days, and was less toxic than pentamidine [39]. The 10-day dosing of pafuramidine gave 93% cure at 3 months follow up, and was selected for a Phase III trial.

The Phase III trial [23], conducted in several centers in the Democratic Republic of the Congo, Angola, and South Sudan recorded a cure rate of 89% at 12 months follow up. The major safety concern noted in these treatment trials was a 7% incidence of increased liver enzymes; however, the incidence of this adverse event was substantially less than in the comparator group treated with pentamidine (77%). A significantly lower percentage (2% vs. 9%) of patients treated with pafuramidine experienced treatment emergent adverse events detected by renal and urinary tract investigations and urinalyses compared to those under pentamidine. Overall, three subjects in the pafuramidine treatment groups were reported to have serious adverse events that could be considered acute renal failure or insufficiency classified as possibly associated with study drugs [23].

As the phase II/III trial was progressing, a further phase I safety trial was conducted in South Africa, necessitated by the increase in the duration of drug administration and the limited number of patients exposed to pafuramidine (unpublished). One hundred healthy sub-Saharan African adult volunteers were treated with 100 mg pafuramidine b.i.d. for 14 days. Generally, a mild and reversible increase of liver enzymes was observed in multiple subjects, which had been anticipated [23]. However, 6 of 100 subjects then experienced delayed renal insufficiency with unclear etiology.

The delayed action might indicate a possible immunological role; HAT is itself immunosuppressive, which could explain why the incidence of kidney injury in treated patients was much lower. Another hypothesis was a genetic origin across a diverse group of individuals, which was supported by a retrospective study on a panel of 34 genetically distinct mouse strains [40]. Urinary secretion of the kidney injury molecule-1 (KIM-1) protein was used as a marker of proximal tubule injury in the kidney. Only a subset of the mice revealed elevated KIM-1. Genetic association studies then showed several genes with alleles associated with the KIM-1 levels. This included PCSK5, a serine peptidase associated with lipid and cholesterol metabolism, and another cholesterol-associated enzyme, sterol O-acyltransferase, among others. Definitive explanations for the kidney injury mechanism, however, remain obscure. DNA from the subjects involved in the clinical trial was not available to determine whether the same genes were associated to kidney damage in humans.

The appearance of unanticipated toxicity with pafuramidine led to the end of clinical development and also a cessation of other activities around the diamidine project. This was unfortunate, since the project had also identified several aza-analogs, including DB820 and DB829 (alongside their respective methoxyamidine prodrugs DB844 and DB868,), which were effective in mouse [41] and vervet monkey (*Chlorocebus pygerythrus*) models of stage 2 infection [42]. Significantly, DB829 accumulated far less (>10 fold) inside mammalian cells than furamidine [43], pointing to a potentially improved safety profile. For HAT, however, the successes that have occurred with other compounds (see below) indicate that the diamidines are unlikely to be resurrected for future work. However, because of their diverse and intriguing biological activities [44], it is likely to see them re-emerging for other conditions in the future [45].

2.2. Pafuramidine: Mode of Action and Resistance Risk

Furamidine, like other diamidines, binds to the minor groove of the DNA double helix [28,45]. The ability to bind is structure-dependent, and intriguing work has aimed to tailor this binding to specific DNA sequences, including regulatory elements [44], with a view to controlling gene expression in, for example, human cancer cells. Furamidine is fluorescent, and its accumulation in trypanosomes shows binding to both the kinetoplast (mitochondrial DNA) and nuclear DNA, as well as its accumulation in vesicles assumed to be acidocalcisomes [46]. The compound accumulates to millimolar concentration, even in cells exposed to low micromolar concentrations over 24 hours [46]. Even a brief exposure (<5 min) to 32 micromolar of the compound, followed by wash out, provoked death 48 hours later [47]. At 3.2 micromolar, exposure time rose to 1 hour to achieve this slow commitment to death. Lanteri also showed a profound decrease in the mitochondrial membrane potential associated with the addition of furamidine to *T. brucei* [48].

The F1Fo ATP synthase complex is an essential mitochondrial complex in trypanosomes. In procyclic forms it acts in a classical fashion, producing ATP as part of the electron transport chain. In bloodstream forms, however, it acts in reverse: consuming ATP in order to maintain the essential mitochondrial membrane potential. All of the F1Fo ATPase subunits are encoded in the nucleus, apart from subunit A6, which is encoded in the kinetoplast. Mutations to the nuclearly-encoded gamma subunit (e.g., L262P substitution or an alanine deletion at amino acid position 281) allow the mitochondrial membrane potential to be generated in bloodstream form trypanosomes without subunit A6, rendering the kinetoplast redundant in this life cycle stage. The kinetoplast can be removed from these cells without apparent impact on viability [49]. The ATPase gamma mutants (now kinetoplast independent) are hundreds of fold resistant to phenanthridine compounds; intriguingly however, only very minor resistance (~ 3-fold) was shown for furamidine [50]. This would indicate that, in contrast to phenanthridines, it is not the kinetoplast per se that is the target of furamidine.

Diamidines also act against yeast mitochondria [51] with *Saccharomyces cerevisiae* that are fermenting glucose, rather than respiring using mitochondrial substrates (e.g., glycerol), being 200-fold less sensitive to pentamidine [52].

Mammalian cells too are vulnerable to diamidines. However, the hypersensitivity of trypanosomes to this class is due to their ability to accumulate diamidines to very high concentrations across their plasma membrane through specific transporters. The P2 aminopurine transporter, *Tb*AT1, which normally carries adenosine and adenine, was the first transporter characterized to carry pentamidine [53]. Subsequently, a high affinity pentamidine transporter [54], later revealed as the aquaglyceroporin *Tb*AQP2 [55], was shown to play a dominant role in uptake [56]. A low affinity pentamidine transporter, whose physiological role remains elusive, was also shown to transport pentamidine [54]. Loss of *Tb*AT1 yields only low-level resistance to pentamidine, while loss of *Tb*AQP2 yields high level resistance [56]. Pentamidine, however, is an exception among the trypanocidal diamidines, having a highly flexible central linker chain. The shorter derivatives (e.g., diminazene, and furamidine plus its aza-analogs), primarily use the *Tb*AT1 aminopurine transporter for uptake [57], and its loss gives high level resistance. Discovering a specific motif found on diamidines, aminopurines and also melaminophenyl arsenicals, all of which can enter via the *Tb*AT1 P2 transporter [58], led to several efforts to create new selective trypanocides to enter via the same carrier protein [59–61].

Diamidines can enter mammalian cells and also cross the blood–brain barrier (BBB) [62]. The human facilitative organic cation transporter 1 (OCT1) is one transporter capable of transporting pentamidine and other diamidines in mammalian cells [63,64]. ATP-dependent pumps (e.g., the P-glycoprotein, P-gp) appear to also be able to efflux pentamidine [62], but not furamidine, nor DB829 [65].

3. Fexinidazole: the First Oral Treatment for HAT

In November 2018, The European Medicines Agency's Committee for Medicinal Products for Human Use (CHMP) offered a positive opinion on the use of oral fexinidazole for the treatment of both stage 1 stage 1 and 2 gambiense HAT [66]. In December 2018 the DRC, the epicenter of the disease, issued marketing authorization allowing use of the drug. Fexinidazole is given once per day for ten days, involving a four-day loading dose of 1.8 g per day followed by six days at 1.2 g per day with 600 mg tablets. The clinical development of fexinidazole is described in an accompanying article in this volume [67].

3.1. Pre-Clinical Development of Fexinidazole

The pathway for fexinidazole to the clinic was both long and disrupted. The drug, a 2-substituted 5-nitroimidazole, was originally synthesized as part of a program seeking anti-infectives by Hoechst in the 1970s [68]. Frank Jennings and George Urquhart at the University of Glasgow extended trypanocidal testing in the 1980s [69]. They could not demonstrate a full cure against the stage 2 disease model in mice which they had developed using the *T. brucei brucei* GVR35 strain which develops a slowly progressing disease in which the parasite enters the brain and establishes a CNS infection, prior to having killed the mice in an acute infection, as most laboratory strains of *T. brucei brucei* do. Administering fexinidazole as a monotherapy (given once a day for four days at 250 mg/kg), it cured 11/14 mice [69], although sequential treatment with a single dose of suramin (20 mg/kg) or diminazene (40 mg/kg), followed by four consecutive daily doses of fexinidazole, was curative. In the case of the suramin followed by a fexinidazole regime, a single dose of suramin, followed by four daily doses of just 30 mg/kg fexinidazole, was curative [69]. It was later shown [70] that five days of fexinidazole monotherapy at 200 mg/kg was curative (7/8 mice) in the stage 2 model, showing the necessity for prolonged exposure.

The finding that many nitroheterocycles were genotoxic and potentially carcinogenic led to a general aversion to this class of molecule for its use as pharmaceuticals for several decades. However, nifurtimox, another nitroheterocycle, entered the anti-trypanosomal armamentarium as a combination partner with eflornithine [4]. The nitroheterocycle known as megazol also showed interesting trypanocidal activity [71], whilst other nitroheterocycles such as PA-824 (now registered as pretomanid for tuberculosis [72]) came to the fore.

Thus, interest in trypanocidal nitroheterocycles was rekindled. A series of 830 nitroimidazoles and related compounds were tested at the Swiss Tropical and Public Health Institute against *T. brucei*. *Trypanosoma cruzi*, *Leishmania donovani*, and mammalian cells *in vitro*. The most active and selective molecules were evaluated in secondary *in vitro* assays and in the mouse models of acute or chronic trypanosomiasis. Based on these data, fexinidazole was singled out as the most promising candidate for further development against HAT [70,73], and a dossier of information was compiled to support the safety and efficacy of the drug [67,74].

3.2. Fexinidazole: Mode of Action and Resistance Risk

Fexinidazole is a prodrug. Its activity depends upon two consecutive electron reductions of the NO_2 group by an NADH-specific nitroreductase (*TbNTR1*) [75]. Diminished NTR activity leads to resistance to fexinidazole [76] and cross-resistance to other nitroheterocycles, including nifurtimox. The fate of the nitro-reduced product is unknown. An orthologous nitroreductase enzyme is also found in *T. cruzi* [75], where it is responsible for the activation of clinically used nitroheterocycles (e.g., benznidazole and nifurtimox). In the case of nifurtimox, *T. cruzi* was shown to reduce the compound to a highly reactive species [77]. Fexinidazole is also under consideration as a new treatment for Chagas disease [78]. For benznidazole, *in vitro* activation also revealed reductive activation and ultimately disintegration of the compound to glyoxal [79]. Another study, however, failed to demonstrate the production of glyoxal in *T. cruzi*, although it revealed a plethora of metabolized products and adducts of these benznidazole breakdown-products [80]. This led to suggestions that, following its activation by *Tc*NTR1, benznidazole ultimately kills through the modification of numerous metabolite and protein targets in *T. cruzi* [80]. The metabolic fate of fexinidazole, following NTR1 mediated reduction, has not been determined, and the mechanism by which it kills trypanosomes is not known. However, a similar "cluster bomb" effect, with the activated fexinidazole product of the nitroreduction hitting multi-targets, seems likely. NTR1 has been proposed to act physiologically as an NADH dehydrogenase involved in reducing ubiquinone to ubiquinol [81], hence its essentiality even in bloodstream form *T. brucei* that requires ubiquinone-based electron transport in its mitochondrial alternative oxidase system [82]. In nifurtimox-treated *T. brucei*, loss of mitochondrial membrane potential and other mitochondrial morphology defects were noted [83]. Other nitroheterocycles, including fexinidazole, may also exert their effects on the mitochondrion, where the drug's activation occurs. Knockout of a single copy of the *TbNTR1* gene (trypanosomes are diploid, hence have two copies of the gene, one on each copy of chromosome 7), led to diminished activity of the drug, albeit by just 1.6–1.9 fold, whilst double knockout was not possible [76]. Parasites resistant to fexinidazole could be selected *in vitro* under the conditions of increasing drug pressure (up to 20-fold resistance), and these parasites lost the 3′ flanking region of one allele of NTR, leading to a 50% reduction in the expression of the gene. The same study selected nifurtimox-resistant parasites, which lost one copy of the gene in developing 6-fold resistance. In both cases, resistance was significantly higher compared to the single NTR1 KO cells, indicating that other, as yet unknown, events beyond partial NTR1 loss, contribute to resistance. A question arises as to whether there is a risk that the current use of nifurtimox could lead to the selection of resistance to fexinidazole and vice versa. However, although diminished nitroreductase activity can yield cross resistance, it is not clear whether parasites, even with diminished nitroreductase, would be viable in the field, if the enzyme were critical in the insect transmitted forms of the parasites. Moreover, with very few cases of gambiense HAT currently reported (fewer than 1000 in 2018), the probability of selecting parasites resistant to either drug under field-settings is currently very low.

NTR1 is a typical enzyme of prokaryote origin. *Salmonella typhimurium*, the bacterium used in the Ames test, possesses nitroreductase genes as well, explaining the positive mutagenicity signal of fexinidazole and its metabolites in the Ames test. In contrast to *T. brucei*, however, nitroreductase activity is dispensable in *S. typhimurium*, and in a nitroreductase null mutant strain fexinidazole was no longer mutagenic [74]. Mammals do not have NTR1 orthologs, and thus, fexinidazole and fexinidazole sulfone were inactive in micronucleus tests with human or mouse cells [74].

4. Acoziborole: A Single Dose Oral Cure for Stage 2 HAT

As the enhanced effort to counter the surging HAT epidemic of the late twentieth century began, the prospect of an orally available drug that was able to cure stage 2, CNS-involved disease with a single administration seemed remote. Yet, as fexinidazole and pafuramidine were entering their first clinical trials, a novel, promising class of antimicrobial agents appeared on the scene: the benzoxaboroles [84]. These compounds are characterized by a core scaffold based around an oxaborole heterocycle fused to a benzene ring. Pursued by the small Californian company Anacor Pharmaceuticals Inc. (incorporated into Pfizer Inc. in 2016), the benzoxaboroles quickly attracted attention due to their numerous bioactivities. Activity against trypanosomes was first reported in 2010 [85], and DNDi selected this class for further work. The US-based pharmaceutical company Scynexis was contracted to initiate an intensive program of the structure-activity-relationship work to seek benzoxaboroles with good activity against trypanosomes. Crucially, these benzoxaboroles were also to demonstrate pharmacokinetic properties suitable to cure stage 2 HAT; i.e., being capable of reaching the CNS and retaining trypanocidal activity levels for long enough to obtain cure [86].

Cyrus Bacchi, the same investigator who had brought eflornithine forward for HAT in the 1980s [87], showed that a 6-carboxamido-based series cured the *T. brucei* strain GVR35 murine model of stage 2 disease. Structure-activity work eventually brought forward SCYX-7158, a gem-dimethyl

4-fluoro-2-trimethylfluoro benzamide derivative, which cured when given orally [88]. Its modest *in vitro* potency against *T. brucei* (IC_{50} around 0.6 μM) [88] was offset by good pharmacokinetic properties, giving a 100% cure in a mouse model of the stage 2 disease following a dosing of 25 mg/kg once a day for 7 days oral dosing [88]. Preclinical testing showed no overt toxicity in mice or dogs with a concentration of no observed adverse event limit (NOAEL) of 15 mg/kg. No binding to key proteins (CYP450), serine/cysteine peptidase or hERG channels emerged [89]. SCYX-7158 was also non-mutagenic in the Ames tests or standard mammalian cell genotoxicity assays [89]. Hence, phase I clinical safety trials were approved, and in 2012, SCYX-7158, or acoziborole, became the first new chemical entity resulting from DNDi's program to enter clinical trials for HAT.

A phase I study that included 128 healthy male subjects of sub-Saharan African origin was conducted in 2015 in France to assess safety, tolerability, pharmacokinetics and pharmacodynamics after single oral, ascending doses [90]. Some adverse effects were noted, including headaches, dizziness and GI tract reactions, as abdominal pain, nausea, vomiting, constipation and diarrhea. However, more serious issues were not identified. This trial led to the selection of a 960 mg dose, given as a single administration in three tablets (each with 320 mg of the active compound). Acoziborole's long half-life (17 days), associated with high protein binding (97.8%) also necessitated safety monitoring in the volunteers for 210 days. Outputs from the phase I trials were good enough to enable progression to phase II/III trials in patients in Africa, which started late in 2016 [91]. The recruitment and dosing of patients is now complete, and follow-up is underway. Final results are eagerly awaited, but early indications (unpublished) suggest that the drug has demonstrated remarkable efficacy and safety profiles.

Acoziborole: Mode of Action and Resistance Risk

The mode of action and resistance mechanisms to benzoxaboroles are emerging. Acoziborole resistance was associated with multiple genetic changes in trypanosomes [92], although it was not possible to assign a specific gene to resistance in that study. However, among the changes in resistant lines was an amplification in the gene copy number of the RNA cleavage and polyadenylation specificity factor subunit 3 (CPSF3) [93]. Subsequently, CPSF3 was identified as a target for benzoxaboroles in apicomplexan parasites *Plasmodium* [93] and *Toxoplasma* [94]. Based on this observation, and the fact that metabolomics experiments had revealed a profound change in the methionine metabolism [95] that might have been related to RNA processing defects, particularly given the multi-methylation of the spliced leader sequence used in trans-splicing in trypanosomes, the effect of over-expression of CPSF3 on sensitivity to the related benzoxaborole, AN7973, was tested [96].

Over-expression of the gene yielded a notable loss of activity [96]. Elegant experiments using a gene over-expression library, followed by a selection of clones over-expressing genes yielding reduced sensitivity to acoziborole itself, also identified CPSF3 [97], and over-expression confirmed loss of sensitivity, pointing to CPSF3 as a target, if not the exclusive target, of these compounds in trypanosomes.

Another trypanocidal benzoxaborole (of the amino-methyl subclass) was shown to be subject to a two-step metabolic processing, involving a primary conversion using amine oxidase in host serum to an aldehyde that is further metabolized to a carboxylate via parasite aldehyde dehydrogenase [98]. Another valinate–amide derivative series shows considerable promise for animal African trypanosomiasis too [99].

5. Conclusions

The twentieth century ended with human African trypanosomiasis epidemics raging across Africa. A disease that had been brought under control in the 1960s was wreaking havoc. This led to a concerted effort across a range of international organizations, including the WHO and newly formed agencies including DNDi and the CPDD. The arrival of the Bill and Melinda Gates Foundation and a re-alignment of many international aid efforts provided key investment to allow the development of new routes to combat HAT. The development of new drugs was central to the process. CPDD produced an orally available cure for stage 1 HAT that ultimately failed. In the meantime, DNDi brought forward an old nitroheterocycle, fexinidazole, and through the combined forces of persistence and diligence worked their way around numerous perceptual hurdles related to the nitroheterocycle class, so as to bring to the clinic the first wholly oral treatment for stage 1 and 2 HAT. As those trials were proceeding, DNDi created a consortium to bring forward a class of compounds, the benzoxaboroles, from Anacor Pharmaceuticals Inc., through to Scynexis and an extended collaborative team. Encouraging clinical results for the leading candidate compound, acoziborole, now promise to deliver a drug that may cure stage 2 HAT with a single oral dose. The ability of non-profit Product Development Partnerships to bring new medicines to market is now proven. The turnaround in the epidemiology of HAT in the twenty first century is a truly remarkable story and a classic model of how to create medical success.

Author Contributions: Writing—review and editing: E.A.D., F.G., M.K.G., P.M., C.B., J.C.M., S.P.S.R., M.P.B. All authors have read and agreed to the published version of the manuscript.

Funding: This research was funded by The Wellcome Trust WT-103024MA.

Conflicts of Interest: The authors declare no conflict of interest. The funders had no role in the design of the study; in the collection, analyses, or interpretation of data; in the writing of the manuscript, or in the decision to publish the results.

References

1. Available online: https://www.who.int/trypanosomiasis_african/en/ (accessed on 12 January 2020).
2. Barrett, M.P.; Boykin, D.W.; Brun, R.; Tidwell, R.R. Human African trypanosomiasis: Pharmacological re-engagement with a neglected disease. *Br. J. Pharmacol.* **2007**, *152*, 1155–1171. [CrossRef] [PubMed]
3. Blum, J.; Nkunku, S.; Burri, C. Clinical description of encephalopathic syndromes and risk factors for their occurrence and outcome during melarsoprol treatment of human African trypanosomiasis. *Trop. Med. Int. Health* **2001**, *6*, 390–400. [CrossRef] [PubMed]
4. Priotto, G.; Kasparian, S.; Mutombo, W.; Ngouama, D.; Ghorashian, S.; Arnold, U.; Ghabri, S.; Baudin, E.; Buard, V.; Kazadi-Kyanza, S.; et al. Nifurtimox-eflornithine combination therapy for second-stage African *Trypanosoma brucei gambiense* trypanosomiasis: A multicenter, randomised, phase III, non-inferiority trial. *Lancet* **2009**, *374*, 56–64. [CrossRef]
5. Fairlamb, A.H.; Horn, D. Melarsoprol resistance in African trypanosomiasis. *Trends Parasitol.* **2018**, *34*, 481–492. [CrossRef] [PubMed]
6. Vincent, I.M.; Creek, D.; Watson, D.G.; Kamleh, M.A.; Woods, D.J.; Wong, P.E.; Burchmore, R.J.; Barrett, M.P. A molecular mechanism for eflornithine resistance in African trypanosomes. *PLoS Pathog.* **2010**, *6*, e1001204. [CrossRef] [PubMed]
7. Sokolova, A.Y.; Wyllie, S.; Patterson, S.; Oza, S.L.; Read, K.D.; Fairlamb, A.H. Cross-resistance to nitro drugs and implications for treatment of human African trypanosomiasis. *Antimicrob. Agents Chemother.* **2010**, *54*, 2893–2900. [CrossRef]
8. Brun, R.; Don, R.; Jacobs, R.T.; Wang, M.Z.; Barrett, M.P. Development of novel drugs for human African trypanosomiasis. *Future Microbiol.* **2011**, *6*, 677–691. [CrossRef]
9. Barrett, M.P. The fall and rise of sleeping sickness. *Lancet* **1999**, *353*, 1113–1114. [CrossRef]
10. Kindermans, J.M.; Matthys, F. Introductory note: The access to essential medicines campaign. *Trop. Med. Int. Health* **2001**, *6*, 955–956. [CrossRef]
11. Burri, C.; Baltz, T.; Giroud, C.; Doua, F.; Welker, H.A.; Brun, R. Pharmacokinetic properties of the trypanocidal drug melarsoprol. *Chemotherapy* **1993**, *39*, 225–234. [CrossRef]
12. Burri, C.; Nkunku, S.; Merolle, A.; Smith, T.; Blum, J.; Brun, R. Efficacy of new, concise schedule for melarsoprol in treatment of sleeping sickness caused by *Trypanosoma brucei gambiense*: A randomised trial. *Lancet* **2000**, *55*, 1419–1425. [CrossRef]
13. Schmid, C.; Nkunku, S.; Merolle, A.; Vounatsou, P.; Burri, C. Efficacy of 10-day melarsoprol schedule 2 years after treatment for late-stage gambiense sleeping sickness. *Lancet* **2004**, *364*, 789–790. [CrossRef]
14. Burri, C.; Brun, R. Eflornithine for the treatment of human African trypanosomiasis. *Parasitol. Res.* **2003**, *90* (Suppl. 1), S49–S52. [CrossRef] [PubMed]

15. Balfour, J.A.; McClellan, K. Topical eflornithine. *Am. J. Clin. Dermatol.* **2001**, *2*, 197–201. [CrossRef] [PubMed]
16. Available online: https://www.theguardian.com/world/2001/may/07/medicalscience.businessofresearch (accessed on 12 January 2020).
17. McKerrow, J.H. Designing drugs for parasitic diseases of the developing world. *PLoS Med.* **2005**, *2*, e210. [CrossRef]
18. Available online: https://www.dndi.org/ (accessed on 12 January 2020).
19. Available online: https://www.finddx.org/ (accessed on 12 January 2020).
20. Tirados, I.; Esterhuizen, J.; Kovacic, V.; Mangwiro, T.N.; Vale, G.A.; Hastings, I.; Solano, P.; Lehane, M.J.; Torr, S.J. Tsetse control and gambian sleeping sickness; implications for control strategy. *PLoS Negl. Trop. Dis.* **2015**, *9*, e0003822. [CrossRef]
21. Ballell, L.; Strange, M.; Cammack, N.; Fairlamb, A.H.; Borysiewicz, L. Open Lab as a source of hits and leads against tuberculosis, malaria and kinetoplastid diseases. *Nat. Rev. Drug Discov.* **2016**, *15*, 292. [CrossRef]
22. Rao, S.P.S.; Barrett, M.P.; Dranoff, G.; Faraday, C.J.; Gimpelewicz, C.R.; Hailu, A.; Jones, C.L.; Kelly, J.M.; Lazdins-Helds, J.K.; Mäser, P.; et al. Drug discovery for kinetoplastid diseases: Future directions. *ACS Infect. Dis.* **2019**, *5*, 152–157. [CrossRef]
23. Pohlig, G.; Bernhard, S.C.; Blum, J.; Burri, C.; Mpanya, A.; Lubaki, J.P.; Mpoto, A.M.; Munungu, B.F.; N'tombe, P.M.; Deo, G.K.; et al. Efficacy and safety of pafuramidine versus pentamidine maleate for treatment of first stage sleeping sickness in a randomized, comparator-controlled, international phase 3 clinical trial. *PLoS Negl. Trop. Dis.* **2016**, *10*, e0004363. [CrossRef]
24. Mesu, V.K.B.K.; Kalonji, W.M.; Bardonneau, C.; Mordt, O.V.; Blesson, S.; Simon, F.; Delhomme, S.; Bernhard, S.; Kuziena, W.; Lubaki, J.F.; et al. Oral fexinidazole for late-stage African *Trypanosoma brucei gambiense* trypanosomiasis: A pivotal multicenter, randomised, non-inferiority trial. *Lancet* **2018**, *391*, 144–154. [CrossRef]
25. Jacobs, R.T.; Plattner, J.J.; Nare, B.; Wring, S.A.; Chen, D.; Freund, Y.; Gaukel, E.G.; Orr, M.D.; Perales, J.B.; Jenks, M.; et al. Benzoxaboroles: A new class of potential drugs for human African trypanosomiasis. *Future Med. Chem.* **2011**, *3*, 1259–1278. [CrossRef] [PubMed]
26. Bray, P.G.; Barrett, M.P.; Ward, S.A.; de Koning, H.P. Pentamidine uptake and resistance in pathogenic protozoa: Past, present and future. *Trends Parasitol.* **2003**, *19*, 232–239. [CrossRef]
27. Peregrine, A.S.; Mamman, M. Pharmacology of diminazene: A review. *Acta Trop.* **1993**, *54*, 185–203. [CrossRef]
28. Paine, M.F.; Wang, M.Z.; Generaux, C.N.; Boykin, D.W.; Wilson, W.D.; De Koning, H.P.; Olson, C.A.; Pohlig, G.; Burri, C.; Brun., R. Diamidines for human African trypanosomiasis. *Curr. Opin. Investig. Drugs* **2010**, *11*, 876–883.
29. Das, B.P.; Boykin, D.W. Synthesis and antiprotozoal activity of 2,5-bis(4-guanylphenyl)furans. *J. Med. Chem.* **1977**, *20*, 531–536. [CrossRef]
30. Zhou, L.; Lee, K.; Thakker, D.R.; Boykin, D.W.; Tidwell, R.R.; Hall, J.E. Enhanced permeability of the antimicrobial agent 2,5-bis(4-amidinophenyl)furan across Caco-2 cell monolayers via its methylamidoidme prodrug. *Pharm. Res.* **2002**, *19*, 1689–1695. [CrossRef]
31. Midgley, I.; Fitzpatrick, K.; Taylor, L.M.; Houchen, T.L.; Henderson, S.J.; Wright, S.J.; Cybulski, Z.R.; John, B.A.; McBurney, A.; Boykin, D.W. Pharmacokinetics and metabolism of the prodrug DB289 (2,5-bis[4-(N-methoxyamidino)phenyl]furan monomaleate) in rat and monkey and its conversion to the antiprotozoal/antifungal drug DB75 (2,5-bis(4-guanylphenyl)furan dihydrochloride). *Drug. Metab. Dispos.* **2007**, *35*, 955–967. [CrossRef]
32. Wang, M.Z.; Saulter, J.Y.; Usuki, E.; Cheung, Y.L.; Hall, M.; Bridges, A.S.; Loewen, G.; Parkinson, O.T.; Stephens, C.E.; Allen, J.L.; et al. CYP4F enzymes are the major enzymes in human liver microsomes that catalyze the O-demethylation of the antiparasitic prodrug DB289 [2,5-bis(4-amidinophenyl)furan-bis-O-methylamidoxime]. *Drug Metab. Dispos.* **2006**, *34*, 1985–1994. [CrossRef]
33. Wang, M.Z.; Wu, J.Q.; Bridges, A.S.; Zeldin, D.C.; Kornbluth, S.; Tidwell, R.R.; Hall, J.E.; Paine, M.F. Human enteric microsomal CYP4F enzymes O-demethylate the antiparasitic prodrug pafuramidine. *Drug Metab. Dispos.* **2007**, *35*, 2067–2075. [CrossRef]

34. Ansede, J.H.; Voyksner, R.D.; Ismail, M.A.; Boykin, D.W.; Tidwell, R.R.; Hall, J.E. In vitro metabolism of an orally active O-methyl amidoxime prodrug for the treatment of CNS trypanosomiasis. *Xenobiotica* **2005**, *35*, 211–226. [CrossRef]

35. Saulter, J.Y.; Kurian, J.R.; Trepanier, L.A.; Tidwell, R.R.; Bridges, A.S.; Boykin, D.W.; Stephens, C.E.; Anbazhagan, M.; Hall, J.E. Unusual dehydroxylation of antimicrobial amidoxime prodrugs by cytochrome b5 and NADH cytochrome b5 reductase. *Drug Metab. Dispos.* **2005**, *33*, 1886–1893. [CrossRef] [PubMed]

36. Ansede, J.H.; Anbazhagan, M.; Brun, R.; Easterbrook, J.D.; Hall, J.E.; Boykin, D.W. O-alkoxyamidine prodrugs of furamidine: *In vitro* transport and microsomal metabolism as indicators of *in vivo* efficacy in a mouse model of *Trypanosoma brucei rhodesiense* infection. *J. Med. Chem.* **2004**, *47*, 4335–4338. [CrossRef] [PubMed]

37. Mdachi, R.E.; Thuita, J.K.; Kagira, J.M.; Ngotho, J.M.; Murilla, G.A.; Ndung'u, J.M.; Tidwell, R.R.; Hall, J.E.; Brun, R. Efficacy of the novel diamidine compound 2,5-Bis(4-amidinophenyl)- furan-bis-O-Methlylamidoxime (Pafuramidine, DB289) against *Trypanosoma brucei rhodesiense* infection in vervet monkeys after oral administration. *Antimicrob. Agents Chemother.* **2009**, *53*, 953–957. [CrossRef] [PubMed]

38. Thuita, J.K.; Karanja, S.M.; Wenzler, T.; Mdachi, R.E.; Ngotho, J.M.; Kagira, J.M.; Tidwell, R.; Brun, R. Efficacy of the diamidine DB75 and its prodrug DB289, against murine models of human African trypanosomiasis. *Acta Trop.* **2008**, *108*, 6–10. [CrossRef] [PubMed]

39. Burri, C.; Yeramian, P.D.; Allen, J.L.; Merolle, A.; Serge, K.K.; Mpanya, A.; Lutumba, P.; Mesu, V.K.; Bilenge, C.M.; Lubaki, J.P.; et al. Efficacy, Safety, and Dose of Pafuramidine, a New Oral Drug for Treatment of First Stage Sleeping Sickness, in a Phase 2a Clinical Study and Phase 2b Randomized Clinical Studies. *PLoS Negl. Trop. Dis.* **2016**, *10*, e0004362. [CrossRef]

40. Harrill, A.H.; Desmet, K.D.; Wolf, K.K.; Bridges, A.S.; Eaddy, J.S.; Kurtz, C.L.; Hall, J.E.; Paine, M.F.; Tidwell, R.R.; Watkins, P.B. A mouse diversity panel approach reveals the potential for clinical kidney injury due to DB289 not predicted by classical rodent models. *Toxicol. Sci.* **2012**, *130*, 416–426. [CrossRef]

41. Wenzler, T.; Boykin, D.W.; Ismail, M.A.; Hall, J.E.; Tidwell, R.R.; Brun, R. New treatment option for second-stage African sleeping sickness: *In vitro* and *in vivo* efficacy of aza analogs of DB289. *Antimicrob. Agents Chemother.* **2009**, *53*, 4185–4192. [CrossRef]

42. Thuita, J.K.; Wang, M.Z.; Kagira, J.M.; Denton, C.L.; Paine, M.F.; Mdachi, R.E.; Murilla, G.A.; Ching, S.; Boykin, D.W.; Tidwell, R.R.; et al. Pharmacology of DB844, an orally active aza analog of pafuramidine, in a monkey model of second stage human African trypanosomiasis. *PLoS Negl. Trop. Dis.* **2012**, *6*, e1734. [CrossRef]

43. Goldsmith, R.B.; Tidwell, R.R. Organ specific accumulation and distribution of structurally related anti-trypanosomal compounds: A possible role in renal toxicity. *Am. J. Trop. Med. Hyg.* **2009**, *81*, 1–50. [CrossRef]

44. Depauw, S.; Lambert, M.; Jambon, S.; Paul, A.; Peixoto, P.; Nhili, R.; Marongiu, L.; Figeac, M.; Dassi, C.; Paul-Constant, C. Heterocyclic diamidine DNA ligands as HOXA9 transcription factor inhibitors: Design, molecular evaluation, and cellular consequences in a HOXA9-dependant leukemia cell model. *J. Med. Chem.* **2019**, *62*, 1306–1329. [CrossRef]

45. Soeiro, M.N.; Werbovetz, K.; Boykin, D.W.; Wilson, W.D.; Wang, M.Z.; Hemphill, A. Novel amidines and analogs as promising agents against intracellular parasites: A systematic review. *Parasitology* **2013**, *140*, 929–951. [CrossRef]

46. Mathis, A.M.; Holman, J.L.; Sturk, L.M.; Ismail, M.A.; Boykin, D.W.; Tidwell, R.R.; Hall, J.E. Accumulation and intracellular distribution of antitrypanosomal diamidine compounds DB75 and DB820 in African trypanosomes. *Antimicrob. Agents Chemother.* **2006**, *50*, 2185–2191. [CrossRef]

47. Ward, C.P.; Wong, P.E.; Burchmore, R.J.; de Koning, H.P.; Barrett, M.P. Trypanocidal furamidine analogs: Influence of pyridine nitrogens on trypanocidal activity, transport kinetics, and resistance patterns. *Antimicrob. Agents Chemother.* **2011**, *55*, 2352–2361. [CrossRef]

48. Lanteri, C.A.; Tidwell, R.R.; Meshnick, S.R. The mitochondrion is a site of trypanocidal action of the aromatic diamidine DB75 in bloodstream forms of *Trypanosoma brucei. Antimicrob. Agents Chemother.* **2008**, *52*, 875–882. [CrossRef]

49. Lanteri, C.A.; Trumpower, B.L.; Tidwell, R.R.; Meshnick, S.R. DB75, a novel trypanocidal agent, disrupts mitochondrial function in *Saccharomyces cerevisiae. Antimicrob. Agents Chemother.* **2004**, *48*, 3968–3974. [CrossRef]

50. Dean, S.; Gould, M.K.; Dewar, C.E.; Schnaufer, A.C. Single point mutations in ATP synthase compensate for mitochondrial genome loss in trypanosomes. *Proc. Natl. Acad. Sci. USA* **2013**, *110*, 14741–14746. [CrossRef]
51. Gould, M.K.; Schnaufer, A. Independence from Kinetoplast DNA maintenance and expression is associated with multidrug resistance in *Trypanosoma brucei in vitro*. *Antimicrob. Agents Chemother.* **2014**, *58*, 2925–2928. [CrossRef]
52. Ludewig, G.; Williams, J.M.; Li, Y.; Staben, C. Effects of pentamidine isethionate on Saccharomyces cerevisiae. *Antimicrob. Agents Chemother.* **1994**, *38*, 1123–1128. [CrossRef]
53. Carter, N.S.; Berger, B.J.; Fairlamb, A.H. Uptake of diamidine drugs by the P2 nucleoside transporter in melarsen-sensitive and -resistant *Trypanosoma brucei brucei*. *J. Biol. Chem.* **1995**, *270*, 28153–28157.
54. De Koning, H.P. Uptake of pentamidine in *Trypanosoma brucei brucei* is mediated by three distinct transporters: Implications for cross-resistance with arsenicals. *Mol. Pharmacol.* **2001**, *59*, 586–592. [CrossRef]
55. Alsford, S.; Eckert, S.; Baker, N.; Glover, L.; Sanchez-Flores, A.; Leung, K.F.; Turner, D.J.; Field, M.C.; Berriman, M.; Horn, D. High-throughput decoding of antitrypanosomal drug efficacy and resistance. *Nature* **2012**, *482*, 232–236. [CrossRef]
56. Baker, N.; Glover, L.; Munday, J.C.; Aguinaga Andrés, D.; Barrett, M.P.; de Koning, H.P.; Horn, D. Aquaglyceroporin 2 controls susceptibility to melarsoprol and pentamidine in African trypanosomes. *Proc. Natl. Acad. Sci. USA* **2012**, *109*, 10996–11001. [CrossRef]
57. Lanteri, C.A.; Stewart, M.L.; Brock, J.M.; Alibu, V.P.; Meshnick, S.R.; Tidwell, R.R.; Barrett, M.P. Roles for the *Trypanosoma brucei* P2 transporter in DB75 uptake and resistance. *Mol. Pharmacol.* **2006**, *70*, 1585–1592. [CrossRef]
58. Barrett, M.P.; Fairlamb, A.H. The biochemical basis of arsenical-diamidine crossresistance in African trypanosomes. *Parasitol. Today* **1999**, *15*, 136–140. [CrossRef]
59. Barrett, M.P.; Gilbert, I.H. Targeting of toxic compounds to the trypanosome's interior. *Adv. Parasitol.* **2006**, *63*, 125–183.
60. Stewart, M.L.; Bueno, G.J.; Baliani, A.; Klenke, B.; Brun, R.; Brock, J.M.; Gilbert, I.H.; Barrett, M.P. Trypanocidal activity of melamine-based nitroheterocycles. *Antimicrob. Agents Chemother.* **2004**, *48*, 1733–1738. [CrossRef]
61. Tye, C.K.; Kasinathan, G.; Barrett, M.P.; Brun, R.; Doyle, V.E.; Fairlamb, A.H.; Weaver, R.; Gilbert, I.H. An approach to use an unusual adenosine transporter to selectively deliver polyamine analogs to trypanosomes. *Bioorg. Med. Chem. Lett.* **1998**, *8*, 811–816. [CrossRef]
62. Sanderson, L.; Dogruel, M.; Rodgers, J.; De Koning, H.P.; Thomas, S.A. Pentamidine movement across the murine blood-brain and blood-cerebrospinal fluid barriers: Effect of trypanosome infection, combination therapy, P-glycoprotein, and multidrug resistance-associated protein. *J. Pharmacol. Exp. Ther.* **2009**, *329*, 967–977. [CrossRef]
63. Ming, X.; Ju, W.; Wu, H.; Tidwell, R.R.; Hall, J.E.; Thakker, D.R. Transport of dicationic drugs pentamidine and furamidine by human organic cation transporters. *Drug Metab. Dispos.* **2009**, *37*, 424–430. [CrossRef]
64. Sekhar, G.N.; Georgian, A.R.; Sanderson, L.; Vizcay-Barrena, G.; Brown, R.C.; Muresan, P.; Fleck, R.A.; Thomas, S.A. Organic cation transporter 1 (OCT1) is involved in pentamidine transport at the human and mouse blood-brain barrier (BBB). *PLoS ONE* **2017**, *12*, e0173474. [CrossRef]
65. Yang, S.; Wenzler, T.; Miller, P.N.; Wu, H.; Boykin, D.W.; Brun, R.; Wang, M.Z. Pharmacokinetic comparison to determine the mechanisms underlying the differential efficacies of cationic diamidines against first- and second-stage human African trypanosomiasis. *Antimicrob. Agents Chemother.* **2014**, *58*, 4064–4074. [CrossRef]
66. Lindner, A.K.; Lejon, V.; Chappuis, F.; Seixas, J.; Kazumba, L.; Barrett, M.P.; Mwamba, E.; Erphas, O.; Akl, E.A.; Villanueva, G.; et al. New WHO guidelines for treatment of gambiense human African trypanosomiasis including fexinidazole: Substantial changes for clinical practice. *Lancet Infect. Dis.* **2020**, *20*, e38–e46. [CrossRef]
67. Neau, P.; Hänel, H.; Lameyre, V.; Strub-Wourgaft, N.; Kuykens, L. Innovative partnerships for the elimination of Human African Trypanosomiasis and the development of fexinidazole. *Trop. Med. Infect. Dis.* **2020**, *5*, 17. [CrossRef]
68. Raether, W.; Hanel, H. Nitroheterocyclic drugs with broad spectrum activity. *Parasitol. Res.* **2003**, *90* (Suppl. 1), S19–S39. [CrossRef]
69. Jennings, F.W.; Urquhart, G.M. The use of the 2 substituted 5-nitroimidazole, Fexinidazole (Hoe 239) in the treatment of chronic *T. brucei* infections in mice. *Z. Parasitenkd.* **1983**, *69*, 577–581. [CrossRef]

70. Kaiser, M.; Bray, M.A.; Cal, M.; Bourdin Trunz, B.; Torreele, E.; Brun, R. Antitrypanosomal activity of fexinidazole, a new oral nitroimidazole drug candidate for treatment of sleeping sickness. *Antimicrob. Agents Chemother.* **2011**, *55*, 5602–5608. [CrossRef]

71. Barrett, M.P.; Fairlamb, A.H.; Rousseau, B.; Chauvière, G.; Perié, J. Uptake of the nitroimidazole drug megazol by African trypanosomes. *Biochem. Pharmacol.* **2000**, *59*, 615–620. [CrossRef]

72. Stover, C.K.; Warrener, P.; VanDevanter, D.R.; Sherman, D.R.; Arain, T.M.; Langhorne, M.H.; Anderson, S.W.; Towell, J.A.; Yuan, Y.; McMurray, D.N.; et al. A small-molecule nitroimidazopyran drug candidate for the treatment of tuberculosis. *Nature* **2000**, *405*, 962–966. [CrossRef]

73. Torreele, E.; Bourdin Trunz, B.; Tweats, D.; Kaiser, M.; Brun, R.; Mazué, G.; Bray, M.A.; Pécoul, B. Fexinidazole—A new oral nitroimidazole drug candidate entering clinical development for the treatment of sleeping sickness. *PLoS Negl. Trop. Dis.* **2010**, *4*, e923. [CrossRef]

74. Tweats, D.; Bourdin Trunz, B.; Torreele, E. Genotoxicity profile of fexinidazole—A drug candidate in clinical development for human African trypanomiasis (sleeping sickness). *Mutagenesis* **2012**, *27*, 523–532. [CrossRef]

75. Wilkinson, S.R.; Taylor, M.C.; Horn, D.; Kelly, J.M.; Cheeseman, I. A mechanism for cross-resistance to nifurtimox and benznidazole in trypanosomes. *Proc. Natl. Acad. Sci. USA* **2008**, *105*, 5022–5027. [CrossRef] [PubMed]

76. Wyllie, S.; Foth, B.J.; Kelner, A.; Sokolova, A.Y.; Berriman, M.; Fairlamb, A.H. Nitroheterocyclic drug resistance mechanisms in *Trypanosoma brucei*. *J. Antimicrob. Chemother.* **2016**, *71*, 625–634. [CrossRef] [PubMed]

77. Hall, B.S.; Bot, C.; Wilkinson, S.R. Nifurtimox activation by trypanosomal type I nitroreductases generates cytotoxic nitrile metabolites. *J. Biol. Chem.* **2011**, *286*, 13088–13095. [CrossRef] [PubMed]

78. Bahia, M.T.; de Andrade, I.M.; Martins, T.A.; do Nascimento, Á.F.; Diniz Lde, F.; Caldas, I.S.; Talvani, A.; Trunz, B.B.; Torreele, E.; Ribeiro, I. Fexinidazole: A potential new drug candidate for Chagas disease. *PLoS Negl. Trop. Dis.* **2012**, *6*, e1870. [CrossRef]

79. Hall, B.S.; Wilkinson, S.R. Activation of benznidazole by trypanosomal type I nitroreductases results in glyoxal formation. *Antimicrob. Agents Chemother.* **2012**, *56*, 115–123. [CrossRef]

80. Trochine, A.; Creek, D.J.; Faral-Tello, P.; Barrett, M.P.; Robello, C. Benznidazole biotransformation and multiple targets in *Trypanosoma cruzi* revealed by metabolomics. *PLoS Negl. Trop. Dis.* **2014**, *8*, e2844. [CrossRef]

81. Hall, B.S.; Meredith, E.L.; Wilkinson, S.R. Targeting the substrate preference of a type I nitroreductase to develop antitrypanosomal quinone-based prodrugs. *Antimicrob. Agents Chemother.* **2012**, *56*, 5821–5830. [CrossRef]

82. Menzies, S.K.; Tulloch, L.B.; Florence, G.J.; Smith, T.K. The trypanosome alternative oxidase: A potential drug target? *Parasitology* **2018**, *145*, 175–183. [CrossRef]

83. Thomas, J.A.; Baker, N.; Hutchinson, S.; Dominicus, C.; Trenaman, A.; Glover, L.; Alsford, S.; Horn, D. Insights into antitrypanosomal drug mode-of-action from cytology-based profiling. *PLoS Negl. Trop. Dis.* **2018**, *12*, e0006980. [CrossRef]

84. Nocentini, A.; Supuran, C.T.; Winum, J.Y. Benzoxaborole compounds for therapeutic uses: A patent review (2010–2018). *Expert. Opin. Ther. Pat.* **2018**, *28*, 493–504. [CrossRef]

85. Ding, D.; Zhao, Y.; Meng, Q.; Xie, D.; Nare, B.; Chen, D.; Bacchi, C.J.; Yarlett, N.; Zhang, Y.K.; Hernandez, V.; et al. Discovery of novel benzoxaborole-based potent antitrypanosomal agents. *ACS Med. Chem. Lett.* **2010**, *1*, 165–169. [CrossRef]

86. Nare, B.; Wring, S.; Bacchi, C.; Beaudet, B.; Bowling, T.; Brun, R.; Chen, D.; Ding, C.; Freund, Y.; Gaukel, E.; et al. Discovery of novel orally bioavailable oxaborole 6-carboxamides that demonstrate cure in a murine model of late-stage central nervous system African trypanosomiasis. *Antimicrob. Agents Chemother.* **2010**, *54*, 4379–4388. [CrossRef]

87. Bacchi, C.J.; Nathan, H.C.; Hutner, S.H.; McCann, P.P.; Sjoerdsma, A. Polyamine metabolism: A potential therapeutic target in trypanosomes. *Science* **1980**, *210*, 332–334. [CrossRef]

88. Jacobs, R.T.; Nare, B.; Wring, S.A.; Orr, M.D.; Chen, D.; Sligar, J.M.; Jenks, M.X.; Noe, R.A.; Bowling, T.S.; Mercer, L.T.; et al. SCYX-7158, an orally-active benzoxaborole for the treatment of stage 2 human African trypanosomiasis. *PLoS Negl. Trop. Dis.* **2011**, *5*, e1151. [CrossRef]

89. Wring, S.; Gaukel, E.; Nare, B.; Jacobs, R.; Beaudet, B.; Bowling, T.; Mercer, L.; Bacchi, C.; Yarlett, N.; Randolph, R. Pharmacokinetics and pharmacodynamics utilizing unbound target tissue exposure as part of a disposition-based rationale for lead optimization of benzoxaboroles in the treatment of Stage 2 Human African Trypanosomiasis. *Parasitology* **2014**, *141*, 104–118. [CrossRef]

90. Available online: https://www.dndi.org/2012/media-center/press-releases/oxa-phasei/ (accessed on 12 January 2020).

91. Available online: https://www.dndi.org/diseases-projects/portfolio/acoziborole/ (accessed on 12 January 2020).

92. Jones, D.C.; Foth, B.J.; Urbaniak, M.D.; Patterson, S.; Ong, H.B.; Berriman, M.; Fairlamb, A.H. Genomic and Proteomic Studies on the Mode of Action of Oxaboroles against the African Trypanosome. *PLoS Negl. Trop. Dis.* **2015**, *9*, e0004299. [CrossRef]

93. Sonoiki, E.; Ng, C.L.; Lee, M.C.; Guo, D.; Zhang, Y.K.; Zhou, Y.; Alley, M.R.; Ahyong, V.; Sanz, L.M.; Lafuente-Monasterio, M.J.; et al. A potent antimalarial benzoxaborole targets a *Plasmodium falciparum* cleavage and polyadenylation specificity factor homologue. *Nat. Commun.* **2017**, *8*, 14574. [CrossRef]

94. Palencia, A.; Bougdour, A.; Brenier-Pinchart, M.P.; Touquet, B.; Bertini, R.L.; Sensi, C.; Gay, G.; Vollaire, J.; Josserand, V.; Easom, E.; et al. Targeting *Toxoplasma gondii* CPSF3 as a new approach to control toxoplasmosis. *EMBO Mol. Med.* **2017**, *9*, 385–394. [CrossRef]

95. Steketee, P.C.; Vincent, I.M.; Achcar, F.; Giordani, F.; Kim, D.H.; Creek, D.J.; Freund, Y.; Jacobs, R.; Rattigan, K.; Horn, D.; et al. Benzoxaborole treatment perturbs S-adenosyl-L-methionine metabolism in *Trypanosoma brucei*. *PLoS Negl. Trop. Dis.* **2018**, *12*, e0006450. [CrossRef]

96. Begolo, D.; Vincent, I.M.; Giordani, F.; Pöhner, I.; Witty, M.J.; Rowan, T.G.; Bengaly, Z.; Gillingwater, K.; Freund, Y.; Wade, R.C.; et al. The trypanocidal benzoxaborole AN7973 inhibits trypanosome mRNA processing. *PLoS Pathog.* **2018**, *14*, e1007315. [CrossRef]

97. Wall, R.J.; Rico, E.; Lukac, I.; Zuccotto, F.; Elg, S.; Gilbert, I.H.; Freund, Y.; Alley, M.R.K.; Field, M.C.; Wyllie, S.; et al. Clinical and veterinary trypanocidal benzoxaboroles target CPSF3. *Proc. Natl. Acad. Sci. USA* **2018**, *15*, 9616–9621. [CrossRef]

98. Zhang, N.; Zoltner, M.; Leung, K.F.; Scullion, P.; Hutchinson, S.; Del Pino, R.C.; Vincent, I.M.; Zhang, Y.K.; Freund, Y.R.; Alley, M.R.K.; et al. Host-parasite co-metabolic activation of antitrypanosomal aminomethyl-benzoxaboroles. *PLoS Pathog.* **2018**, *14*, e1006850. [CrossRef]

99. Akama, T.; Zhang, Y.K.; Freund, Y.R.; Berry, P.; Lee, J.; Easom, E.E.; Jacobs, R.T.; Plattner, J.J.; Witty, M.J.; Peter, R.; et al. Identification of a 4-fluorobenzyl l-valinate amide benzoxaborole (AN11736) as a potential development candidate for the treatment of Animal African Trypanosomiasis (AAT). *Bioorg. Med. Chem. Lett.* **2018**, *28*, 6–10. [CrossRef]

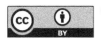

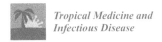

Tropical Medicine and
Infectious Disease

Article

Anti-Trypanosomal Proteasome Inhibitors Cure Hemolymphatic and Meningoencephalic Murine Infection Models of African Trypanosomiasis

Srinivasa P S Rao [1,*], Suresh B Lakshminarayana [1], Jan Jiricek [1], Marcel Kaiser [2,3], Ryan Ritchie [4], Elmarie Myburgh [5], Frantisek Supek [6], Tove Tuntland [6], Advait Nagle [6], Valentina Molteni [6], Pascal Mäser [2,3], Jeremy C Mottram [7], Michael P Barrett [4] and Thierry T Diagana [1]

[1] Novartis Institute for Tropical Diseases, 5300 Chiron Way, Emeryville, CA 94608, USA; suresh.b_lakshminarayana@novartis.com (S.B.L.); jan.jiricek@novartis.com (J.J.); thierry.diagana@novartis.com (T.T.D.)

[2] Swiss Tropical and Public Health Institute, Socinstrasse 57, 4501 Basel, Switzerland; marcel.kaiser@swisstph.ch (M.K.); pascal.maeser@swisstph.ch (P.M.)

[3] Department of Epidemiology and Public Health, University of Basel, Petersplatz 1, 4000 Basel, Switzerland

[4] Wellcome Centre for Integrative Parasitology, Institute of Infection, Immunity and Inflammation, College of Medical, Veterinary and Life Sciences, University of Glasgow, Glasgow G12 8TA, UK; Ryan.Ritchie@glasgow.ac.uk (R.R.); Michael.Barrett@glasgow.ac.uk (M.P.B.)

[5] York Biomedical Research Institute, Hull York Medical School, University of York, Wentworth Way, Heslington, York YO10 5DD, UK; elmarie.myburgh@york.ac.uk

[6] Genomics Institute of the Novartis Research Foundation, 10675 John Jay Hopkins Drive, San Diego, CA 92121, USA; fsupek@gnf.org (F.S.); tovetuntland@outlook.com (T.T.); anagle@gnf.org (A.N.); vmolteni@gnf.org (V.M.)

[7] York Biomedical Research Institute, Department of Biology, University of York, Wentworth Way, Heslington, York YO10 5DD, UK; jeremy.mottram@york.ac.uk

* Correspondence: srinivasa.rao@novartis.com

Received: 9 January 2020; Accepted: 14 February 2020; Published: 17 February 2020

Abstract: Current anti-trypanosomal therapies suffer from problems of longer treatment duration, toxicity and inadequate efficacy, hence there is a need for safer, more efficacious and 'easy to use' oral drugs. Previously, we reported the discovery of the triazolopyrimidine (TP) class as selective kinetoplastid proteasome inhibitors with in vivo efficacy in mouse models of leishmaniasis, Chagas Disease and African trypanosomiasis (HAT). For the treatment of HAT, development compounds need to have excellent penetration to the brain to cure the meningoencephalic stage of the disease. Here we describe detailed biological and pharmacological characterization of triazolopyrimidine compounds in HAT specific assays. The TP class of compounds showed single digit nanomolar potency against *Trypanosoma brucei rhodesiense* and *Trypanosoma brucei gambiense* strains. These compounds are trypanocidal with concentration-time dependent kill and achieved relapse-free cure in vitro. Two compounds, GNF6702 and a new analog NITD689, showed favorable in vivo pharmacokinetics and significant brain penetration, which enabled oral dosing. They also achieved complete cure in both hemolymphatic (blood) and meningoencephalic (brain) infection of human African trypanosomiasis mouse models. Mode of action studies on this series confirmed the 20S proteasome as the target in *T. brucei*. These proteasome inhibitors have the potential for further development into promising new treatment for human African trypanosomiasis.

Keywords: sleeping sickness; drug discovery; *Trypanosoma* growth inhibitors

Trop. Med. Infect. Dis. **2020**, *5*, 28

1. Introduction

Human African trypanosomiasis (HAT) is a neglected tropical disease caused by the protozoan parasites *Trypanosoma brucei gambiense* and *Trypanosoma brucei rhodesiense*. The disease is endemic to sub-Saharan Africa and transmitted by tsetse flies (*Glossina* spp.). Over the last decade, there has been a significant reduction in the number of new cases of HAT, reaching below ~1000 reported new cases per annum in 2018 [1]. HAT comprises hemolymphatic (stage 1) and meningoencephalic (stage 2) infections. The successful introduction of nifurtimox–eflornithine combination therapy (NECT) for the treatment of gambiense HAT significantly helped in achieving a cure in stage 2 HAT patients [2]. Although NECT is effective, it requires long infusions and continuous monitoring. The introduction of fexinidazole, as an oral drug capable of curing stage 1 and stage 2 disease, offers great potential, and a further orally available drug, acoziborole, is currently being evaluated in late-stage clinical trials [3]. For treatment of rhodesiense HAT, suramin and melarsoprol (a highly toxic arsenical) are still used. New drugs remain desirable if we are to assure no repeat of the historical re-emergence of HAT, following a successful campaign in the mid-twentieth century where cases had dropped to the low thousands, only to resurge to an estimated 300,000 cases by the turn of the century [4]. Recent publications showing that trypanosomes dwell in adipose tissue [5] and skin [6], along with several reports of possible animal reservoirs of gambiense trypanosomes and latent human infections, all point out potential threats to the elimination of HAT [7].

Novartis, in collaboration with academic partners, embarked to find novel, safe short-course therapies for treatment of all forms of HAT. Previously, we reported [8] the discovery of the triazolopyrimidine (TP) chemical class as growth inhibitors of *Leishmania donovani*, *Trypanosoma cruzi* and *T. b. brucei* and identified the 20S proteasome as the target responsible for the pharmacological activity. Furthermore, exemplar from this class (GNF6702) demonstrated efficacy in the murine models for the three indications [8]. An earlier study had shown in vitro growth inhibition activity of TP cpds against *T. b. brucei* and GNF6702's stage 2 efficacy at highest dosing regimen of 100 mg/kg once daily [8]. Here, we describe detailed biological, chemical and pharmacological characterization of the three TP class of inhibitors (GNF3849, GNF6702 and NITD689) in various HAT-specific assays. The TPs are active against disease causing *T. b. gambiense* and *T. b. rhodesiense* strains, as well as drug-resistant (melarsoprol and pentamidine) isolates. These compounds inhibit the chymotrypsin activity of the 20S proteasome and are trypanocidal showing concentration-time dependent kill. Stage 2 HAT treatment requires compounds to have unique properties that enable them to cross the blood–brain barrier in order to be efficacious against CNS-resident parasites. Two compounds, GNF6702 and the newer analog NITD689, had favorable physicochemical and pharmacokinetic properties amenable for oral dosing and achieving free brain concentrations required for stage 2 efficacy. They also achieve relapse-free cure in mouse models of stage 1 and 2 trypanosomiasis, in a dose-dependent manner, suggesting the potential to treat all forms of HAT.

2. Materials and Methods

2.1. Parasites, Cell Culture and Growth Inhibition Assays

The *T. b. brucei* strain Lister 427 (bloodstream form) parasites were continuously grown in complete HMI-9 medium supplemented with 10% Serum Plus and 10% heat-inactivated fetal bovine serum (FBS) [8]. All other parasite strains were cultured as described elsewhere [9].

For determination of 50% growth inhibition, all compounds were dissolved in DMSO, and 200 nL of threefold serially diluted compounds were added into solid-bottom 384-well white plates (Greiner Bio-One, Kremsmunster, Austria) by an Echo 555 acoustic liquid-handling system. Forty microliters of 10^4 cells/mL of *T. b. brucei* parasites was added into each well, and the plates were incubated in a 5% CO_2 incubator at 37 °C for 48 h. Viability of parasites were determined by measuring intracellular ATP levels, using CellTiter-Glo (CTG) luminescent cell viability reagent (Promega, Madison, Wisconsin WI, USA). The EC_{50} values were determined by using GraphPad Prism software. Growth inhibition assays for all clinical isolates were carried out as described earlier [9]. All experiments had two technical replicates and three biological replicates. Appropriate statistical tests were used for evaluating significance, and mean ± SEM is represented in the tables.

2.2. HepG2 Cytotoxicity Assay

The HepG2 (human hepatocellular carcinoma) cells were obtained from ATCC (American Type Culture Collection) and grown in RPMI media. Cytotoxicity assay was performed in 384-well format, and 25 μL, approximately 1.6×10^4 cells/mL, suspension was added to clear-bottom 384-well Griener plates and incubated in 5% CO_2 incubator, at 37 °C for 24 h. Once the cells adhered, 125 nL of threefold serially diluted compounds in DMSO was added. Plates were incubated for 96 h, at 37 °C, in a 5% CO_2 incubator. Plates were read for viability by adding 10 μL of CCK-8 reagent (APExBIO) into each well, followed by 3 h incubation and absorbance reading at 450 nM, using an Envision plate reader. Absorbance values were used for determination of cytotoxic concentration (CC_{50}) required to inhibit growth by 50%, using GraphPad Prism software. Puromycin was used as a positive control. All experiments had two technical replicates and three biological replicates. Appropriate statistical tests were used for evaluating significance, and mean ± SEM is represented in the tables.

2.3. Determination of Solubility, PAMPA, Plasma Protein Binding, Brain Tissue Binding and Microsomal Clearance

Test compounds' solubility was determined in a high-throughput thermodynamic solubility assay, as described previously [10]. The PAMPA (parallel artificial membrane) assays were carried out, using a standard protocol [11]. Plasma protein binding was determined by using mouse blood [12], whilst brain tissue binding was determined by using rat brain tissue homogenate. Intrinsic metabolic clearances were determined in mouse liver microsomes, using the compound depletion approach and LC–MS/MS quantification [13].

2.4. Time to Kill and Reversibility Assays

Time-to-kill experiments were carried out to determine the ability of compounds to kill bloodstream form of *T. b. brucei* Lister 427 at 6, 24 and 48 h post-compound treatment. Viability of parasites were assessed by measuring ATP content as a surrogate. The assay was conducted in 384-well format, in a similar manner as the growth inhibition assay stated above, but with minor modifications. Compound-containing plates were incubated with 40 μL of approximately 1×10^5 parasites per mL, and at each time point, CTG reagent was added to lyse the parasites, and luminescence was measured after 30 min of incubation, using a Tecan M1000 plate reader.

Reversibility assessment to establish time and concentration required to achieve irreversible (relapse-free) growth inhibition in vitro was carried out as described elsewhere [14]. The AC_{cure} is the absolute concentration required to achieve sterile cure under in vitro conditions with incubation of compound for 24, 48 and 72 h, respectively.

All experiments had two technical replicates and three biological replicates. Appropriate statistical tests were used for evaluating significance, and mean ± SEM was represented.

2.5. In Vivo Pharmacokinetic (PK) Analysis

Determination of intravenous (i.v.) and per oral (p.o.) pharmacokinetics (PK) were carried out by using male BALB/c mice. For i.v. PK studies, compounds were formulated at a concentration of 2.5 mg/mL in 75% PEG300 and 25% D5W (5% dextrose in distilled water). To avoid any granular material, the solution was filtered, using a 0.45 μm syringe filter. The filtered solutions were dosed intravenously to mice via the lateral tail vein, at 5 mg/kg, with a dosing volume of 2 mL/kg. For all the p.o. PK studies, compounds were resuspended in 0.5% *v/v* methyl cellulose in 0.5 % *v/v* tween 80 solution. For 20 mg/kg dosing, 200 μL of compounds was administered orally to mice. Six blood samples of 50 μL each were collected serially from each animal, up to 24 h after dosing. Blood samples were collected into heparin microtainers and centrifuged, and then plasma was separated and frozen until analysis. Plasma samples (20 μL) were extracted with acetonitrile:methanol (3:1) containing internal standard. The samples were vortexed and then centrifuged in an Eppendorf centrifuge 5810R, at a setting of 4000 rpm, for 5 min, at 4 °C. The supernatant was transferred to a 96-well analysis plate and analyzed, using optimized LC/MS/MS conditions. For every experiment, 3 mice were used per compound, per dose. The plasma concentration-time profile was obtained by plotting the mean value from the three animals at each time point. Various PK parameters, such as C_{max} (maximum concentration), area under curve (AUC) and oral bioavailability (F) for compounds, were calculated by non-compartmental regression analysis, using an in-house fitting program developed at GNF [8]. All the in-life studies were carried out under protocols approved by the Animal Care and Use Committee (IACUC), following animal ethics guidelines of GNF.

For measurement of the brain-to-plasma drug concentration ratio, mice were dosed intravenously with 1 mg/kg compounds. Mice were euthanized at 5 and 60 min post-dosing, and blood and brains were collected. The compound concentrations in plasma and brains were measured, following the protocol described above.

2.6. Hemolymphatic Mouse Model (Stage 1 HAT Efficacy Model)

The *T. b. brucei* STIB795 acute mouse model mimics the hemolymphatic stage of the sleeping sickness disease. We used six female NMRI mice per experimental group, divided into two cages. Heparinized blood from a donor mouse with approximately 5×10^6 per mL parasitemia was suspended in phosphate saline glucose (PSG), to obtain a parasite suspension of 1×10^5 per mL. Each mouse was injected with 0.25 mL of parasite suspension (10^4 bloodstream forms of *T. b. brucei* STIB795) intraperitoneally. All compounds were formulated in 0.5% methylcellulose and 0.5% Tween80. Three days post-infection, test compounds were administered orally on four consecutive days, in a volume of 100 μL/10 g. Three mice served as infected–untreated controls. The control mice were not injected with the vehicle, because we have established in our labs that this vehicle does not affect parasitemia or the mice. Until 31 days post-infection, parasitemia was monitored microscopically by tail-blood examination twice a week. Mice were considered cured when there was no parasitemia detected in the tail blood. All the results from the individual experiments were reported as number of mice cured over total number of mice treated. A Kaplan–Meier plot was used for representing the number of mice cured at different treatment doses.

In vivo efficacy studies in mice were conducted at the Swiss Tropical and Public Health Institute (Basel) (License number 2813), according to the rules and regulations for the protection of animal rights ("Tierschutzverordnung") of the Swiss "Bundesamt für Veterinärwesen". They were approved by the veterinary office of Canton Basel-Stadt, Switzerland.

2.7. Meningocephalic Mouse Model (Stage 2 HAT Efficacy Model)

The GVR35 mouse CNS model mimics the second (meningoencephalic) stage of African trypanosomiasis. Female CD1 mice (~8 weeks old, from Charles River) were injected intraperitoneally (i.p.) with 3×10^4 *T. b. brucei* (GVR35-VSL2) bloodstream-form parasites [15]. As controls, a group of three untreated mice and another group of three mice treated with diminazene aceturate (DA) were included. The DA is a known anti-trypanosomal compound, which lacks brain penetration; hence, they clear only the blood parasitemia, leaving behind the parasites in brain. Mice treated with DA usually relapse after 42 days post-infection. Groups of six infected mice were dosed with TP compounds by oral gavage, once daily, from day 21 or 22 post-infection, for seven days.

Blood parasitemia was quantified weekly from day 21/22, by microscopy of blood from the tail vein. Mice were imaged for bioluminescence using an in vivo imaging system (IVIS) prior to treatment on day 21/22, and weekly after treatment, as described previously [8,15]. Briefly, mice, in groups of three, were injected i.p. with 150 mg of D-luciferin (Promega) per kilogram body weight in PBS and imaged after 10 min, using an IVIS Spectrum (PerkinElmer, Waltham, Massachusetts MA, USA). Living

Image Software (PerkinElmer) was used for acquisition and analysis of bioluminescence imaging data. Bioluminescence in the same rectangular region of interest (ROI) on whole-body mouse images was quantified and is shown in total flux (photons per second). Images were cropped to the ROIs and composites of images from representative mice are shown. Uncured mice were euthanized within 1 or 2 days of parasite detection in the blood. Cured mice were euthanized between day 92 and 101 post-infection. All the results from the individual experiments were reported as number of mice cured over total number of mice treated. A Kaplan–Meier plot was used for representing the number of mice cured at different treatment doses.

All animal protocols and procedures were reviewed and approved by the UK Home Office (Project License PPL60/4442 entitled "Molecular Genetics of Trypanosomes and Leishmania") and University of York and University of Glasgow Ethics Committees, and was done in accordance with the Animals (Scientific Procedures) Act 1986 (ASPA).

3. Results

3.1. Extended Characterization of TP Series of Kinetoplastid Proteasome Inhibitors for Treatment of Human African Trypanosomiasis

Previously, we described our efforts to identify novel chemotypes for the treatment of HAT. These efforts led the identification of GNF6702, a prototypical pan-kinetoplastid inhibitor that was efficacious in the mouse models for all three kinetoplastid diseases [8].

All the three TP compounds (GNF3849, GNF6702 and NITD689) showed potent growth inhibition (EC_{50} < 70 nM) against *T. b. brucei* with varying cytotoxicity profile (Figure 1). Further evaluation of triazolopyrimidine analogues for the optimal blood–brain barrier penetration properties, such as lipophilicity (cLogP) and polar surface area, led to prioritization of NITD689, in addition to GNF3849 and GNF6702. All three compounds exhibited good membrane permeability, low mouse liver microsomal clearance and moderate lipophilicity (Figure 1). While GNF3849 had favorable potency against *T. brucei*, it was cytotoxic against HepG2 cells. Moreover, it also suffered from poor solubility and high plasma protein binding, indicating that higher total exposure might be needed to observe efficacy in in vivo. As reported previously [8], replacement of a phenyl group of GNF3849 with a pyridine moiety (GNF6702) improved solubility, lowered PPB and also created a molecule with a better cytotoxicity. Medicinal chemistry optimization by increasing SP^3 fraction within the molecule by replacing pyridine group with a tertiary butyl group led to the identification of NITD689. The NITD689 showed improved solubility, reduced plasma protein binding and retained non-cytotoxic profile, with 30 nM potency against *T. b. brucei* (Figure 1 and Table 1).

Table 1. Biological, physicochemical and in vitro pharmacokinetic properties of the triazolopyrimidine inhibitors.

Assays/Properties *	GNF3849 [#]	GNF6702 [#]	NITD689 [$]
T. b. brucei EC_{50} (nM)	22 ± 4	70 ± 3	30 ± 4
HepG2 CC_{50} (µM)	1.1 ± 0.2	>20	>20
Solubility pH 6.8 (g/L)	<0.002	0.009	0.071
LogD/Mol Wt/PSA	3.31/428/98	2.32/429/103	3.05/408/98
MPO	3.4	3.7	3.6
PAMPA Permeability (% FA)	96	92	99.1
Mouse liver microsomal clearance (µL/min/mg)	15.2	34.1	7.41
Mouse plasma protein binding (%)	>99	95.1	90.5

Note: All EC_{50} and CC_{50} values correspond to mean ± SEM (n = 4 biological replicates); * LogD: measured octanol water co-efficient; Mol wt: molecular weight; PSA: polar surface area; MPO: multi-parametric optimization; PAMPA: parallel artificial membrane permeability assay; FA: fraction absorbed. [#] Khare et al., Nature 2016 [8]; [$] patent US 2019/0000852 A1.

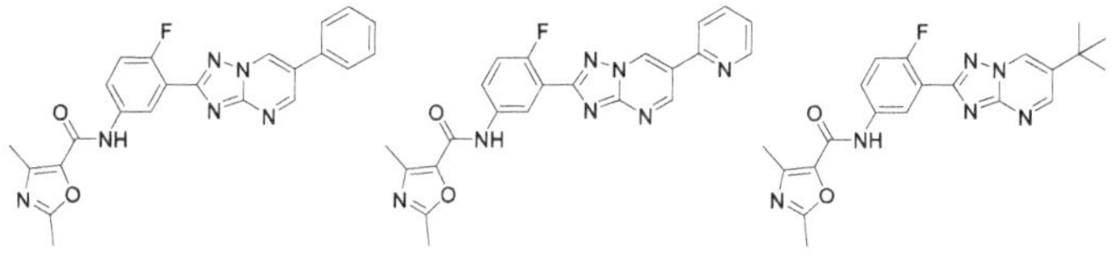

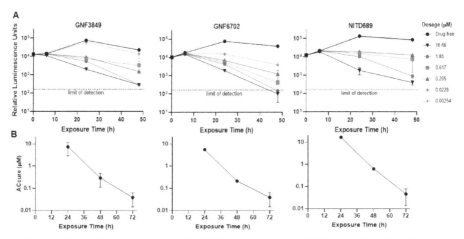

GNF3849   GNF6702   NITD698

Figure 1. Chemical structure of the triazolopyrimidine class of inhibitors.

3.2. Biological Profiling of the TP Class of Inhibitors

Triazolopyrimidines were evaluated for their potential to kill parasites under in vitro conditions. Time-to-kill assessment showed that all the three compounds were trypanocidal. At an early time point (6 h post exposure), no significant cidality was seen compared to the untreated control, even at the highest concentration tested (16.7 μM). However, at 24 and 48 h post-incubation, with compounds, significant kill was evident, suggesting this class of inhibitors requires 24 h in order to show cidality. All three compounds showed concentration and time-dependent lethality (Figure 2A).

Figure 2. Biological characterization of the TP class of compounds. (**A**) Time-to-kill profile indicating concentration-time dependent kill. (**B**) To achieve sterile cure without relapse under in vitro conditions. All experiments were carried out three times, independently, and mean ± SEM was plotted.

In order to evaluate the ability of TP compounds to kill all parasites without recrudescence (sterile cidality), we carried out drug wash-out assays. All the three TP compounds achieved sterile cure with ACcure (Absolute concentration of drug required to kill parasites without relapse) values of <100 nM, after a 72-h compound treatment and subsequent wash-out. The ACcure values also decreased as the time of exposure increased, indicating exposure-driven sterile cure (Figure 2B).

3.3. The TP Class of Inhibitors Are Active against Clinical Isolates

GNF3849 and GNF6702 were also tested for their ability to inhibit growth of clinical isolates of *T. b. gambiense* and *T. b. rhodesiense*. Our compounds showed single-digit nM potency against all strains tested. The compounds were also active against pentamidine- and melarsoprol-resistant strains of *T. b. rhodesiense*, as well as *T. b. brucei* (Table 2), suggesting a distinct mechanism of action, at least in terms of drug uptake, since resistance to these drugs relates to loss of transporters specific for their uptake [16,17].

Table 2. Growth inhibitory profile of the triazolopyrimidine class of compounds against various parasite strains.

Parasite	Strain	GNF3849	GNF6702	Melarsoprol	Pentamidine
T. b. gambiense (EC_{50} in nM)	STIB930	4.5 ± 1	3.7 ± 2	7.1 ± 2.7	1.4 ± 0.9
	K048	4.8 ± 1.1	3.5 ± 1.4	10.2 ± 1.9	33.9 ± 16
	R130	1.9 ± 1	2.3 ± 1.1	7.7 ± 3.1	13.5 ± 4
T. b. rhodesiense (EC_{50} in nM)	STIB900	1.4 ± 1	1.6 ± 0.9	3.9 ± 2	2.1 ± 0.7
	STIB900 Pent^R	1.7 ± 1	1.2 ± 0.3	46.8 ± 19	203 ± 54
	STIB900 Mel^R	0.6 ± 3	0.7 ± 0.2	95.5 ± 24	217 ± 86
T. b. brucei (EC_{50} in nM)	BS221	1.9 ± 0.8	0.9 ± 0.3	4.7 ± 1.8	0.3 ± 0.1
	BS221 (P2 KO)	4.0 ± 2.5	3.5 ± 1.2	37.7 ± 14.8	3.1 ± 0.4
	STIB950	0.9 ± 0.2	1.2 ± 0.5	16.9 ± 8.8	0.5 ± 0.2

Note: All EC_{50} values correspond to mean $\pm$ SD (n = 3 biological replicates).

3.4. The TP Class of Compounds Are Proteasome Inhibitors

The TP class of inhibitors is active against both *T. cruzi* and *T. brucei*. Resistance selection in *T. brucei* proved difficult; hence, we generated *T. cruzi* resistant isolates, using a classical resistant mutant generation approach. Whole-genome sequencing identified single nucleotide polymorphisms in F24L and I29M of β4 subunit of 20S proteasome. Further validation of the proteasome as a target for the TP class of compounds has been described elsewhere [8]. *T. brucei* parasites modified to express an F24L mutant β4 subunit of the 20S proteasome were previously shown to be resistant to the parent proteasome inhibitor. Here, we used the same strain to demonstrate its resistance to the new TP compounds, confirming that they, too, target the proteasome (Table 3). Meanwhile, bortezomib, a known chymotrypsin proteasome inhibitor, was equipotent against both wild-type and F24L mutant of *T. brucei*, suggesting that bortezomib and TP compounds interact differently by binding into different pockets within 20S proteasome.

Table 3. Mutations in F24L in the 20S proteasome β4 subunit confers resistance to TP class of compounds.

Strain	*T. brucei* PSMB4^{WT} (EC_{50} = nM)	*T. brucei* PSMB4^{F24L} (EC_{50} = nM)
GNF3849	10 ± 3	2200 ± 20
GNF6702	18 ± 1.8	1200 ± 13
NITD689	20 ± 4	1900 ± 20
Bortezomib	0.94 ± 0.05	1.1 ± 0.26

Note: All EC_{50} values correspond to mean $\pm$ SEM (n = 3 biological replicates); PSMB^{WT}: *T. brucei* ectopically expressing wild-type copy of 20S proteasome β4 subunit; PSMB^{F24L}: *T. brucei* ectopically expressing F24L mutant copy of 20S proteasome β4 subunit.

3.5. In Vivo Pharmacokinetic Properties of TP Class of Compounds

In vivo mice PK profiling was carried out, using intravenous and oral routes (Table 4). Following intravenous administration, all three TP compounds displayed a moderate volume of distribution (V_{ss}: 1.2 to 1.5 L/kg), low total systemic clearance (2.5 to 15% of hepatic blood flow) and moderate-to-long elimination half-life (1.6 to 7 h). Following oral administration at 20 mg/kg, all three TP compounds showed good oral exposure, with bioavailability ranging from 34% to 100%. The dose-normalized total exposure was highest for GNF6702 in terms of AUC, followed by GNF3849 and NITD689. Although

NITD689 had the lowest exposure in terms of total concentration, it had the highest free C_{max} and better free AUC compared to GNF3849, due to low plasma protein binding (Figure 1 and Table 4).

Table 4. In vivo pharmacokinetics properties of the TP class of compounds.

Parameters	Units	GNF3849	GNF6702	NITD689
I.V. PK				
Dose	mg/kg	5	5	5
V_{ss}	L/kg	1.2	1.2	1.5
CL	mL/min/kg	2.46	2.26	13.48
$T_{1/2}$	H	6.5	7.0	1.6
P.O. PK				
Dose	mg/kg	20	20	20
C_{max}	nM	7160 (<71.6)	13,668 (669.7)	12,170 (1156.2)
T_{max}	H	3	7.67	0.5
AUC	nM*h	107,510 (<1075.1)	271,489 (13,303)	89,692 (8235.7)
F	%	34	79	100

Note: I.V. PK: intravenous pharmacokinetics in mouse; P.O. PK: per oral pharmacokinetics in mouse; V_{ss}: Volume of distribution at steady state; CL: total systemic clearance; $T_{1/2}$: Elimination half-life; C_{max}: maximum concentration reached in blood, values in parenthesis represent free fraction; T_{max}: time to reach maximum concentration; AUC: exposure between 0 to infinity, values in parenthesis represent free fraction; F: oral bioavailability.

3.6. TP Class of Compounds Is Efficacious against Hemolymphatic Infection in a Stage 1 HAT Mouse Model

Since all three TP compounds showed promising in vivo PK properties in mice, they were evaluated for their ability to achieve cure in a mouse model of stage 1 (hemolymphatic) disease. GNF3849 achieved complete cure at all doses (7.5, 25 and 75 mg/kg, once daily, for four days). The other two compounds, GNF6702 and NITD689, showed dose-dependent cure, with increasing doses showing better cure (Figure 3). Minimum efficacious doses for GNF6702 and NITD689 were 1 and 10 mg/kg QD dosing for four days, respectively (Table 5).

Table 5. In vivo efficacy of GNF3849, GNF6702 and NITD689 in a HAT hemolymphatic mouse model.

Compound ID	Dose (mg/kg)	Dose Frequency	Mice Cured/Total	Mean day of Relapse	% Cured
GNF3849	7.5	QD	6/6	>31	100
	25	QD	6/6	>31	100
	75	QD	6/6	>31	100
GNF6702	0.1	QD	0/6	6.83	0
	0.3	QD	2/6	19	33.3
	1	QD	6/6	>31	100
	3	QD	6/6	>31	100
	10	QD	6/6	>31	100
NITD689	1	QD	0/6	19.5	0
	1.5	BID	1/6	21	16.7
	3	QD	3/6	21	50
	10	QD	6/6	>31	100

NOTE: Mean day of relapse refers to days post infection; QD = once daily; BID = twice daily.

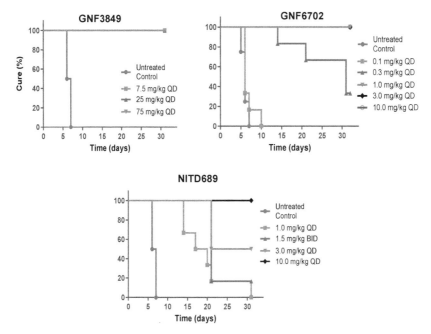

Figure 3. In vivo efficacy of GNF3849, GNF6702 and NITD689 in a HAT hemolymphatic mouse model. Six mice each were orally treated for four days, with varying doses of compounds, three days post-infection. Mice were monitored for 30 days post-infection, and cure plot (Kaplan–Meier plot) showing percentage of animals cured over time are shown.

3.7. Assessment of Brain Permeability, Tissue Binding and Partitioning of TP Compounds

In order to evaluate potential of brain permeability, all three compounds were tested in an MDR1-MDCK permeability assay. Compounds with better A to B permeability and reduced efflux ratio have good potential to reach high concentrations in the brain. Those that have a high efflux ratio are generally substrates for Pgp transporters, thereby having a higher propensity to be excluded from the brain. All three compounds had reasonable permeability and an efflux ratio of <3.5 (Table 6). To assess directly the TP compounds' ability to penetrate brain, mice were dosed with compound, and plasma and brains were collected after 5 and 60 min following intravenous dosing. GNF3849 had the highest brain-to-plasma ratio (B/P ratio), followed by GNF6702 and NITD689 (Table 6). Although GNF3849 had a better B/P ratio based on total concentration, it had high brain tissue protein binding (>99%), whereas GNF6702 and NITD689 had lower brain tissue binding (94.7% and 96.5%, respectively). This implies that the free concentration available at the site of infection could be lower for GNF3849 compared to the other two TP compounds.

Table 6. Assessment of brain permeability, tissue binding and partitioning of TP compounds.

Compound ID	BTB (%)	MDR1-MDCK		Efflux Ratio	B/P Ratio	
		A–B	B–A	B–A/A–B	5 min	60 min
GNF3849	>99	4.5	14.1	3.2	0.22	0.28
GNF6702	94.7	8.3	22.1	2.7	0.13	0.17
NITD689	96.5	32.6	29.2	0.9	0.12	0.12

Note: BTB: rat brain tissue binding; MDR1-MDCK = Multi Drug Resistant 1 overexpressing Madin–Darby canine kidney cells; A–B = Apical to Basolateral; B–A = Basolateral to Apical; B/P ratio = brain-to-plasma ratio.

3.8. TP Class Compounds Are Efficacious against Meningoencephalic Infection in HAT Mouse Model

Having demonstrated brain permeation, all three compounds were evaluated in a stage II (meningoencephalic) mouse model of HAT, with various doses (Figure 4). The recrudescence of bioluminescent parasites was monitored by using an in vivo imaging system over a period of three months (Figure 5). GNF6702, which had the best exposure and longest half-life, was dosed by oral gavage at 3, 10, 30 and 100 mg/kg, once daily. A dose-dependent increase in cure rate was noticed, with 30 and 100 mg/kg showing complete cure, and 10 mg/kg showing partial cure, with four out of six mice achieving relapse-free cure (Table 7). GNF3849 was the next best molecule, with reasonable exposure (~2.5 fold less than GNF6702) and a long half-life of 6.5 hours. Hence, they were dosed at 7.5 and 75 mg/kg, once daily. GNF3849 failed to achieve complete cure at either dose with 75 mg/kg, showing only 50% cure. GNF3849 had high plasma protein (>99%) and brain tissue binding (>99%), which could have resulted in significantly lower free concentration of compounds required to achieve 100% relapse-free cure.

NITD689 had promising physicochemical properties, better permeability and the lowest efflux ratio, although the exposure was lower than GNF6702 (Tables 2, 4 and 6). NITD689 also had a moderate half-life of 1.6 h; hence, we adopted both a once-daily and twice-daily dosing schedule. Both doses of 15 mg/kg twice daily and 30 mg/kg once daily failed to cure, suggesting that the time and concentrations reached were not sufficient to kill all parasites in the brain. However, 30 mg/kg twice daily and 60 mg/kg once daily of NITD689 achieved complete cure, without relapse.

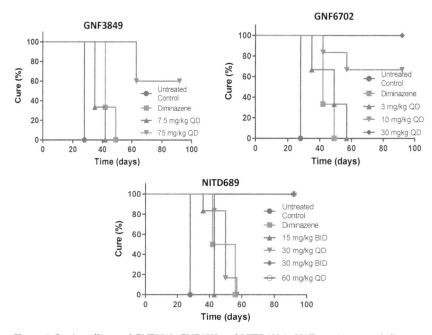

Figure 4. In vivo efficacy of GNF3849, GNF6702 and NITD689 in HAT meningoencephalic mouse model. Six mice each were orally treated for seven days, with varying doses compounds, 21or 22 days post-infection. Mice were monitored for 92–94 days post-infection, and cure plots (Kaplan–Meier plots) showing percentage of animals cured over time are shown. Three mice each were dosed with vehicle control and diminazene aceturate. Note the early parasite recrudescence in mice treated with diminazene aceturate.

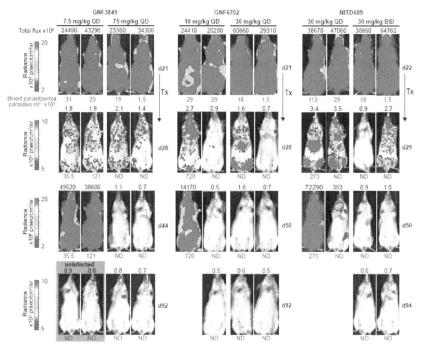

Figure 5. Bioluminescence imaging of mice infected with *T. b. brucei*. Dose-dependent clearance of parasites from triazolopyrimidine class of inhibitors. In vivo quantification of bioluminescent *T. b. brucei* (GVR35–VSL2) in infected mice before and after treatment; day 21/22, start of treatment; day 28/29, 24 h after last dose; day 44/50 and day 92/94, parasite recrudescence or cure in mice treated with GNF3849, GNF6702 and NITD689 (images of two representative mice from a total of six mice are shown). Blood parasitemia (in parasites/mL, red font below image) and whole mouse total flux (in photons per second, black font above image) values of each animal are shown; QD, once daily; BID, twice daily; N.D., not detectable; Tx, treatment. The same two representative mice are shown for all time points. Mice with detectable parasites were euthanized and are therefore not shown at day 92/94. Images from uninfected mice, aged-matched for day 21, that were collected independently, using the same acquisition settings, are shown in the gray box (two of three mice are shown).

Table 7. In vivo efficacy of GNF3849, GNF6702 and NITD689 in a HAT meningoencephalic mice model.

Compound ID	Dose (mg/kg)	Dose Frequency	Mice Cured/Total	Mean Day of Relapse	% Cured
GNF3849	7.5	QD	0/6	37	0
	75	QD	3/6	60 (>92 *)	50
GNF6702	3	QD	0/6	47	0
	10	QD	2/6	50 (>92 *)	66
	30	QD	6/6	>92	100
	100	QD	6/6	>92	100
NITD689	15	BID	0/6	42	0
	30	QD	0/6	50	0
	30	BID	6/6	>94	100
	60	QD	6/6	>94	100
Diminazene	40	QD	0/3	42	0

NOTE: Mean day of relapse refers to days post infection; * mean values shown are for the mouse which relapsed; values in parenthesis are for mice which did not relapse; QD = once daily; BID = twice daily.

4. Discussion

Several research groups have been working on the development of anti-trypanosomal compounds with a potential to treat HAT. The most significant challenge has been achieving brain penetration for chemical molecules, which is critical for killing brain stage parasites to achieve complete cure in stage 2 infection. For example, N-myristoyltransferase inhibitors have been shown to be potent trypanocides and curative of stage 1 models of the disease, but failed to achieve reasonable brain concentrations, thereby leading to failure to cure stage 2 models of HAT [18]. Attempts to screen compound libraries specifically inhibiting kinases [19] and proteases [20] also identified potent trypanocides which failed to achieve complete cure in mouse models, due to lack of adequate brain penetration. Our attempts to find novel trypanocides led to the identification of potent growth inhibitors. Further medicinal chemistry optimization of compounds led to brain-penetrant derivatives belonging to TP class (GNF6702 and NITD689) which completely cured both stages of infection.

We had previously reported that the TP class of molecules are chymotrypsin proteasome inhibitors with pan-kinetoplastid activity [8]. All the compounds described in the current manuscript also inhibited chymotrypsin activity of the 20S proteasome in *T. brucei*. The *T. b. brucei* strain overexpressing F24L mutation in β4 subunit of 20S proteasome showed greater than 60-fold shift in growth inhibition concentration for the TP compounds, confirming on-target activity. Recently, Wyllie and co-workers also described proteasome inhibitors with the potential to treat visceral leishmaniasis [21]. The proteasome inhibitors described here demonstrate great potency against clinical isolates of *T. b. gambiense* (EC_{50} = < 10 nM), compared to fexinidazole (EC_{50} = 0.95–3.3 µM) [9] and acoziborole (EC_{50} = 0.18–1 µM) [14]. Our compounds also showed concentration and time-dependent cidality and relapse-free kill of all parasites in wash-out assays in vitro, at concentrations below 100 nM. These cidality properties are essential for achieving cure in HAT mouse models [22]. Extensive medicinal chemistry optimization helped in improving PK properties required to achieve moderate brain penetration, which proved essential to cure brain infection. Both GNF6702 and NITD689 completely cured a stage 2 infection in a HAT mouse model, at 30 and 60 mg/kg dose, respectively. In addition, the exposures reached in the animal models were higher than their respective ACcure concentrations required for sterilization in vitro. Furthermore, these doses were lower than the curative dose of fexinidazole [9] (200 mg/kg) and comparable to that of acoziborole (25 mg/kg) [14]. A detailed structure activity relationship of TP class of compounds against both *T. brucei* and *T. cruzi* has been described by Nagendar and co-workers [23]. Although, one of their compounds, compound **20**, had a brain-to-plasma ratio of 0.23, it was not profiled in the stage 2 HAT model, due to higher plasma protein binding (98.5%), which might affect free concentration in brain required for achieving stage 2 efficacy.

While other developments in the treatment of HAT have been very promising, the TP class of proteasome inhibitors has significant potential for further progress. Other than acoziborole, which is in phase II studies for HAT, the proteasome inhibitors described here are the most advanced compounds with drug-like properties. They not only have promising in vitro and in vivo potency in disease relevant HAT models, but also have favorable pharmacokinetic properties, with potential for further development.

Author Contributions: Conceptualization: S.P.S.R., F.S., A.N., P.M., J.C.M., M.P.B. and T.T.D.; data curation: S.P.S.R. S.B.L., E.M. and T.T.; formal analysis, S.P.S.R., S.B.L., J.J., R.R. and E.M.; funding acquisition, S.P.S.R., P.M., J.C.M., M.P.B. and T.T.D.; methodology, S.P.S.R., S.B.L., A.N., T.T., R.R., E.M.; project administration, S.P.S.R., J.J., V.M., P.M., J.C.M., M.P.B. and T.T.D.; resources, J.J., M.K., F.S., T.T., E.M.; supervision, S.P.S.R., S.B.L., J.J., M.K., E.M., F.S., A.N., V.M., P.M., J.C.M., M.P.B. and T.T.D.; writing—original draft, S.P.S.R. and M.P.B.; Writing—review and editing, S.P.S.R., S.B.L., E.M., A.N., P.M., J.C.M., M.P.B. and T.T.D. All authors have read and agreed to the published version of the manuscript.

Funding: This research was funded by Wellcome Trust, United Kingdom, grant number WT-103024MA and WT-104976.

Acknowledgments: Authors would like to thank Manoharan V., Wong J., Koh H., Vachaspati V., Karuna R., Wan K.H., Patra D., Biggart A., Lai Y.H., Liang F., Davis L.C., Mathison C.J., Liu X., Ballard J., Yeh V., Groessl T., Shapiro

M., Smith P., Beer D. from Novartis and Cal M., Rocchetti R., Keller-Märki S., Riccio G. and Braghiroli C., from Swiss TPH for their technical assistance.

Conflicts of Interest: The authors declare no conflicts of interest. Some of the authors (S.P.S.R., S.B.L., J.J., F.S., T.T., A.N., V.M. and T.T.D.) are Novartis Employees.

References

1. WHO. *World Health Organization: Human African Trypanosomiasis*; WHO: Rome, Italy, 2019.
2. Yun, O.; Priotto, G.; Tong, J.; Flevaud, L.; Chappuis, F. Nect is next: Implementing the new drug combination therapy for *Trypanosoma brucei gambiense* sleeping sickness. *PLoS Negl. Trop. Dis.* **2010**, *4*, e720. [CrossRef] [PubMed]
3. Drugs for Neglected Diseases initiative. *Sleeping Sickness: Current Treatments*; Drugs for Neglected Diseases initiative: Geneva, Switzerland, 2019.
4. Franco, J.R.; Simarro, P.P.; Diarra, A.; Jannin, J.G. Epidemiology of human African trypanosomiasis. *Clin. Epidemiol.* **2014**, *6*, 257–275. [PubMed]
5. Trindade, S.; Rijo-Ferreira, F.; Carvalho, T.; Pinto-Neves, D.; Guegan, F.; Aresta-Branco, F.; Bento, F.; Young, S.A.; Pinto, A.; Van Den Abbeele, J.; et al. *Trypanosoma brucei* parasites occupy and functionally adapt to the adipose tissue in mice. *Cell Host Microbe* **2016**, *19*, 837–848. [CrossRef]
6. Capewell, P.; Cren-Travaille, C.; Marchesi, F.; Johnston, P.; Clucas, C.; Benson, R.A.; Gorman, T.A.; Calvo-Alvarez, E.; Crouzols, A.; Jouvion, G.; et al. The skin is a significant but overlooked anatomical reservoir for vector-borne african trypanosomes. *Elife* **2016**, *5*, e17716. [CrossRef] [PubMed]
7. Buscher, P.; Cecchi, G.; Jamonneau, V.; Priotto, G. Human African trypanosomiasis. *Lancet* **2017**, *390*, 2397–2409. [CrossRef]
8. Khare, S.; Nagle, A.S.; Biggart, A.; Lai, Y.H.; Liang, F.; Davis, L.C.; Barnes, S.W.; Mathison, C.J.; Myburgh, E.; Gao, M.Y.; et al. Proteasome inhibition for treatment of leishmaniasis, Chagas disease and sleeping sickness. *Nature* **2016**, *537*, 229–233. [CrossRef] [PubMed]
9. Kaiser, M.; Bray, M.A.; Cal, M.; Bourdin Trunz, B.; Torreele, E.; Brun, R. Antitrypanosomal activity of fexinidazole, a new oral nitroimidazole drug candidate for treatment of sleeping sickness. *Antimicrob. Agents Chemother.* **2011**, *55*, 5602–5608. [CrossRef]
10. Zhou, L.; Yang, L.; Tilton, S.; Wang, J. Development of a high throughput equilibrium solubility assay using miniaturized shake-flask method in early drug discovery. *J. Pharm. Sci.* **2007**, *96*, 3052–3071. [CrossRef]
11. Faller, B. Artificial membrane assays to assess permeability. *Curr. Drug Metab.* **2008**, *9*, 886–892. [CrossRef]
12. Waters, N.J.; Jones, R.; Williams, G.; Sohal, B. Validation of a rapid equilibrium dialysis approach for the measurement of plasma protein binding. *J. Pharm. Sci.* **2008**, *97*, 4586–4595. [CrossRef]
13. Kalvass, J.C.; Tess, D.A.; Giragossian, C.; Linhares, M.C.; Maurer, T.S. Influence of microsomal concentration on apparent intrinsic clearance: Implications for scaling in vitro data. *Drug Metab. Dispos.* **2001**, *29*, 1332–1336. [PubMed]
14. Jacobs, R.T.; Nare, B.; Wring, S.A.; Orr, M.D.; Chen, D.; Sligar, J.M.; Jenks, M.X.; Noe, R.A.; Bowling, T.S.; Mercer, L.T.; et al. Scyx-7158, an orally-active benzoxaborole for the treatment of stage 2 human African trypanosomiasis. *PLoS Negl. Trop. Dis.* **2011**, *5*, e1151. [CrossRef] [PubMed]
15. Myburgh, E.; Coles, J.A.; Ritchie, R.; Kennedy, P.G.; McLatchie, A.P.; Rodgers, J.; Taylor, M.C.; Barrett, M.P.; Brewer, J.M.; Mottram, J.C. In vivo imaging of trypanosome-brain interactions and development of a rapid screening test for drugs against cns stage trypanosomiasis. *PLoS Negl. Trop. Dis.* **2013**, *7*, e2384. [CrossRef] [PubMed]
16. Bernhard, S.C.; Nerima, B.; Maser, P.; Brun, R. Melarsoprol- and pentamidine-resistant *Trypanosoma brucei rhodesiense* populations and their cross-resistance. *Int. J. Parasitol.* **2007**, *37*, 1443–1448. [CrossRef]
17. Graf, F.E.; Ludin, P.; Arquint, C.; Schmidt, R.S.; Schaub, N.; Kunz Renggli, C.; Munday, J.C.; Krezdorn, J.; Baker, N.; Horn, D.; et al. Comparative genomics of drug resistance in *Trypanosoma brucei rhodesiense*. *Cell Mol. Life Sci.* **2016**, *73*, 3387–3400. [CrossRef]
18. Frearson, J.A.; Brand, S.; McElroy, S.P.; Cleghorn, L.A.; Smid, O.; Stojanovski, L.; Price, H.P.; Guther, M.L.; Torrie, L.S.; Robinson, D.A.; et al. N-myristoyltransferase inhibitors as new leads to treat sleeping sickness. *Nature* **2010**, *464*, 728–732. [CrossRef]

19. Diaz, R.; Luengo-Arratta, S.A.; Seixas, J.D.; Amata, E.; Devine, W.; Cordon-Obras, C.; Rojas-Barros, D.I.; Jimenez, E.; Ortega, F.; Crouch, S.; et al. Identification and characterization of hundreds of potent and selective inhibitors of *Trypanosoma brucei* growth from a kinase-targeted library screening campaign. *PLoS Negl. Trop. Dis.* **2014**, *8*, e3253. [CrossRef]
20. Cleghorn, L.A.; Albrecht, S.; Stojanovski, L.; Simeons, F.R.; Norval, S.; Kime, R.; Collie, I.T.; De Rycker, M.; Campbell, L.; Hallyburton, I.; et al. Discovery of indoline-2-carboxamide derivatives as a new class of brain-penetrant inhibitors of *Trypanosoma brucei*. *J. Med. Chem.* **2015**, *58*, 7695–7706. [CrossRef]
21. Wyllie, S.; Brand, S.; Thomas, M.; De Rycker, M.; Chung, C.W.; Pena, I.; Bingham, R.P.; Bueren-Calabuig, J.A.; Cantizani, J.; Cebrian, D.; et al. Preclinical candidate for the treatment of visceral leishmaniasis that acts through proteasome inhibition. *Proc. Natl. Acad. Sci. USA* **2019**, *116*, 9318–9323. [CrossRef]
22. De Rycker, M.; O'Neill, S.; Joshi, D.; Campbell, L.; Gray, D.W.; Fairlamb, A.H. A static-cidal assay for *Trypanosoma brucei* to aid hit prioritisation for progression into drug discovery programmes. *PLoS Negl. Trop. Dis.* **2012**, *6*, e1932. [CrossRef]
23. Nagendar, P.; Gillespie, J.R.; Herbst, Z.M.; Ranade, R.M.; Molasky, N.M.R.; Faghih, O.; Turner, R.M.; Gelb, M.H.; Buckner, F.S. Triazolopyrimidines and imidazopyridines: Structure-activity relationships and in vivo efficacy for trypanosomiasis. *ACS Med. Chem. Lett.* **2019**, *10*, 105–110. [CrossRef] [PubMed]

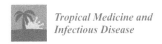
Tropical Medicine and Infectious Disease

MDPI

Article

Phenotypic Drug Discovery for Human African Trypanosomiasis: A Powerful Approach

Frederick S. Buckner [1],*, Andriy Buchynskyy [2], Pendem Nagendar [2], Donald A. Patrick [3], J. Robert Gillespie [1], Zackary Herbst [1], Richard R. Tidwell [3] and Michael H. Gelb [2]

[1] Center for Emerging and Reemerging Infectious Diseases, Department of Medicine, University of Washington, Seattle, WA 98109, USA; jrgilles@uw.edu (J.R.G.); zherbst@uw.edu (Z.H.)

[2] Department of Chemistry, University of Washington, Seattle, WA 98195, USA; andriyb@uw.edu (A.B.); pendem2@uw.edu (P.N.); gelb@chem.washington.edu (M.H.G.)

[3] Department of Pathology and Laboratory Medicine, University of North Carolina, Chapel Hill, NC 27599, USA; donald_patrick@med.unc.edu (D.A.P.); tidwell@med.unc.edu (R.R.T.)

* Correspondence: fbuckner@uw.edu; Tel.: +1-206-616-9214

Received: 31 December 2019; Accepted: 2 February 2020; Published: 5 February 2020

Abstract: The work began with the screening of a library of 700,000 small molecules for inhibitors of *Trypanosoma brucei* growth (a phenotypic screen). The resulting set of 1035 hit compounds was reviewed by a team of medicinal chemists, leading to the nomination of 17 chemically distinct scaffolds for further investigation. The first triage step was the assessment for brain permeability (looking for brain levels at least 20% of plasma levels) in order to optimize the chances of developing candidates for treating late-stage human African trypanosomiasis. Eleven scaffolds subsequently underwent hit-to-lead optimization using standard medicinal chemistry approaches. Over a period of six years in an academic setting, 1539 analogs to the 11 scaffolds were synthesized. Eight scaffolds were discontinued either due to insufficient improvement in antiparasitic activity (5), poor pharmacokinetic properties (2), or a slow (static) antiparasitic activity (1). Three scaffolds were optimized to the point of curing the acute and/or chronic *T. brucei* infection model in mice. The progress was accomplished without knowledge of the mechanism of action (MOA) for the compounds, although the MOA has been discovered in the interim for one compound series. Studies on the safety and toxicity of the compounds are planned to help select candidates for potential clinical development. This research demonstrates the power of the phenotypic drug discovery approach for neglected tropical diseases.

Keywords: *Trypanosoma brucei*; human African trypanosomiasis; drug discovery; high-throughput screening; blood–brain barrier; brain permeability; pharmacology; phenotypic drug screening

---

1. Introduction

Two *Trypanosoma brucei* subspecies, *gambiense* and *rhodesiense*, cause human African trypanosomiasis (HAT). Natural transmission occurs in 36 countries of sub-Saharan Africa via the bite of infected tse-tse flies. After the initial cutaneous inoculation, early stage (hemolymphatic) infection occurs. In the Central/West-African form (Gambian HAT), the early stage can last for months to years before progressing to late-stage infection in the central nervous system (CNS). In the East-African form (Rhodesian HAT), the early stage lasts only a few weeks to months before causing late-stage disease. Once the parasites enter the CNS, patients suffer neuropsychiatric effects that culminate in coma and death if untreated (hence the name "sleeping sickness"). Optimal treatments for HAT will address the infection in the CNS, necessitating that drugs have the ability to penetrate the blood–brain barrier (BBB).

The therapeutic landscape for HAT has recently been upgraded with the approval of fexinidazole for the treatment of both the first-stage and second-stage of HAT due to *T. b. gambiense* in adults and children aged ≥6 years [1]. Fexinidazole represents the first all oral therapy for this disease and will likely be a major advancement over nifurtimox-eflornithine combination therapy (NECT), which requires parenteral administration (usually in a hospital setting) for the eflornithine component [2]. As much as fexinidazole is a welcome advancement, there continues to be a need for drug discovery for HAT in order to strengthen the therapeutic armamentarium: (1) for patients that cannot tolerate fexinidazole; (2) to address the inevitable risk of drug resistance; (3) to eliminate the need for a staging spinal tap before initiating therapy [3]; and (4) to respond to the unmet need of safe and effective drugs for Rhodesian HAT. Toward this end, our research group is conducting a drug discovery campaign to identify compounds that are distinct from nitroheterocycle drugs such as nifurtimox and fexinidazole, and that will meet the target product profile of an oral drug with activity for late stage HAT [4].

A high throughput phenotypic screen, performed at the Genomics Institute of the Novartis Research Foundation (GNF), formed the basis of this drug discovery campaign [5]. The compound library of 700,000 compounds consisted of a collection of small-molecules with druglike properties and structural diversity. The library had been previously profiled in more than 60 high throughput screens (both biochemical and cell-based), allowing for the identification and elimination of compounds with a "frequent hitter profile". The phenotypic assay measured the inhibition of bloodstream-form *T. brucei* cultures at a single compound concentration of 3.6 μM. The screen resulted in 3889 primary hits with an inhibition of greater than 50% for a 0.6% hit rate (Z' score > 0.6). The primary hits were further tested in dose-response assays in order to measure EC_{50} values. In parallel, the cytotoxicity (CC_{50}) of the hit compounds was measured against cultures of the human hepatoma cell line (Huh7). A final set of compounds was compiled with *T. brucei* EC_{50} < 3.6 μM and CC_{50} > 10 μM, consisting of 1035 molecules that could be grouped into 115 distinct scaffolds [5]. This paper summarizes the progress to date of our drug discovery campaign to identify preclinical candidates for HAT, starting from this phenotypic screen.

2. Materials and Methods

The methods employed in this paper have been described in detail in previous publications as follows. All murine experiments were approved by the University of Washington Institutional Animal Care and Use Committee, IACUC approval code 4248-01 (animal welfare approval number A3464-01).

2.1. Phenotypic Screen for T. brucei Growth Arrest

Compound libraries were screened against the bloodstream form of the *T. brucei* isolate, Lister 427 [5]. Parasites were grown in 1536-well plates in 5.5 μL of HMI-9 medium in the presence of library compounds. All wells including negative controls contained a final of 0.4% dimethyl sulfoxide. Plates were incubated at 37 °C for 48 h and the parasite density was determined using the CellTiter-Glo reagent (Promega, Madison, Wisconsin WI, USA), a firefly luciferase assay system that measures the amount of cellular adenosine triphosphate present in plate wells.

2.2. In Vitro Parasite Growth Arrest Assay

Follow up compounds were tested for antiparasitic activity on *T. brucei brucei* (strain BF427) [5]. Parasites were tested in triplicate in the presence of serial dilutions of compound, and growth was quantified with AlamarBlue. Pentamidine isothionate (Aventis, Dagenham, U.K.) was included as a positive control in each assay (EC50 = 1.2 ± 0.3 nM).

2.3. Mammalian Cell Cytotoxicity Assay

Compounds were tested for cytotoxicity against CRL-8155 cells (human lymphoblasts) [5]. Cells were grown in culture with serial dilutions of compounds for 48 h and cytotoxicity was assayed using AlamarBlue (Life Technologies, Carlsbad, California CA, USA). Each dilution was assayed in quadruplicate with the standard error of the mean values averaging < 15%. Concentrations causing 50% growth inhibition (CC50) were calculated by nonlinear regression using GraphPad Prism software (San Diego, CA, USA).

2.4. Solubility Measurement

Solubility was measured in pH 7.4, pH 6.5, and pH 2.0 aqueous buffers in a two-tier system via LC-MSMS. In Tier 1 testing, 1 μL of DMSO stock (20 mM) was measured with a Hamilton syringe and diluted to 400 μL with the respective buffer, giving a final concentration of 50 μM test compound with 0.25% DMSO. The buffer solutions were capped and incubated while shaking at 37 °C for 24 h until equilibrium was reached. Buffer solutions were centrifuged at 14,000× *g* for 15 min and two aliquots are taken from the supernatant. The concentration of the test compound in each aliquot was determined by liquid chromatography-mass spectrometry/mass-spectrometry analysis and by calculations using a linear regression of the test compound standards made over a range of known concentrations. Solubility was reported as the final concentration in the supernatant. If the concentration in the supernatant was determined to be 50 μM (maximum solubility for Tier 1), then a Tier 2 test was carried out. In Tier 2 testing, 5 μL of the test compound's 20 mM DMSO stock was transferred to a microcentrifuge tube with a Hamilton syringe. The DMSO was then removed in a Speed-Vac concentrator and the test compound was diluted with 100 μL of the respective buffer, giving a final concentration of 1 mM test compound with negligible DMSO. The sample was heated and agitated by vortexing and by pipetting up and down to ensure the test compound was completely exposed to the buffer. The sample was then capped and incubated for 24 h while shaking at 37 °C. Buffer solutions were centrifuged at 14,000× *g* for 15 min and two aliquots were taken from the supernatant. The concentration of the test compound in the aliquots was determined by LC-MSMS, as described above.

2.5. Permeability Across Monolayers of MDCKII-MDR1 Cells

This assay utilizes Madin–Darby canine kidney cells that were transfected with the human MDR1 (P-gp) gene [5,6]. Permeability across these monolayers was measured in triplicate. The assay was performed with and without the addition of GF-120918, an inhibitor of the MDR1 efflux pump, to determine if the compound was a pump substrate. Propranolol was used as a permeable, non-MDR1 substrate control, and amprenavir was used as a permeable, MDR1 substrate control.

2.6. Pharmacokinetic Studies in Mice

Test compounds were administered to mice by oral gavage followed by blood sampling at intervals of 30, 60, 120, 240, 360, 480, and 1440 min [5,7]. Compounds were dosed orally at 50 mg/kg in 0.2 mL of dosing solution (7% Tween 80, 3% ethanol, 5% DMSO, 0.9% saline). Experiments were performed with groups of three mice per compound as published. Plasma was separated and extracted with acetonitrile for measurements of the compound concentrations by liquid chromatography/tandem mass spectrometry.

2.7. Brain Permeability Studies

Test compounds were injected (ip) at 5 mg/kg to three mice in a vehicle consisting of DMSO (5%), Tween 80 (7%), and EtOH (3%) in physiological saline (0.9%) solution [8]. At 1 h post injection, blood was collected, and plasma was separated by centrifugation. Simultaneously, the brain was removed and homogenized in acetonitrile. Concentrations of compound in the plasma and brain were determined via liquid chromatography/tandem mass spectrometry. Calculations of brain levels accounted for 3% volume/weight of blood in the brain.

2.8. Anti-Parasite Efficacy Studies in Mice (Acute Model)

Female Swiss-Webster mice age 6–8 weeks (group size = 5) were infected with 2×10^4 *T. brucei rhodesiense* STIB 900 strain on day 0, then administered the compound or vehicle for five days [5,8]. Treatments were administered orally in the same vehicle described above at a dose and schedule anticipated to maintain plasma concentrations well above the EC_{50}. The first dose was 48 h after parasite injection, and dosing was 12 or 24 h apart. Parasitemia was monitored for 60 days by microscopic analysis of blood collected from tail bleeds. Cures were defined by sustained clearance of microscopic parasitemia through the end of the 60-day observation period. Mice were euthanized when parasitemia was evident on the peripheral blood slides.

2.9. Anti-Parasite Efficacy Studies in Mice (Chronic Model)

Groups of six to eight mice were infected with 1×10^4 *T. b. brucei* (strain TREU667) to establish a chronic infection [8]. Treatment began on day 21 post-infection, and mice received 50 mg/kg test compound orally twice per day for 10 days (total of 20 doses) in a 200 µL volume of vehicle. A control group received the vehicle with no compound and another control group received a single intraperitoneal dose of diminazene aceturate at 10 mg/kg on day 21. The diminazene aceturate clears parasites from the blood, but because it does not cross the BBB, the blood is later repopulated from parasites in the CNS. After dosing, parasitemia was monitored via microscopic examination of tail blood slides until 180 days post-infection. Mice were removed from the experiment when parasites were detected in the blood.

2.10. Chemical Synthesis Procedures

For compound series 1, 2, 4, and 9, the synthesis methods are in the references. The methods for the synthesis of the initial hit compounds for compound series 3, 5, 6, 7, 8, 10, and 11 are provided in the Supplementary Materials (Figures S1–S7). Compounds were purified to > 95% purity by high performance liquid chromatography (Varian Prep star system) using a reverse phase C18 semi-preparative column (YMC S5 ODS-A 20 × 100 mm column) and a solvent program of methanol/water or acetonitrile/water with 0.1% trifluoroacetic acid.

2.11. Metabolite Identification

A 90-min incubation in 0.5 mg/mL mouse liver microsomes preceded liquid chromatography-mass spectrometry/mass-spectrometry analysis for each compound of interest. After incubation, aliquots drawn at various time points in the incubation period were prepared for LC-MSMS analysis alongside a microsome mixture blank containing no compound. A Thermo LTQ Orbitrap Tandem Hybrid Mass Spectrometer combined with an Acquity UPLC system was used for analysis and the MS/MS data were analyzed using MZMine 2.30 software. Peaks from the blank were compared with peaks from the microsome incubation mixture aliquots taken at different timepoints in order to determine whether the detected analyte was a product of the background components or a metabolic product of the compound in question.

3. Results

3.1. Selection of Hit Compounds

The set of 1035 active/selective compounds was further curated by a committee of three medicinal chemists involved in the project. The following filters were applied, resulting in 17 selected compounds of different chemical scaffolds: (1) compliance with the Lipinski's rule of 5 (MW < 500, Log P not > 5, not more than 5 H-bond donors, not more than 10 H-bond acceptors) [9]; (2) avoidance of compounds with structural alerts for toxicity (e.g., avoiding alkylating agents, etc.) [10]; (3) avoidance of molecules with > 1 chiral center (to help simplify synthesis and control costs of goods); (4) avoidance of singletons, which meant excluding compounds for which analogs of the same scaffold in the library were inactive as this suggested that further optimization would be difficult to accomplish; and (5) emphasis on chemical tractability as judged by the expertise of the medicinal chemists. The structures, chemical properties, and screening results of the 16 selected hit compounds are shown in Table 1a,b.

Table 1. a. Structures, properties, and screening results of the 17 selected hit compounds. b. Structures, properties, and screening results of the 17 selected hit compounds.

a.

Scaffold	Structure	MW (g/mol)	Clog P	T. brucei EC50 (nM)	Mammalian CC50 (nM) *	B/P Ratio (Mouse) **
1		339.7	3.21	217.6	>50,000	0.547
2		308.4	3.77	480	>50,000	0.3
3		349.4	3.56	873.7	37,968	2.86

Table 1. *Cont.*

Scaffold	Structure	MW (g/mol)	Clog P	T. brucei EC50 (nM)	Mammalian CC50 (nM) *	B/P Ratio (Mouse) **
4		363.6	3.48	790	15,860	2.00
5		443.4	3.69	657.5	>100,000	0.845
6		328.4	2.02	306.9	>100,000	0.727

Table 1. *Cont.*

Scaffold	Structure	MW (g/mol)	Clog P	T. brucei EC50 (nM)	Mammalian CC50 (nM) *	B/P Ratio (Mouse) **
7		468.9	2.87	656.6	>50,000	0.587
8		294.3	2.4	214.4	14,300	7.11
9		346.8	3.72	346	>50,000	0.743 ***

Table 1. *Cont.*

b.

Scaffold	Structure	MW (g/mol)	Clog P	*T. brucei* EC50 (nM)	Mammalian CC50 (nM) *	B/P Ratio (Mouse) **
10	Racemic	428.5	3.67	2438		0.224
11		413.376	5.11	3089		0.09
12		438.54	4.17	1700	>100,000	0.267

Table 1. *Cont.*

Scaffold	Structure	MW (g/mol)	Clog P	T. brucei EC50 (nM)	Mammalian CC50 (nM) *	B/P Ratio (Mouse) **
13		391.49	2.66	1000	>100,000	0.02
14	Racemic	510.565	5.5	707.5	>100,000	0.01
15		505.618	8.15	1500	33,000	0

Table 1. *Cont.*

Scaffold	Structure	MW (g/mol)	Clog P	T. brucei EC50 (nM)	Mammalian CC50 (nM) *	B/P Ratio (Mouse) **
16		487.57	6.37	650	>100,000	No plasma exposure
17		465.57	6.17	3500	>100,000	0

* Mammalian cell cytotoxicity done with lymphocytic cell line CRL–8155. ** B/P ratio = brain to plasma ratio at 60 min following IP dose (except Scaffold 8 at 15 min). *** Scaffold 9 parent had poor ionization in MS. B: P ratio data are for close analog (see [11]).

3.2. Screening for Brain Permeability

The long-term goal of the project was to develop a drug for treatment of HAT including late-stage disease involving the central nervous system. For this reason, we included an early screen in our compound triage process to identify hit compounds that demonstrated at least moderate brain permeability in mice. To assess this, the sixteen hit compounds were injected subcutaneously and mice were sacrificed at 60 min (n = 3 mice) for the simultaneous collection of plasma and whole brains for the quantification of compound concentrations. The ratios of brain to plasma levels are shown in Table 1. Eleven compounds (**1–10, 12**) had brain levels of at least 25% of plasma levels and were considered candidates for development. One compound (**11**) had modest brain permeability of 9%, but was included for further chemistry despite this marginal activity. Four compounds (**13–15, 17**) had minimal concentrations in the brain (< 2% of plasma levels) and were no longer pursued. One compound (**16**) had nearly undetectable plasma and brain levels at the 60-min time point and was also considered unsuitable for further development.

3.3. Hit-to-Lead Optimization

The program supported three medicinal chemists through a six-year period. Eleven hit compounds representing different scaffolds were pursued with a total of 1539 compounds synthesized. Lead optimization was generally performed on 2–3 scaffolds at a time due to the available manpower. Since the molecular targets or mechanisms of action were unknown for all the hit compounds at the start of the project, new compounds were designed using standard medicinal chemistry principles [12]. For illustration, compounds such as **2** were divided into regions where small changes were discretely introduced by synthetic methods (Figure 1). New compounds were made on a 3–5 milligram scale at >95% purity by HPLC, nuclear magnetic resonance, and mass spectrometry analysis.

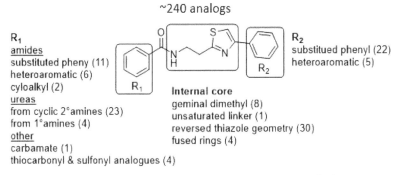

Figure 1. Medicinal chemistry strategy for optimization of Scaffold 2.

New compounds had *T. brucei* EC_{50}, mammalian host cell cytotoxicity (CC_{50}), and aqueous solubility assayed per our screening cascade (Figure 2). The cut-off values for further advancement are shown. For most compound series, an initial major focus was to improve activity against *T. brucei* cells to an $EC_{50} < 200$ nM before concentrating on pharmacokinetic (PK) activity. The screening results were continuously reviewed by the chemistry group to define structure activity relationships (SAR). Changes in different regions of the molecule that resulted in improved activities were combined in subsequent molecules. As compounds were identified with substantially improved potency against *T. brucei* (and retained selectivity compared to mammalian cells), they were tested in a single dose PK assay in mice. Mice were administered compounds by oral gavage at 50 mg/kg and whole blood samples were collected on blotting cards at serial time points. The parameters of maximum blood concentration (C_{max}) and the concentration of compound integrated over time (area under curve, AUC) were of primary interest. The general rule was to attain plasma concentrations 10 times above the *T. brucei* EC_{50}

value for at least eight hours. For some series, we performed in vitro microsome stability assays prior to the PK experiments (Figure 3), although our experience was that microsome studies were just as expensive and labor intensive as "shotgun" PK experiments and provided less information, particularly about oral bioavailability. In order to improve the PK profile of compounds, substitutions were introduced that were associated with improved metabolic stability such as introducing fluorine groups to protect possible oxidation sites or introduction of N-cycloalkyl groups (pyrrolidine, piperidine) to decrease oxidative N-demethylation [12,13]. Selected compounds were subjected to metabolite identification studies to define metabolic weak points to inform the design of the next round of compounds to improve the metabolic profile (see Methods). Compounds that matched the selection criteria for antiparasitic activity and PK properties were next subjected to brain permeability studies in mice according to the flow chart (Figure 2). A brain-to-plasma ratio of 0.3 was the minimum value as a go/no-go requirement for further advancement. The compounds passing all of the above testing criteria were upscaled (75 mg synthesis) for efficacy studies in the *T. brucei* acute infection model in mice. Compounds showing cures in the acute infection model were then tested in the more challenging chronic infection model that requires clearing parasites from the CNS. Three compound series remained active in our program, having passed the different levels of our screening cascade (discussed below).

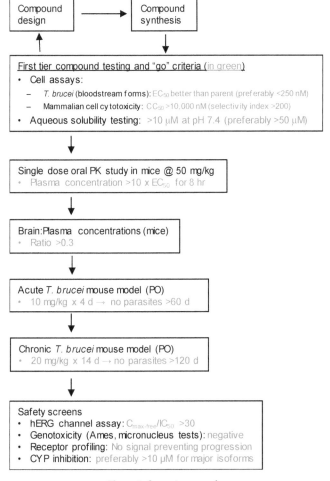

Figure 2. Screening cascade.

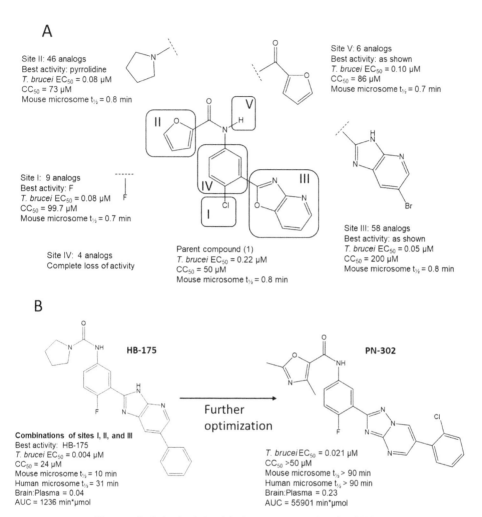

Figure 3. Optimization (**A**) and further optimization (**B**) of Scaffold 1.

When roadblocks prevented progress for specific scaffolds, they were discontinued and replaced with new scaffolds from the list of 17 candidates in Table 1. The reasons for discontinuing various compound series are summarized in Table 2. One candidate scaffold (12) has yet to be pursued.

Table 2. Summary of progress in hit-to-lead campaigns for the 12 compound series.

Compound Series	# Analogs Made	Status	Reason for Discontinuation	Reference
1	253	Active		[5,14]
2	249	Active		[8,15,16]
3	131	Stopped	Insufficient improvement in EC50	
4	141	Stopped	Slow killing activity ("static")	[17]
5	102	Stopped	Poor solubility. Poor PK.	
6	41	Stopped	Insufficient improvement in EC50	
7	138	Stopped	Poor metabolic stability; Poor PK	

Table 2. *Cont.*

Compound Series	# Analogs Made	Status	Reason for Discontinuation	Reference
8	91	Stopped	Insufficient improvement in EC50	
9	280	Active		[11]
10	66	Stopped	Insufficient improvement in EC50	
11	47	Stopped	Insufficient improvement in EC50	
12	0	Not started		
Total	**1539**			

3.4. Active Compound Series (Highlights)

Three scaffolds (1, 2, and 9) have been developed to the level of lead compounds ready for late preclinical studies [5,8,11,14–16]. The optimization of hit compound 1 is shown in Figure 3. The different regions of the molecule (I-V) are indicated in the center structure. The number of variants made and tested, and the optimal substitution at each region are indicated in the surrounding structures. At the bottom left (Figure 3), the partially optimized compound (HB-175) is shown, which combines the best substituents of regions I, II, and III [5]. The changes included efforts to improve metabolic stability by making the following modifications: (a) replacing the furan amide with mono or di-substituted fluoro pyrrolidine ureas, or with dimethyloxazole amide; (b) by substitution at C6 of the pyridine/pyrimidine ring; and (c) replacing azabenzofurans with imidazopyridines. Subsequent work was dedicated to further improve metabolic stability and brain permeability, leading to the current lead compound PN-302. The changes included altering the core ring system from an imidazopyridine to a triazolopyrimidine [14].

The strategy for optimizing Scaffold 2 is illustrated in Figure 1. Changes that improved antiparasitic activity, metabolic stability, and brain permeability included: (1) substitution of the phenyl group on the left side with 3-fluoropyrrolidine; (2) rigidifying the linker with a benzthiazole as opposed to an alkyl-linked thiazole; and (3) fluorination of the right-sided phenyl group. Of note, the stereochemistry of the fluorine substituent on the pyrrolidine was critical for activity [8]. The illustrated lead compound, 45DAP076, has excellent metabolic stability and excellent brain permeability properties (Figure 4). Importantly, it was shown to have *curative* activity in the chronic *T. brucei* infection model [8], putting it in a category of very few compounds with such high potential for development for HAT.

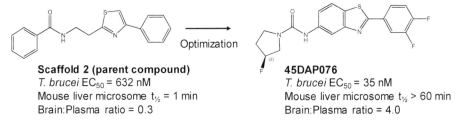

Scaffold 2 (parent compound)
T. brucei EC$_{50}$ = 632 nM
Mouse liver microsome t$_{1/2}$ = 1 min
Brain:Plasma ratio = 0.3

45DAP076
T. brucei EC$_{50}$ = 35 nM
Mouse liver microsome t$_{1/2}$ > 60 min
Brain:Plasma ratio = 4.0

Figure 4. Scaffold 2: Optimization of hit "thiazole" compound to lead compound 45DAP076.

The third compound series that remained active in the program was Scaffold 9, the thiohydantoins (Figure 5). Changes to the central thiohydantoin moiety itself abrogated antiparasitic activity, so this portion of the molecule was held constant. However, through making systematic substitutions in the two terminal rings systems, we identified highly potent inhibitors (EC$_{50}$ as low as 2 nM) and excellent brain permeability (brain:plasma = 1.68). Compound BA-738 cured mice with acute *T. brucei* infection [11], but only gave partial cures (20% of mice) in the chronic infection model (unpublished). Further optimization will be necessary before advancing this series for late-preclinical studies such as the safety screens shown in Figure 2.

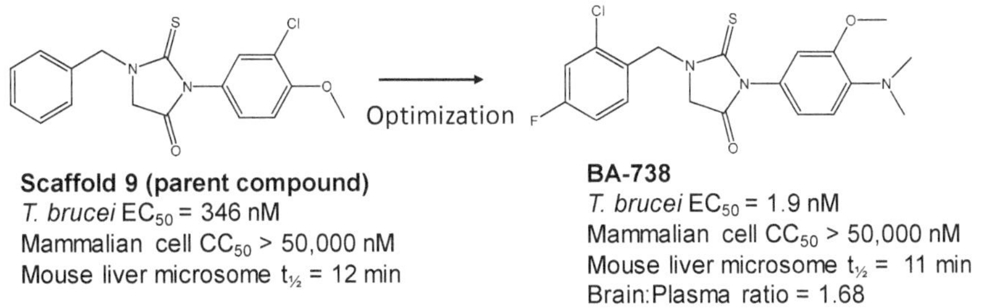

Figure 5. Scaffold 9: Optimization of hit "thiohydantoin" compound to lead compound BA-738.

4. Discussion

This paper summarizes the results of a drug discovery campaign to identify preclinical candidates for HAT starting from a phenotypic screen. Detailed results relating to four of the scaffolds have been published (see references in Table 2), but an overview of the general strategy and complete results has not been previously reported. Some helpful points can be learned by studying the failed scaffolds as well as by studying the successful ones. As indicated, 17 compounds representing distinct scaffolds (Table 1) were selected from the original hit list of 1035 compounds. By definition, these compounds had activity against *T. brucei* cells and thus demonstrated sufficient cell permeability to reach intracellular targets. This feature of the cell-based screen provided a theoretical advantage over biochemical (acellular) screens where hit compounds subsequently have to be tested for (and perhaps optimized for) cell permeability properties. Similarly, the screening protocol included a counter screen against mammalian cells that eliminated compounds with cytotoxicity. A whole-cell cytotoxicity assay identified any type of cellular toxicity and thus was broader than a counter screen against, for example, a mammalian homolog in an enzymatic screen. Thus, these features illustrate the potential advantages of phenotypic screens over target-based screening with the acknowledged disadvantage that the target of activity is unknown. As a result, the hit-to-lead optimization was done agnostically to the target. For most of the project, we chose not to divert time and resources to the effort of target identification. Hit-to-lead chemical optimization was done using standard medicinal chemistry approaches without guidance from protein crystal structures. The target of compound series **1** (the trypanosome proteasome) has subsequently been identified [18], but this did not contribute to designing or synthesizing the current lead compounds (Figure 3). The results of the program to-date are that three of 11 scaffolds (27%) have been optimized to the point of giving cures in the murine model of *T. brucei* infection. More work needs to be done before compounds are brought to clinical trials, but the output of this campaign shows strong promise for delivering clinical candidates, particularly when compared to the results of target-based screening efforts for other microbial pathogens. For example, GlaxoSmithKline reported the outcome of 70 high-throughput screening campaigns (67 target based and three whole cell) for antibiotic development with only five leads delivered, translating to a 7% success rate [19].

As mentioned, the target product profile for HAT dictates that the final drug be administered orally [4], thus we filtered the hit list for compounds that were compliant with Lipinski's rule of five [9]. There were some examples (e.g., compounds 14 and 15) for which the rules were slightly relaxed, although this proved to be disadvantageous as those compounds were terminated due to poor brain permeability. The decision to triage compounds early in the campaign based on brain permeability was done for the following reasons. First, it has been reported that 98% of small molecule drugs do not cross through the BBB [20], meaning the BBB is a major obstacle for developing drugs intended for CNS diseases. Furthermore, the predictive tools to design changes in molecules to improve brain permeability are unreliable when applied to diverse sets of compounds. Thus, we reasoned that it would be helpful to identify compounds with at least moderate brain permeability properties at the start, rather than struggling to try to build in this property later in the process. In order to improve the probability of brain penetrant compounds, we favored molecules with MW < 450 as this has been shown to be an approximate cut off for BBB permeability [21]. A caveat to the brain permeability studies was that the measurements were of total, rather than free, concentrations of the compounds. Thus, it is possible that some compounds were concentrated in the brain due to high tissue binding (e.g., from lipophilicity), and could be inaccessible to bind targets in the trypanosomes. With only one exception (compound **7** with MW of 469 g/mol), all the compounds that passed the permeability test of a brain to plasma ratio of > 0.25 had MWs < 450 g/mol (Table 1). In contrast, the remaining compounds that failed the permeability test had a MW > 450 g/mol with the exception of **12**, which had a MW of 391 g/mol. Amongst the 11 scaffolds that were further developed, only one (compound series **7**, which had the highest starting MW) failed to advance due to the inability to maintain or improve adequate brain permeability. The results indicate that the strategy to select compounds for good brain permeability early in the process was effective.

As noted above, the synthesis of new compounds was not guided by structure-based drug design. Rather, design and synthesis were guided by standard medicinal chemistry approaches [12]. Specifically, hit molecules were divided into specific regions and substitutions were systematically introduced (Figure 1) to provide analogs for biological testing as per our screening cascade (Figure 2). The results of the biological testing were returned to our chemistry group to generate SAR that informed iterative rounds of synthesis and optimization. As regions of the scaffolds were improved, the various substitutions were combined, often leading to additive or multiplicative improvements. The pharmacological properties of the compounds were evaluated early in the screening process given the importance of optimizing this parameter. The "shotgun PK" experiments provided C_{max} and AUC values for initial insights into the absorption, distribution, metabolism, and elimination (ADME) of the compounds. Some scaffolds were also analyzed in microsome stability assays to help track the rates of metabolic degradation by CYP450 enzymes [8,11]. When typical methods such as fluorination did not adequately help with metabolic stability, we performed metabolite identification studies with qualitative mass spectrometry (using incubations of compound in liver microsomes) to understand the molecular targets of degradation so that new analogs could be designed to overcome the weaknesses. In rapid succession, the compounds matching our "go" criteria were then tested for in vivo CNS permeability in mice. At an early stage in the program, we utilized an in vitro trans-well methodology using MDR1-MDCK cells [5] to model permeability across the BBB [6]. Although this method has been widely used, we had specific examples in which the results of the MDR1-MDCK assay were not consistent with the in vivo brain-permeability data (not shown). We also determined that in vivo brain-permeability studies could be efficiently performed with three mice per compound at a single harvest time of 60 min post-dose (5 mg/kg IP). The combination of fewer specimens for mass spectrometry analysis plus greater predictive accuracy made the in vivo experiments preferable to the MDR1-MDCK model in our view.

The reasons for scaffold failures are indicated in Table 2. The most common reason for discontinuation (five scaffolds) was failure to make significant improvement in anti-*T. brucei* activity (EC_{50}). There were no absolute criteria, but if EC_{50} values of < 200 nM could not be achieved, a compound series was stopped. The number of compounds made in these failed series were 41, 47, 66, 91, and 131, respectively. Obviously, it was a judgement decision as to when to no longer expend resources on a scaffold due to failure to achieve the sufficient target efficacy, but the listed scaffolds that failed typically involved the work of one chemist over a period of approximately one year. The next most common reason for failure (Scaffolds 5 and 7) involved difficulties achieving the desired PK endpoints. This primarily involved the failure to achieve robust plasma exposure of the compounds so that in vivo antiparasitic activity was unlikely to be achievable. The underlying problem with Scaffold 5 was presumably related to poor aqueous solubility (< 1 µM at pH 7.4 and pH 2.0). For Scaffold 7, it was poor metabolic stability that precluded its further development. Finally, Scaffold 4 was discontinued because of a "static" killing mechanism [17]. This became apparent during in vivo efficacy experiments when administration of the compound resulted in temporary suppression of parasites followed by rebound. The "static mechanism could be recapitulated in vitro in "washout" experiments [17], which was latter incorporated into our screening routine to avoid repeating the problem.

As mentioned, the biochemical targets of the compounds were unknown at the start of the program. Work through collaborators at Genomics Institute of the Novartis Research Foundation (with contributions from the University of Washington group) led to the discovery of the target of Scaffold 1 as the trypanosome proteasome [18]. Research against the closely related *Leishmania* parasites further confirmed that proteasome inhibition was the mechanism of action for this compound series [22]. At this more advanced stage in the program, more resources will now be committed for target identification of the remaining two scaffolds. This work could help with further optimization toward inhibiting the parasite target, for example, by allowing us to develop an enzyme assay or to obtain a crystal structure, but more importantly, the information may be useful for guiding future safety studies on the compound. If the parasite target is identified and it has human orthologs, then directed efforts can be made to optimize compounds that avoid or minimize activity on the human orthologs. The information could also guide future animal studies (and clinical trials) to help predict potential toxicities in mammalian hosts.

5. Conclusions

Three compound series stemming from a high-throughput phenotypic screen remained viable in this program for HAT drug development. The lead compounds demonstrated curative activity in murine models of *T. brucei* infection. The compounds are now undergoing safety studies as indicated in the bottom of the screening cascade (Figure 2). Dose/response studies in mice are also underway to establish the optimal doses and dosing schedules that will define the pharmacodynamic parameters of the leads. Subsequent investigations will include rat toxicity studies to determine the toxicities resulting from high doses of compounds. For all three series, back up compounds are available in case we encounter significant problems with toxicity or other setbacks. The described drug discovery campaign, conducted in academic centers, remains on track for producing at least one or more late preclinical candidates for HAT.

Supplementary Materials: The following are available online at http://www.mdpi.com/2414-6366/5/1/23/s1, Synthetic Schemes and Procedures for the Synthesis of Compound Series 3, 5, 6, 7, 8, 10, and 11. Figure S1: Synthetic scheme for compound series 3. Figure S2: Synthetic scheme for compound series 5. Figure S3: Synthetic scheme for compound series 6. Figure S4: Synthetic scheme for compound series 7. Figure S5: Synthetic scheme for compound series 8. Figure S6: Synthetic scheme for compound series 10. Figure S7: Synthetic scheme for compound series 11.

Author Contributions: Conceptualization, M.H.G., F.S.B., and R.R.T.; Methodology, M.H.G., F.S.B., R.R.T., A.B., D.A.P., P.N., Z.H., and J.R.G.; Writing—original draft preparation, F.S.B.; Writing—review and editing, F.S.B., M.H.G., R.R.T., A.B., D.A.P., P.N., Z.H., and J.R.G.; Project administration, M.H.G., F.S.B., and R.R.T.; Funding acquisition, M.H.G., F.S.B., and R.R.T. All authors have read and agreed to the published version of the manuscript.

Funding: The research was supported by the National Institutes of Health (grant R01AI106850 and R01AI147504).

Acknowledgments: For the chemical synthesis, we are thankful for the contributions by Hari Babu Tatipaka, Naveen K. Chennamaneni, Praveen K. Suryadevara, Elizabeth Raux, Moloy Banerjee, Amit Thakkar, Neil R. Norcross, Patrick Weiser, Kishore Kumar, GV Reddy, Stanislav Bakunov, Svetlana Bakunova, and Daniel G. Silva. For the analytical chemistry, we thank Joshua McQueen. For contributions to in vitro and in vivo biological experiments we thank Matthew Hulverson, Ranae Ranade, Uyen Nguyen, Sharon Creason, Nicole Duster, Jennifer Arif, Nora Molasky, and Aisha Mushtaq. Finally, we acknowledge contributions from David Boykin.

Conflicts of Interest: The authors declare no conflicts of interest.

References

1. Deeks, E.D. Fexinidazole: First global approval. *Drugs* **2019**, *79*, 215–220. [CrossRef]
2. Lutje, V.; Seixas, J.; Kennedy, A. Chemotherapy for second-stage Human African trypanosomiasis. *Cochrane Database Syst. Rev.* **2013**, *6*, CD006201. [CrossRef]
3. WHO Interim Guidelines for the Treatment of Gambiense Human African Trypanosomiasis. Available online: https://apps.who.int/iris/handle/10665/326178 (accessed on 4 February 2020).
4. DNDi. HAT Target Product Profile. Available online: https://www.dndi.org/diseases-projects/hat/hat-target-product-profile/ (accessed on 4 February 2020).

5. Tatipaka, H.B.; Gillespie, J.R.; Chatterjee, A.K.; Norcross, N.R.; Hulverson, M.A.; Ranade, R.M.; Nagendar, P.; Creason, S.A.; McQueen, J.; Duster, N.A.; et al. Substituted 2-phenylimidazopyridines: A new class of drug leads for human African trypanosomiasis. *J. Med. Chem.* **2014**, *57*, 828–835. [CrossRef] [PubMed]

6. Evers, R.; Cnubben, N.H.; Wijnholds, J.; Van Deemter, L.; Van Bladeren, P.J.; Borst, P. Transport of glutathione prostaglandin A conjugates by the multidrug resistance protein 1. *FEBS Lett.* **1997**, *419*, 112–116. [CrossRef]

7. Suryadevara, P.K.; Olepu, S.; Lockman, J.W.; Ohkanda, J.; Karimi, M.; Verlinde, C.L.; Kraus, J.M.; Schoepe, J.; Van Voorhis, W.C.; Hamilton, A.D.; et al. Structurally simple inhibitors of lanosterol 14alpha-demethylase are efficacious in a rodent model of acute Chagas disease. *J. Med. Chem.* **2009**, *52*, 3703–3715. [CrossRef] [PubMed]

8. Patrick, D.A.; Gillespie, J.R.; McQueen, J.; Hulverson, M.A.; Ranade, R.M.; Creason, S.A.; Herbst, Z.M.; Gelb, M.H.; Buckner, F.S.; Tidwell, R.R. Urea derivatives of 2-aryl-benzothiazol-5-amines: A new class of potential drugs for human African trypanosomiasis. *J. Med. Chem.* **2017**, *60*, 957–971. [CrossRef] [PubMed]

9. Lipinski, C.A.; Lombardo, F.; Dominy, B.W.; Feeney, P.J. Experimental and computational approaches to estimate solubility and permeability in drug discovery and development settings. *Adv. Drug Deliv. Rev.* **2001**, *46*, 3–26. [CrossRef]

10. Macherey, A.C.; Dansette, P. Chemical mechanisms of toxicity: Basic knowledge for designing safer drugs. In *The Practice of Medicinal Chemistry*, 2nd ed.; Wermuth, C.G., Ed.; Elsevier Academic Press: Amsterdam, The Netherlands, 2003; pp. 545–560.

11. Buchynskyy, A.G.; Gillespie, J.R.; Herbst, Z.; Ranade, R.; Buckner, F.S.; Gelb, M.H. 1-Benzyl-3-aryl-2-thiohydantoin derivatives as anti-*Trypanosoma brucei* agents: SAR and in-vivo efficacy. *ACS Med. Chem. Lett.* **2017**, *8*, 886–891. [CrossRef] [PubMed]

12. Wermuth, C.G. *The Practice of Medicinal Chemistry*, 2nd ed.; Academic Press: San Diego, CA, USA, 2003.

13. Muller, K.; Faeh, C.; Diederich, F. Fluorine in pharmaceuticals: Looking beyond intuition. *Science* **2007**, *317*, 1881–1886. [CrossRef] [PubMed]

14. Nagendar, P.; Gillespie, J.R.; Herbst, Z.M.; Ranade, R.M.; Molasky, N.M.R.; Faghih, O.; Turner, R.M.; Gelb, M.H.; Buckner, F.S. Triazolopyrimidines and imidazopyridines as antitrypanosomal agents: Structure-activity relationships and in vivo efficacy. *ACS Med. Chem. Lett.* **2018**, *10*, 105–110. [CrossRef] [PubMed]

15. Patrick, D.A.; Wenzler, T.; Yang, S.; Weiser, P.T.; Wang, M.Z.; Brun, R.; Tidwell, R.R. Synthesis of novel amide and urea derivatives of thiazol-2-ethylamines and their activity against *Trypanosoma brucei rhodesiense*. *Bioorg. Med. Chem.* **2016**, *24*, 2451–2465. [CrossRef] [PubMed]

16. Silva, D.G.; Gillespie, J.R.; Ranade, R.M.; Herbst, Z.M.; Nguyen, U.T.T.; Buckner, F.S.; Montanari, C.A.; Gelb, M.H. New class of antitrypanosomal agents based on imidazopyridines. *ACS Med. Chem. Lett.* **2017**, *8*, 766–770. [CrossRef] [PubMed]

17. Buchynskyy, A.; Gillespie, J.R.; Hulverson, M.A.; McQueen, J.; Creason, S.A.; Ranade, R.M.; Duster, N.A.; Gelb, M.H.; Buckner, F.S. Discovery of *N*-(2-aminoethyl)-*N*-benzyloxyphenyl benzamides: New potent *Trypanosoma brucei* inhibitors. *Bioorg. Med. Chem.* **2017**, *25*, 1571–1584. [CrossRef] [PubMed]

18. Khare, S.; Nagle, A.S.; Biggart, A.; Lai, Y.H.; Liang, F.; Davis, L.C.; Barnes, S.W.; Mathison, C.J.; Myburgh, E.; Gao, M.Y.; et al. Proteasome inhibition for treatment of leishmaniasis, Chagas disease and sleeping sickness. *Nature* **2016**, *537*, 229–233. [CrossRef] [PubMed]

19. Payne, D.J.; Gwynn, M.N.; Holmes, D.J.; Pompliano, D.L. Drugs for bad bugs: Confronting the challenges of antibacterial discovery. *Nat. Rev. Drug Discov.* **2007**, *6*, 29–40. [CrossRef] [PubMed]

20. Pardridge, W.M. The blood-brain barrier: Bottleneck in brain drug development. *NeuroRx* **2005**, *2*, 3–14. [CrossRef] [PubMed]

21. Van de Waterbeemd, H.; Camenisch, G.; Folkers, G.; Chretien, J.R.; Raevsky, O.A. Estimation of blood-brain barrier crossing of drugs using molecular size and shape, and H-bonding descriptors. *J. Drug Target.* **1998**, *6*, 151–165. [CrossRef] [PubMed]

22. Wyllie, S.; Brand, S.; Thomas, M.; De Rycker, M.; Chung, C.-W.; Pena, I.; Bingham, R.P.; Bueren-Calabuig, J.A.; Cantizani, J.; Cebrian, D.; et al. Preclinical candidate for the treatment of visceral leishmaniasis that acts through proteasome inhibition. *Proc. Natl. Acad. Sci. USA* **2019**, *116*, 9318–9323. [CrossRef] [PubMed]

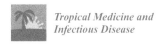

Tropical Medicine and
Infectious Disease

Review

The Trypanosomal Transferrin Receptor of Trypanosoma Brucei—A Review

Christopher K. Kariuki [1,2,*], **Benoit Stijlemans** [1,3] **and Stefan Magez** [1,4,*]

1   Laboratory of Cellular and Molecular Interactions (CMIM), Vrije Universiteit Brussels, Brussels, 1050 Ixelles, Belgium; Benoit.Stijlemans@vub.be
2   Department of Tropical and Infectious Diseases, Institute of Primate Research (IPR), 00502 Nairobi, Kenya
3   Myeloid Cell Immunology Lab, VIB Center for Inflammation Research, Brussels, 9052 Gent, Belgium
4   Laboratory for Biomedical Research, Ghent University Global Campus, Yeonsu-Gu, Incheon 219220, Korea
*   Correspondence: Christopher.kariuki@vub.be (C.K.K.); Stefan.magez@ghent.ac.kr (S.M.);
     Tel.: +322-629-1975 (C.K.K.); +82-32626-4207 (S.M.)

Received: 9 September 2019; Accepted: 25 September 2019; Published: 1 October 2019

Abstract: Iron is an essential element for life. Its uptake and utility requires a careful balancing with its toxic capacity, with mammals evolving a safe and bio-viable means of its transport and storage. This transport and storage is also utilized as part of the iron-sequestration arsenal employed by the mammalian hosts' 'nutritional immunity' against parasites. Interestingly, a key element of iron transport, i.e., serum transferrin (Tf), is an essential growth factor for parasitic haemo-protozoans of the genus *Trypanosoma*. These are major mammalian parasites causing the diseases human African trypanosomosis (HAT) and animal trypanosomosis (AT). Using components of their well-characterized immune evasion system, bloodstream *Trypanosoma brucei* parasites adapt and scavenge for the mammalian host serum transferrin within their broad host range. The expression site associated genes (ESAG6 and 7) are utilized to construct a heterodimeric serum Tf binding complex which, within its niche in the flagellar pocket, and coupled to the trypanosomes' fast endocytic rate, allows receptor-mediated acquisition of essential iron from their environment. This review summarizes current knowledge of the trypanosomal transferrin receptor (TfR), with emphasis on the structure and function of the receptor, both in physiological conditions as well as in conditions where the iron supply to parasites is being limited. Potential applications using current knowledge of the parasite receptor are also briefly discussed, primarily focused on potential therapeutic interventions.

Keywords: trypanosomosis; iron; transferrin; transferrin receptor; nutritional immunity; flagellar pocket

---

1. Trypanosomes and Their Need for Iron during a Mammalian Infection

Iron is an essential requirement for life [1–3]. Iron's biological utility lies in its cycling between two oxidation states, namely ferrous (Fe^{2+}) and ferric (Fe^{3+}) [4]. Thus, iron can serve as redox catalyst, which accepts and donates electrons [4]. As a result of this redox capability, once absorbed from the environment via the mammalian duodenum, iron is not circulated freely in mammalian tissues, as it readily catalyzes conversion of H_2O_2 into toxic free radicals via the Fenton reaction [1,5].

Under conditions of neutral pH and high oxygen tension of most physiological fluids, such as mammalian serum, iron exists predominantly in its ferric (Fe^{3+}) form [3]. Given its high hydrolytic propensity, under these conditions, ferric iron (Fe^{3+}) in excess of 2.5×10^{-18} M readily polymerizes, resulting in an insoluble and bio-inert form [6]. Therefore, to keep ferric iron (Fe^{3+}) soluble, bio-available, and render it non-toxic, vertebrates such as mammals store and transport iron via specific iron sequestering molecules [3,6,7]. Storage of iron is achieved using two formats; in an soluble form as a mobilizable reserve by ferritin and an insolubly form as hemosiderin [3,8]. Transport of ferric iron

(Fe^{3+}) in the mammalian serum is usually as a tight, but reversible association, with an abundant serum carrier protein family, the transferrins [3,7,9,10].

Serum transferrin/serotransferrin (Tf) is the transporter of ferric iron (Fe^{3+}) in the blood serum of vertebrates, acting as the connection between the ferritin storing hepatocytes to the diverse cellular population of the vertebrate body [9,10]. Serum transferrin, i.e., a 80 kDa glycoprotein, has been structurally resolved, indicating a bi-lobed tertiary structure (N- and C-lobes) with a short connecting loop between them as well as possessing two domains per lobe, with the ferric iron (Fe^{3+}) binding sites located within the inter-domain clefts of each lobe [11]. In the presence of an anion, e.g., bicarbonate or carbonate, and at a physiological serum pH range, serum transferrin can bind either mono- or di-ferric iron atoms, transforming from apo- (iron-free) to holo- (iron-laden) transferrin [3,11]. Though both lobes bind ferric iron (Fe^{3+}), there is a difference in binding capability as the C-terminal lobe binds Fe^{3+} more tightly and releases it more slowly [12]. Mammalian serum Tf is expressed in the liver, central nervous system (CNS), reproductive organs, spleen, and kidneys [13].

The rich resource of bio-available iron is a prized target for parasites, particularly those that reside in the bloodstream, such as the trypanosome species, *T. brucei*, thus leading to the diseases, human African trypanosomosis (HAT) and animal trypanosomosis (AT).

Animal trypanosomosis (also known as animal trypanosomiasis) is a parasitic disease of veterinary importance in the tropical world [14]. From its cradle in Africa, through the steppes of Asia to the far ends of the Americas, the disease has devastatingly negative economic and societal impacts [15,16].

In domestic livestock, AT is a wasting disease assigned by various names such as '*Nagana*', '*Derrengadera*', '*Dourine*', '*Mals de coits*', or '*Surra*', depending on the causative *Trypanosoma* species [17]. Five of the most important species, namely, *T. vivax*, *T. evansi*, *T. congolense*, *T. equiperdum*, and *T. brucei* cause AT in all domestic animals [16]. These trypanosome species are considered heteroxenous (Figure 1) [18]. Of note, the *T. brucei* (sub-genus *Trypanozoon*) clade can be further divided into strictly animal infecting parasites (*T. brucei brucei*) and parasites able to infect also humans and higher primates, namely the zoonotic *T. brucei rhodesiense* and the anthroponotic *T. brucei gambiense* [19,20]. This is attributed to the fact that these latter parasites acquired the ability to resist trypanolytic molecular complexes, expressed by humans and higher primates as part of the innate immune system [20–24]. Due to this reason, and its implications for human medicine, the *T. brucei* clade has received greater attention and is better characterized, despite being it having a lower, though still potent, worldwide impact on veterinary economy, than for example *T. congolense* (Sub-genus *Nannomonas*) or *T vivax* (Sub-genus *Dutonella*) [25].

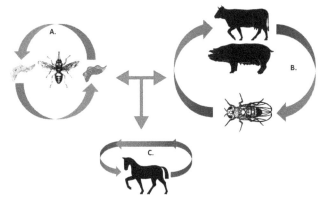

Figure 1. The trypanosomes' lifecycle. (**A**) Cyclical transmission of *T. brucei* and *T. congolense* (causing 'Nagana') occurs in the Tsetse fly (*Glossina* species), in grey is a representation of the procyclic form and in red is the representation of the bloodstream form (BSF); (**B**) mechanical transmission via tabanids

Trop. Med. Infect. Dis. **2019**, *4*, 126

leading to trypanosomosis caused by *T. vivax* and *T. evansi*; (**C**) sexual transmission occurs in equines for *T. equiperdum* during the course of dourine [26–28].

By parasitizing the haemo-lymphatic environment, trypanosomes must reconcile two seemingly conflicting requirements, namely, to avoid the immune responses of the mammalian host by rapid variation of their plasma membrane as well as efficiently acquire potentially scarce nutritive resources from their environment via the same plasma membrane [29].

2. Expression Sites; the Trypanosomal Swiss Army Knife for Host Adaptation

Trypanosomes exemplify the general survival strategy of phenotypic variation, a mechanism by which diverse parasitic organisms, from viruses to eukaryotes, contain a subset of contingency genes hypermutating as a rapid adaptation to hostile or changing environments [30]. This is the classically described paradigm of antigenic variation of the major trypanosome surface glycoproteins, the variable surface glycoprotein (VSG) [31,32]. Antigenic variation in trypanosomes occurs when a subset of a trypanosome population randomly switches the expression of a particular set of VSG genes, thus displaying a different surface coat of VSGs [29,30,33]. Contrary to avoiding the mammalian hosts' immune system, VSGs are highly immunogenic, with surface epitopes that are highly recognizable by the mammalian hosts' immune system [29]. When the immune system clears the parasite population bearing the recognized VSG by the humoral response, there is the emergence of sub-population of the haemo-protozoans with a different surface coat of VSG homodimers, against which the immune system has to prepare another humoral response [30]. The ebb and rise of different populations of trypanosomes is reflected on the parasitemia pattern observed microscopically and confers to the parasite an advantage of establishing a controlled but chronic host infection [29].

The active *T. brucei* spp. bloodstream form (BSF) VSG gene is obtained from an arsenal of more than 1500 VSG genes, most of which are pseudogenes in sub-telomeric silent arrays [34–36]. For expression, the VSG gene has to be relocated to a devoted genomic environment, aptly termed the expression site (ES), at the telomeric regions of one of the large chromosomes [37–40]. In the ES, specifically the bloodstream form expression site (BES), transcription occurs in a polycistronic manner, with VSG genes always the last gene of the unit, separated from the other genes, by 70 bp repeats (Figure 2A) [39,41,42]. The polycistronic nature of transcription allows a tightly regulated expression of the VSG gene from only 1 of the 20 telomeric expression sites (ESs), in conjunction with associated proteins within the ES, namely the expression site associated genes (ESAGs) [35,43]. The polycistronic mRNA is transcribed from a highly conserved BES promoter, that has also been shown to be sensitive to temperature changes, and which is considered a specificity signal that triggers the activation of the BES upon encountering the bloodstream of a mammalian host [42].

With only one type of VSG being expressed at a time, a portion of the trypanosome population is guaranteed invisibility from the host's immune system at any given time [35,43–47]. Variation within the VSG is achieved by homologous DNA recombination such as gene conversion, targeted to the active VSG ESs (Figure 2B,C) or by either transcriptional switching (in-situ activation and in-activation (Figure 2D) between the VSG ESs) [40].

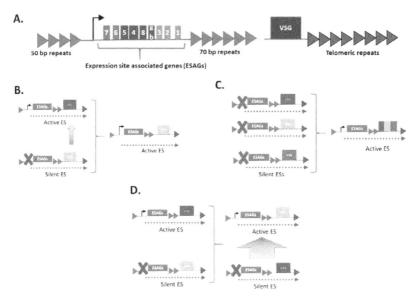

Figure 2. Modes of variable surface glycoprotein (VSG) gene switching. (**A**) The expression site (ES) of VSG including the proximal promoter, expression site-associated genes (ESAGs), the VSG, and their associated repeats. Transcription occurs in a polycistronic manner, with the ESAGs 7 and 6 being most proximally located and the VSG most distally located on the expression sites. (**B**) Mechanism of gene conversion: A VSG gene conversion event occurs when a VSG gene from a silent ES is copied (via homologous recombination) into an active ES where it is expressed. (**C**) Mechanism of segmental gene conversion: Various VSG gene recombination events occurring in the silent ES, leading to formation of a novel and mosaic VSG gene, which is copied via homologous recombination into the active ES. (**D**) Mechanism of transcriptional switching (in-situ (in)-activation): A non-recombination event occurs that activates a new (previously silent) ES while inactivating a previously active ES [48].

This immune evasion tactic also serves a rather utilitarian purpose for the parasite. As stated previously, in addition to successfully evading the host's immune system, the extracellular parasite must somehow combine the antigenic variation of its homogenous and over-arching surface coat, with the uptake of different substrates that it requires for its survival [49]. The parasite approaches this possible problem using a specific set of genes, namely the expression site associated genes (ESAGs). Within the *T. brucei* ES's, the BSF trypanosome also has a more limited repertoire of ESAGs (Figure 3) [43]. Most of the ESAGs encode predicted proteins that contain N-terminal signal sequences as well as putative hydrophobic membrane spanning segments, indicative of surface exposed proteins, such as the integral membrane proteins such as the receptor-like transmembrane adenylyl cyclase (ESAG4), a surface transporter (ESAG10), and the glycosyl phosphatidyl inositol (GPI)-anchored heterodimeric trypanosomal transferrin receptor (ESAG6/7) and serum-associated resistance antigen (SRA) [50–52]. Several ESAGs have been found to belong to multigene families including pseudogenes and members that are not transcribed within the ESs, aptly named "genes related to ESAGs" (GRESAGs) [51]. In total, within the *T. brucei* clade, sequencing has revealed about 12 polymorphic genes comprising the ESAGs, and approximately 20 different variants of each ESAG [43,45,46,51,53]. In comparison, there are relatively fewer homologs or orthologs in the closely related *T. congolense* or *T. vivax* [54]. An analysis of the cell-surface phylome for the trypanosomes revealed that for some ESAGs, e.g., ESAG1, there are neither homologs nor orthologs, indicating recent innovation by the *T. brucei* clade [54]. Other ESAGs, for example the ESAG6 and 7, encoding the trypanosomal transferrin receptor and that are considered essential for bloodstream iron scavenging in the *T. brucei* spp., are missing from *T. vivax* but are present in *T. congolense*, which is indicative of a more recently shared ancestry between *T. congolense* and *T. brucei* [54].

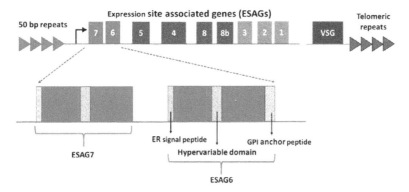

Figure 3. The ESAG 6 and 7 genes (forming the pESAG 6 and 7 heterodimeric transferrin receptor) are transcribed as part of the polycistronic VSG mRNA. The polycistronic VSG mRNA is transcribed from the active subtelomeric expression site (ES) (only 1 of the 20 available ES is active at a time). The gene products appear to have a similar structure except for the glycosyl phosphatidyl inositol (GPI) peptide on ESAG 6 [35,45–47].

Some genes in the expression site, i.e., ESAG 6, 7, and SRA, share an evolutionary origin with the VSGs, and may thus confer an increased capacity for the parasite to adapt to various mammalian hosts [51,52,55]. Given that some of the ESAGs are involved in substrate capture, it therefore seems plausible that the transcriptional switching between multiple expression sites would offer the parasite antigenic variation for these minor surface proteins [40,50].

More importantly, the transcriptional switching of BESs would also allow the selection and expression of the appropriate ESAG 6 and 7 genes for efficient capture of the requisite host transferrin molecule, which would enable the trypanosome to adapt not only to the different mammalian host range that is available to the *T. brucei* spp., but as well to the mammalian hosts' "nutritional immunity" [56,57].

3. The Trypanosomal Transferrin Receptor: A Structural Review

As indicated previously, ESAG 6 and 7 genes (encoding the trypanosomal heterodimeric transferrin receptor) are transcribed in a polycistronic mRNA together with the current VSG from an upstream promoter (Figure 3) [58,59].

However, given that both ESAG 6 and 7 genes are situated nearest to the ES promoter site with the end of ESAG 6 being approximately +5.3 kB from this promoter, there is a low but detectable transcription occurring from 'inactive' ESs in bloodstream form (BSF) trypanosomes [60,61]. It has been estimated that up to 20% of ESAG 6 mRNA originates from 'inactive' ESs [60]. This promoter-proximal position of the two genes provides the parasite with a flexibility in the regulation of the genes, providing a competitive edge, especially during periods of limited transferrin uptake, e.g., during the switch to another host.

Different but homologous pESAG6-7 heterodimers encoded by the different ESs are present in the BSF trypanosomes (Figure 4), differing in sequence identity by only 1–10% [60]. The proteins pESAG6 and 7 have been shown to be synthesized individually, containing N-terminal signal sequences that are not present in the matured protein forms [62].

In *T. brucei*, the two genes (ESAG 6 and 7) give rise to heterogeneously glycosylated proteins between 50–60 kDa and 40–42 kDa, respectively [63,64]. Only heterodimeric complexes (with a 1:1 stoichiometry) of the products from the two genes form a functional *T. brucei* trypanosomal TfR, indicating that there is a combination of elements, specific to each subunit, that are required for the transferrin binding site [65,66]. Though the protein subunits are glycosylated, the pESAG 6/pESAG 7 heterodimer can function just as well without this post-translational modification [64]. Small amino acid switches in the surface exposed loops of the pESAG 6-pESAG 7 complex, forming the transferrin binding site, brings about differences in affinity of the various TfRs for their respective Tf ligands in different hosts (ranging from 2 nM to 1 μM), all lying within the reported physiological range of Tf (30–40 μM) in the mammalian serum [67]. This allows rapid adaptation of the parasites' Tf scavenging capacity in different hosts, particularly in the presence of host antibodies [68–70]. This high affinity for Tf combined with the rapid recycling of the TbTfR enables the bloodstream parasites to actively compete, despite efforts by the mammalian host immune system, for the limited substrate until a novel higher affinity TfR is expressed [61].

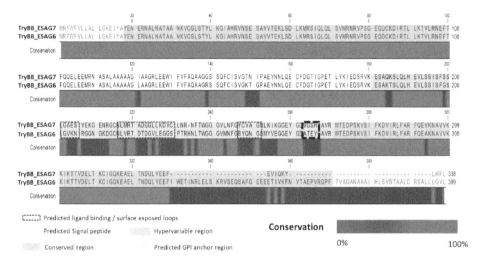

Figure 4. The products of ESAG 6 gene (pESAG6) and ESAG 7 (pESAG7) in *T. b. brucei* Strain 427 (UniProt ID Q8WPU1_9TRYP and Q8WPU2_9TRYP respectively) are similar along their N-terminus, differing only at their C-terminal end (GPI anchor peptide).

The ESAG 6 and 7 products (pESAG6 and pESAG7, respectively) are nearly identical in sequence, especially in their N-termini, which also contain the ligand binding sites, differing only in their C-termini [65]. The two proteins also share significant homology (20% identity and 60% similarity) with an A domain type VSG N-terminus, indicating a possible structural design requirement for accommodation within the dense VSG protein coat as well as an evolutionary relationship between the two ESAGs and the VSG N-terminal domain [51,65,66,71]. The pESAG6 and 7 appear to have a number of the structurally conserved features of the N-terminus of the VSG class A, whereby, especially, the ESAG 7 gene appears to be a VSG gene conversion domain [66]. Salmon et al. [63] showed that the ESAG 7/6 can be aligned to VSG (sharing significant similarity) and hypothesized that the binding sites are most likely to occur on the surface exposed loops of the heterodimeric protein (Figure 4), i.e., in the dashed boxes (where they align with the surface exposed regions of VSG gene products). Sequence secondary structure predictions e.g., JPRED indicates that these regions are most likely in loops. Prediction of ligand binding regions using the Kolaskar and Tongaonkar method [64] indicates their surface accessibility (again confirming the VSG linkage). In fact, a VSG-based chimeric TfR has been constructed and shown to effectively bind Tf [66]. This was achieved by grafting the C-termini of either ESAG 6 or 7 with the N-terminus of a MiTat 1.5 VSG [66]. The heterogeneously expressed chimeric VSG-ESAG 6 and VSG-ESAG 7 gave a heterodimeric receptor that bound Tf equally well as the native pESAG6/7 heterodimer (1.2 ± 0.27 μM vs. 0.97 ± 0.36 μM, respectively) in *Xenopus* oocytes [65,66].

The pESAG6 has a hydrophobic C-terminus that is eventually replaced by a GPI-anchor, making it the plasma-membrane bound member for the heterodimeric TfR [63,65,66,72]. An alignment of publicly available ESAG 6 gene sequences reveals the gene's homology within the *T. brucei* subspecies (Figure 5A), particularly indicative of the reported close phylogenetic relation between *T. brucei* and *T. evansi* [25,73]. In contrast, the pESAG7 has no such modification, therefore it is hypothesized to bind non-covalently with the ESAG6 [63]. Between the two proteins, there are differences in residues within the stretches forming the ligand binding site, i.e., positions 205–215 and 223–238 of pESAG6 and 7, respectively [65,66]. These amino acid stretches, especially on pESAG6, have been mapped to surface exposed loops by modeling on the resolved N-terminal VSG crystal structure (Figure 5B) [66]. Switching, by site-directed mutagenesis, of key amino acid within these stretches of pESAG6 and 7, resulted in a predicted enhancement of the Tf binding capacity [66]. Further proof was obtained from the site-directed mutagenesis of residues immediately outside each of the four domains, which resulted in loss of the Tf binding capacity, predictably due to loss of the surface exposed loop structure [66]. Despite the endeavors to model the TfR by various groups [66,74], there has been no actual structure (via X-ray crystallography or NMR) resolved yet, not for the pESAG6 neither the pESAG 7 nor the pESAG6/7 heterodimer.

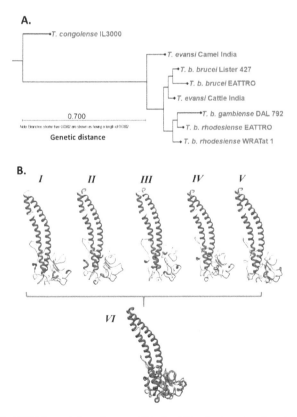

Figure 5. (A) The ESAG 6 gene is homologous within the *T. brucei* subspecies. A protein BLAST query for ESAG6 (which is the GPI-anchored partner of the ESAG7/6 heterodimer) revealed approximately 100 sequences from *T. brucei*, *T. evansi*, and *T. congolense*. The results were then assembled to make an alignment and a phylogenetic tree. Alignment was done using the program MUSCLE, and the phylogenetic tree was

constructed via Neighbor joining algorithm with a JTT (Jones-Taylor-Thornton) protein substitution model: (**B**) Modelled ESAG6 is similarly structured between the different *T. brucei* subspecies i.e., I. *T. b. rhodesiense*, II. *T. b. gambiense*, III. *T. b. brucei*, IV. *T. evansi*, and V. *T. equiperdum*. (VI.) An overlay model built from a structural alignment of all the models indicates that the predicted binding site is on surface exposed loops (red ribbons) and occurs similarly in all the proteins. Helices are denoted by the blue ribbons, while the brown ribbons denote loops and the magenta ribbons denote beta sheets. Modelling was done on the *T. b. brucei* VSG ILTat 1.24 (PDB ID: 2VSG) using the SWISS-MODEL homology modelling server (https://swissmodel.expasy.org/) [75–79] with the 2.7 Å X-ray diffraction structure of ILTat 1.24 (2VSG.pdb) as a template [80].

4. Fishing from a Hole; the Flagellar Pocket and the Quest for Iron

Iron is already a tightly controlled resource within the mammalian body fluids, with iron chelation molecules, i.e., serum transferrin (in blood and lymph) and lactoferrin (in external secretions), restricting the amount of bio-available ferric iron (Fe^{3+}) in body fluids to about 10^{-18} M [81,82].

Iron availability is a key component employed by mammals to minimize the parasite burden and increase the hosts' fitness [83]. By coupling of the mammalian immunosurveillance apparatus to iron metabolism, immunocompetence is associated with iron regulation [56,83]. Thus, the presence of parasites, indicated by their concomitant biochemical signals, signals a hazard to the mammalian system leading to the triggering of the acute-phase immune response [56]. A consequence of this is the sequestration of iron, thus limiting the bio-availability of this essential nutrient for circulating pathogens, a host-defense strategy known as 'nutritional immunity' [56]. Additionally, this also serves in strengthening specific immune effector mechanisms including the proliferation and functionality of immune cells, activation of cytokines, nitric oxide (NO) formation, activation of cellular proteins/peptides, and hormones that are dependent on iron availability [84,85].

Therefore, to sidestep nutritional immunity and obtain ferric iron (Fe^{3+}) from their hosts body fluids, parasites have to either compete against these chelates by devising their own iron chelation molecules, e.g., bacterial siderophores, or cleave the mammalian iron chelates by releasing proteases, e.g., bacterial reductases, or scavenge for these chelates by using specific receptors, e.g., trypanosomal transferrin receptors [63].

Transferrin (Tf) acquisition is the main route of iron uptake for BSF trypanosomes, particularly *T. brucei* spp., which are exclusively extracellular within the bloodstream and which has been the model organism for studying Tf uptake [13,57,65,86–88]. Tf uptake has been shown to be saturable, indicative of receptor mediated endocytosis (RME) with the ligand in this case, holo-/apo-Tf, being specifically competed out from its receptor, the trypanosomal TfR [57,65].

Binding of Tf and recycling of the trypanosomal TfR occurs in a process quite different to that observed in mammalian cells (Table 1) [7,89]. The main route of iron uptake in trypanosomes is localized within the trypanosomal flagellar pocket (FP) [57,90].

The trypanosomal FP, a membrane invagination surrounding the base of the flagellum, is a specialized organelle with multiple roles in the trypanosome [91,92]. This region is uniquely excluded from the sub-pellicular microtubule array under the parasites' plasma membrane [93,94]. The FP is also delineated from the rest of the plasma membrane by the FP collar, an electron-dense annulus, without which the FP is lost [93,95]. This collar encloses the FP lumen, a space filled with a carbohydrate-rich matrix with a poorly defined composition and unknown function [91]. The FP is the main turnover point for parasite nutrition [91]. As the only site of exo- and endocytosis by the trypanosome, the FP is part of a multi-organelle intracellular complex comprised of the Golgi complex, the endoplasmic reticulum as well as secretory and endocytic organelles, making it an important cog in the trypanosome's virulence and protein trafficking [92,95]. The efficiency of the FP protein trafficking is comparable to that of mammalian cells, which is quite remarkable, given that it covers about 2–5% of the total surface of the trypanosome [88]. In BSF trypanosomes, the FP is a site of high protein trafficking, with infectivity tied closely to a high rate of endocytosis [95]. Efficient nutrient scavenging occurs in the FP via selective retention of many of the invariant or variant host-associated nutrient receptors within its lumen by yet-unknown mechanisms but, mostly postulated to be the dynamic result of the high endocytic rate [95]. It is within the FP that the trypanosomal TfR binds iron laden transferrin (holo-Tf) as well as iron free transferrin (apo-Tf) as a GPI-anchored heterodimeric complex (Figure 6) [57,86].

Table 1. Features of the transferrin receptors (TfR) of *T. brucei* and human cells. [86].

Features	Trypanosome TfR	Human TfR
Subunit organization	Heterodimer of ESAG6 (50–60 kDa) and ESAG7 (40–42 kDa)	Homodimer of 90-kDa subunits
Post-translational modifications	ESAG6: 2–5 N-linked glycans ESAG7: 2–3 N-linked glycans	Per subunit: 3 N-linked glycan 1 Phosphorylation (Ser 24) 1 Acylation (Cys 62)
Membrane anchorage	GPI-anchor at the C-terminus of ESAG6	1 Transmembrane domain per subunit
Copy number per cell	3000	20000–700000
Ligand/receptor stoichiometry	1 Transferrin molecule per heterodimer	1 Transferrin molecule per monomer

Reprinted from Steverding, D. The transferrin receptor of Trypanosoma brucei. Parasitol. Int. 2000, 48, 191–198 doi:10.1016/S1383-5769(99)00018-5, with permission from Elsevier.

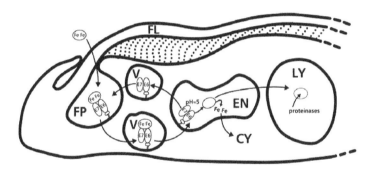

Figure 6. The trypanosomal transferrin receptor is located in the flagellar pocket and is internalized via receptor mediated endocytosis. The transferrin receptor of T. brucei (TbTfR) binds one molecule of Tf [86]. The parasite internalizes host transferrin by transferrin receptor-mediated endocytosis, facilitated by TbRab5. Holo- and apo-transferrin are bound at pH 7 and released at pH 5. Iron is incorporated into the cell cytosol and Tf is degraded by the lysozyme [19]. **Key: E7/E6**, heterodimeric transferrin receptor; **ellipse with Fe**, holo-transferrin; **empty ellipse**, apo-transferrin; **FP**, flagellar pocket; **FL**, flagellum; **V**, endo- and exocytotic vesicles; **EN**, endosome; **LY**, lysosome; **CY**, cytosol. Reprinted from Steverding, D. The transferrin receptor of Trypanosoma brucei. Parasitol. Int. 2000, 48, 191–198 doi:10.1016/S1383-5769(99)00018-5, with permission from Elsevier.

The TfR–ligand complex is endocytosed via a clathrin-dependent pathway [12,96]. Invagination of clathrin-coated vesicles leads to internalization of the receptor–ligand complex and subsequent discharge into the intracellular tubular system [95,96]. The endocytosis process has been hypothesized to involve the cleavage of the intracellular GPIs by the GPI-phospholipase leading to production of DAG and inositol-phosphoglycan [97–99]. DAG is an intracellular second messenger for signaling in eukaryotes [97]. Its role in stimulating endocytosis of Tf in the BSF trypanosome is proposed to be an adaptation of *T. brucei* to compete effectively with the mammalian host cells for Tf, as it does not have the same effect in mammalian Tf endocytosis [97]. Binding of DAG to its cognate receptors leads to their activation with the subsequent downstream activation of the protein tyrosine kinase (PTK)-dependent DAG signaling pathway [97]. The PTK is responsible for the phosphorylation and activation of the other proteins of the endocytic system including clathrin, actin, adaptins, and other components [97].

Once in the endosome, the acidic pH (6.5–4.5) enhances the release of the iron bound to the holo-Tf:TfR complex leading to formation of apo-Tf:TfR complex (Table 2) [57,86]. However, at the low (acidic) pH, the trypanosomal TfR, in contrast to the mammalian TfR, loses affinity for apo-Tf [19]. The apo-Tf is in turn delivered to the lysosomes for proteolytic degradation by the *T. brucei* cathepsin B-like protease (TbcatB) [100,101]. The resulting fragments are transported out of the cell via the TbRAb11 positive recycling vesicles [102]. TbRAB11 is specifically present in endosomal structures with recycling cargo molecules [102].

Table 2. K_d-values of ligand–receptor complexes for apo- and holo-transferrin at pH 7 and pH 5 [86].

Transferrin Receptor (nM)	Transferrin	pH	K_d-Value	Reference
T. brucei strain 427	Holo bovine	7	2.6–3.6	[57,69]
		5	12	[19]
	Apo bovine	7	20	[103]
		5	1100	[19]
Human cells	Holo human	7	1.9–7.7	[104]
		5	13	[104]
	Apo human	7	>700	[104]
		5	13–21	[104]

Reprinted from Steverding, D. The transferrin receptor of Trypanosoma brucei. Parasitol. Int. 2000, 48, 191–198 doi:10.1016/S1383-5769(99)00018-5, with permission from Elsevier.

The iron released from holo-Tf is initially converted from Fe^{3+} (insoluble) to Fe^{2+} (soluble) via two ferric reductases, i.e., a cytochrome b561-type (Tb927.6.3320) and a NADPH-dependent flavoprotein (Tb11.02.1990), before being imported into the cytoplasm in cooperation with the divalent cation transporter, *T. brucei* Mucolipin-like protein (TbMLP) [105]. The TbMLP, a protein of the endocytic system, is expressed both in the bloodstream and insect stages of the parasite, with high expression in the lysosomes [105]. However, other iron transport mechanisms such as ferric reductase and putative divalent metal transporters containing ZIP domains might also be involved [105,106]. Once in the cytosol, it is presumed that excess iron is stored in a storage compartment and released when cytosolic iron levels decline, which in turn is a possible signal for the TfR upregulation [107].

During periods of acute iron scarcity (which has only been documented using in vitro cultivated trypanosomes), mirroring those expected during the switch from one host to another or during chronic infection in the mammalian host, it has been shown that the TfR can be found outside of the FP [107]. The receptor then exists as islands within the VSG coat and was initially hypothesized to allow the parasite to utilize a wider surface area to capture any Tf [61,71]. This spillover is precipitated by an approximately 3- to 5-fold upregulation of the transcription of the receptor [61]. The upregulation of the *TfR* gene is not triggered by an increase in serum concentrations of the apo-Tf, as the receptor does not discriminate between holo- and apo-Tf [68,108]. Rather, upregulation has recently been shown to be mediated via the 3′ untranslated region (UTR) of the *TfR* gene that gets activated upon a reduction in the cytosolic iron concentration [107,109]. This signal triggers the upregulation long before the depletion of the iron stores in the parasite, thus allowing division of the parasite with the subsequent cycling and selection of a suitable high affinity TfR from the ESAGs [107]. The TfR has also been modelled to spread out from the surrounding VSG molecules, which previously was presumed to allow adequate contact and capture of Tf [74]. However, this hypothesis has recently been contradicted by evidence that the TfR outside of the FP is not functional, as it is composed of an ESAG6 homodimer, rather than an ESAG6/7 heterodimer [110]. The GPI valence in trypanosomes has been shown to be a critical determinant of intracellular sorting, with molecular complexes with two GPIs (GPI^2) being trafficked out of the FP, one GPI (GPI²) being retained within the FP, and non-GPI-anchored complexes being degraded in the lysosome [110]. Given that ESAG6 is the GPI-anchored partner in the complex, when over-expressed as homodimer during iron starvation, its GPI valence allows its escape from the FP [110].

5. The Trypanosomal Transferrin Receptor as A Target for Chemotherapeutic Purposes

Given the differences between the mammalian and the trypanosomal iron uptake in the form of Tf, it seems feasible to selectively target this pathway for chemotherapeutic purposes [106]. The mammalian host-trypanosome interaction is characterized by a macrophage hyper-activation, which through enhanced erythrophagocytosis cascades to anemia [111,112]. This iron deficiency represents a key challenge to the BSF trypanosomes, a situation further exacerbated by the release of various cytokines and hormones, such as the hepatocyte-derived hepcidin [113]. Hepcidin helps to further accentuate iron deficiency, by down-regulating the iron-exporting ferroportin-1, limiting the contribution of cellular iron to the blood [56,113]. As the parasite has to survive in already limiting conditions, interfering with its otherwise efficient scavenging of iron from the host, may represent a new strategy for treatment of AT [84].

The use of iron chelators to deprive parasites of iron and therefore limit the parasites' growth within the mammalian host represents an interesting chokepoint [56,63,106,114]. In another haemo-protozoan parasite, *Plasmodium*, the iron metabolism has been a successful in vivo target for many compounds, with iron chelation being a consistently applied therapy [115–117]. One iron chelator in particular, a desferrithiocin analogue, has been already applied in human trials for mitigation of iron mediated damage in transfusional iron overload [118,119]. While not curative in nature, the chelation of iron from the incorporation into apolipoproteins or even into Fe^{3+}-containing enzymes, e.g., ribonucleotide reductase, by chelators such as deferoxamine, has been shown to limit in vitro the growth of trypanosomes [104,120]. Given that the BSF parasite population needs to rapidly divide to keep up with the high rate of clearance by the immune system, this approach seems useful [121]. However, the use of these chelators is limited by both their water solubility, as well as their cytotoxicity, when applied in vitro on mammalian cells [120]. The potential for these drugs, however, is in the reduction of these unsuitable traits, e.g., by making lipophilic iron-chelating agents with reduced toxicity and in using these in conjunction with currently available anti-trypanosomal drugs [84,120].

Blocking the uptake of Tf by selectively targeting the trypanosomal TfR has been proposed severally as an alternative to controlling parasitemia in mammals [58,84]. It has already been shown that the TfR can be targeted by antibodies, with the main problem being delivery of the antibodies to the FP in sufficient quantities to achieve a therapeutic effect [57]. The question then arises whether a smaller targeting molecule, such as a single-domain antibody (sdAb) could work to target the receptor and block it. Such sdAbs do exist as nanobodies (Nbs), i.e., nanometer-sized camelid derived single-domain antibody fragments, which have been used for such cryptic targets as beta-lactamase enzyme active sites amongst other targets [122–124]. In addition, the specificity of nanobodies for the trypanosomes' unique and cryptic sites on their surface proteins has been previously applied to deliver toxic molecules into trypanosomes [125]. Hereby, a nanobody against the conserved region of VSG and conjugated to a trypanolytic molecule, i.e., human ApoL1, allowed to target and kill ˆT. b. brucei and T. b. rhodesiense parasites [125]. In addition, nanobodies against the variable part of VSG have also been successfully raised that block the endocytic machinery or target drugs to the trypanosome thereby causing its lysis and death [126,127]. Despite these properties, no experiments with nanobodies have been published with regards to the Tf uptake. Though Tf uptake is a potentially lucrative target, the BSF parasite in vivo would be surrounded by adequate ligand, even in the anemic state, thus requiring a considerable dose of a very high affinity nanobody to block, appreciably, the trypanosomal TfR. In addition, the rapid in vivo half-life of nanobodies, due to their size (15 kDa), which is below the renal cut-off (>50 kDa), might further hamper their applicability [122]. Yet, this might be circumvented by increasing their in vivo retention time by generating half-life extended constructs [128–130].

6. Conclusions

Understanding the trypanosomal transferrin receptor promises to provide unique insights into the trypanosome physiology. As an adaptation to the iron-scavenging lifestyle of the parasite, this molecular complex represents an interesting interface between the host and parasite [106]. Though there has been great progress made in unravelling the working mechanisms of this molecule, there has not been a diagnostic application based on the receptor, nor has there been development of chemotherapeutic agents targeting this essential parasite molecule. There are also gaps in understanding the function of this receptor particularly in the in vivo disease state. This is mainly attributed to the lack of suitable models to fit this context. It is of interest to unravel, in particular, the relevance of the TfR for the BSF trypanosome in this context (in vivo disease state), especially when faced by the fact that the *T. vivax* parasite survives just as well in the host bloodstream without any homologue of the *T. brucei* or *T. congolense* TfR.

Nonetheless, the TfR is a necessary element for the successful *T. brucei* parasitization of the mammalian host. It is also a relatively invariant molecule in comparison to its homologue, the VSG. Specifically targeting this heterodimeric molecule, at least for chemotherapeutic purposes, provides a novel way to deliver trypanocides or even to slow down parasite growth. This would allow parasite clearance by the infected mammalian host's immune system, thus controlling parasitemia as well as the inflammation that ensues.

Author Contributions: All authors contributed equally to the manuscript.

Funding: The authors acknowledge the financial support of the Interuniversity Attraction Pole Program (PAI-IAP N. P7/41, http://www.belspo.be/belspo/iap/index_en.stm), and the FWO G015016N (Characterization of the cellular and molecular mechanisms leading to the development of inflammation-driven immunopathologies in African Trypanosome infection). BS is a research fellow supported by the Strategic Research Programs: targeting inflammation linked to infectious diseases and cancer (Nanobodies for Health, SRP3) and Molecular Imaging and TARgeting of Macrophages in Inflammation (ITARMI, SRP47).

Conflicts of Interest: The authors declare no conflict of interest. The funders had no role in the design of the study; in the collection, analyses, or interpretation of data; in the writing of the manuscript, or in the decision to publish the results.

References

1. Aggett, P.J. Iron. In *Present Knowledge in Nutrition*; Erdman, J.W., Jr., Macdonald, I.A., Zeisel, S.H., Eds.; John Wiley & Sons, Inc.: Hoboken, NJ, USA, 2012; pp. 506–520. ISBN 9780470959176.

2. Hentze, M.W.; Muckenthaler, M.U.; Galy, B.; Camaschella, C. Two to Tango: Regulation of Mammalian Iron Metabolism. *Cell* **2010**, *142*, 24–38. [CrossRef] [PubMed]

3. Aisen, P.; Listowsky, I. Iron Transport and Storage Proteins. *Annu. Rev. Biochem.* **1980**, *49*, 357–393. [CrossRef] [PubMed]

4. Cassat, J.E.; Skaar, E.P. Iron in infection and immunity. *Cell Host Microbe* **2013**, *13*, 509–519. [CrossRef] [PubMed]

5. Fenton, H.J.H. Oxidation of tartartc acid in presence of iron. *J. Chem. Soc. Trans.* **1894**, *65*, 899–910. [CrossRef]

6. Kosman, D.J. Iron metabolism in aerobes: Managing ferric iron hydrolysis and ferrous iron autoxidation. *Coord. Chem. Rev.* **2013**, *100*, 130–134. [CrossRef]

7. Anderson, G.J.; Vulpe, C.D. Mammalian iron transport. *Cell. Mol. Life Sci.* **2009**, *66*, 3241–3261. [CrossRef]

8. Brissot, P.; Ropert, M.; Le Lan, C.; Loréal, O. Non-transferrin bound iron: A key role in iron overload and iron toxicity. *Biochim. Biophys. Acta Gen. Subj.* **2012**, *1820*, 403–410. [CrossRef]

9. Williams, J. The evolution of transferrin. *Trends Biochem. Sci.* **1982**, *7*, 394–397. [CrossRef]

10. Morgan, E.H. Transferrin, biochemistry, physiology and clinical significance. *Mol. Asp. Med.* **1981**, *4*, 1–123. [CrossRef]

11. Mizutani, K.; Toyoda, M.; Mikami, B. X-ray structures of transferrins and related proteins. *Biochim. Biophys. Acta Gen. Subj.* **2012**, *1820*, 203–211. [CrossRef]

12. Reyes-López, M.; Piña-Vázquez, C.; Serrano-Luna, J. Transferrin: Endocytosis and Cell Signaling in Parasitic Protozoa. *Biomed. Res. Int.* **2015**, *2015*, 641392. [CrossRef] [PubMed]

13. Macedo, M.F.; de Sousa, M. Transferrin and the transferrin receptor: Of magic bullets and other concerns. *Inflamm. Allergy Drug Targets* **2008**, *7*, 41–52. [CrossRef] [PubMed]

14. OIE. OIE Animal Trypanosomoses. In *Manual of Diagnostic Tests and Vaccines for Terrestrial Animals*; OIE: Paris, France, 2018; Volume 91, pp. 399–404. ISBN 978-92-95108-18-9.

15. Giordani, F.; Morrison, L.J.; Rowan, T.G.; De Koning, H.P.; Barrett, M.P. The animal trypanosomiases and their chemotherapy: A review. *Parasitology* **2016**, *143*, 1862–1889. [CrossRef] [PubMed]

16. Morrison, L.J.; Vezza, L.; Rowan, T.; Hope, J.C. Animal African Trypanosomiasis: Time to Increase Focus on Clinically Relevant Parasite and Host Species. *Trends Parasitol.* **2016**, *32*, 599–607. [CrossRef] [PubMed]

17. Vokaty, S.; Desquesnes, M. *Proceedings of First Symposium on New World Trypanosomes*; Vokaty, S., Desquesnes, M., Eds.; Biblioteca Orton IICA: Bridgetown, Barbados, 1999; ISBN 0253-4746.

18. Achcar, F.; Kerkhoven, E.J.; Barrett, M.P. Trypanosoma brucei: Meet the system. *Curr. Opin. Microbiol.* **2014**, *20*, 162–169. [CrossRef] [PubMed]

19. Maier, A.; Steverding, D. Low affinity of Trypanosoma brucei transferrin receptor to apotransferrin at pH 5 explains the fate of the ligand during endocytosis. *FEBS Lett.* **1996**, *396*, 87–89. [CrossRef]

20. Thomson, R.; Genovese, G.; Canon, C.; Kovacsics, D.; Higgins, M.K.; Carrington, M.; Winkler, C.A.; Kopp, J.; Rotimi, C.; Adeyemo, A.; et al. Evolution of the primate trypanolytic factor APOL1. *Proc. Natl. Acad. Sci. USA* **2014**, *111*, E2130–E2139. [CrossRef] [PubMed]

21. Pays, E.; Vanhollebeke, B.; Vanhamme, L.; Paturiaux-Hanocq, F.; Nolan, D.P.; Pérez-Morga, D. The trypanolytic factor of human serum. *Nat. Rev. Microbiol.* **2006**, *4*, 477–486. [CrossRef]

22. Currier, R.B.; Cooper, A.; Burrell-Saward, H.; MacLeod, A.; Alsford, S. Decoding the network of Trypanosoma brucei proteins that determines sensitivity to apolipoprotein-L1. *PLoS Pathog.* **2018**, *14*, e1006855. [CrossRef]

23. Cooper, A.; Capewell, P.; Clucas, C.; Veitch, N.; Weir, W.; Thomson, R.; Raper, J.; MacLeod, A. A Primate APOL1 Variant That Kills Trypanosoma brucei gambiense. *PLoS Negl. Trop. Dis.* **2016**, *10*, e0004903. [CrossRef]

24. Hajduk, S.L.; Moore, D.R.; Vasudevacharya, J.; Siqueira, H.; Torri, A.F.; Tytler, E.M.; Esko, J.D. Lysis of Trypanosoma brucei by a toxic subspecies of human high density lipoprotein. *J. Biol. Chem.* **1989**, *264*, 5210–5217. [PubMed]

25. Radwanska, M.; Vereecke, N.; Deleeuw, V.; Pinto, J.; Magez, S. Salivarian Trypanosomosis: A Review of Parasites Involved, Their Global Distribution and Their Interaction with the Innate and Adaptive Mammalian Host Immune System. *Front. Immunol.* **2018**, *9*, 1–20. [CrossRef] [PubMed]

26. Claes, F.; Büscher, P.; Touratier, L.; Goddeeris, B.M. Trypanosoma equiperdum: Master of disguise or historical mistake? *Trends Parasitol.* **2005**, *21*, 316–321. [CrossRef] [PubMed]

27. Touratier, L. Challenges of non-tsetse transmitted animal trypanosomoses (NTTAT). An outline and some perspectives. *Ann. N. Y. Acad. Sci.* **2000**, *916*, 237–239. [CrossRef] [PubMed]

28. Desquesnes, M.; Yangtara, S.; Kunphukhieo, P.; Jittapalapong, S.; Herder, S. Zoonotic trypanosomes in South East Asia: Attempts to control Trypanosoma lewisi using human and animal trypanocidal drugs. *Infect. Genet. Evol.* **2016**, *44*, 514–521. [CrossRef] [PubMed]

29. Pays, E.; Nolan, D.P. Expression and function of surface proteins in Trypanosoma brucei. *Mol. Biochem. Parasitol.* **1998**, *91*, 3–36. [CrossRef]

30. David Barry, J.; McCulloch, R. Antigenic variation in trypanosomes: Enhanced phenotypic variation in a eukaryotic parasite. *Adv. Parasitol.* **2004**, *49*, 1–70. [CrossRef]

31. Borst, P.; Frasch, A.C.C.; Bernards, A.; Hoeijmakers, J.H.; van der Ploeg, L.H.; Cross, G.A.M. The genes for variant antigens in trypanosomes. *Am. J. Trop. Med. Hyg.* **1980**, *29*, 1033–1036. [CrossRef]

32. Pays, E.; Vanhamme, L.; Pérez-Morga, D. Antigenic variation in Trypanosoma brucei: Facts, challenges and mysteries. *Curr. Opin. Microbiol.* **2004**, *7*, 369–374. [CrossRef]

33. Rudenko, G. African trypanosomes: The genome and adaptations for immune evasion. *Essays Biochem.* **2015**, *51*, 47–62. [CrossRef]

34. Cross, G.A.M.; Kim, H.S.; Wickstead, B. Capturing the variant surface glycoprotein repertoire (the VSGnome) of Trypanosoma brucei Lister 427. *Mol. Biochem. Parasitol.* **2014**, *195*, 59–73. [CrossRef] [PubMed]

35. Graham, S.V.; Barry, J.D. Expression site-associated genes transcribed independently of variant surface glycoprotein genes in Trypanosoma brucei. *Mol. Biochem. Parasitol.* **1991**, *47*, 31–41. [CrossRef]

36. Berriman, M.; Ghedin, E.; Hertz-Fowler, C.; Blandin, G.; Renauld, H.; Bartholomeu, D.C.; Lennard, N.J.; Caler, E.; Hamlin, N.E.; Haas, B.; et al. The genome of the African trypanosome Trypanosoma brucei. *Science* **2005**, *309*, 416–422. [CrossRef] [PubMed]

37. Pays, E.; Vanhamme, L.; Pérez-Morga, D. Antigenic variation in Trypanosoma african: Memorandum. *Bull. World Health Organ.* **1978**, *56*, 389–401.

38. Pays, E.; Vanhollebeke, B.; Uzureau, P.; Lecordier, L.; Pérez-Morga, D. The molecular arms race between African trypanosomes and humans. *Nat. Rev. Microbiol.* **2014**, *12*, 575–584. [CrossRef]

39. Kassem, A.; Pays, E.; Vanhamme, L. Transcription is initiated on silent variant surface glycoprotein expression sites despite monoallelic expression in Trypanosoma brucei. *Proc. Natl. Acad. Sci. USA* **2014**, *111*, 8943–8948. [CrossRef]

40. Pays, E. The variant surface glycoprotein as a tool for adaptation in African trypanosomes. *Microbes Infect.* **2006**, *8*, 930–937. [CrossRef]

41. Vanhamme, L.; Lecordier, L.; Pays, E. Control and function of the bloodstream variant surface glycoprotein expression sites in Trypanosoma brucei. *Int. J. Parasitol.* **2001**, *31*, 523–531. [CrossRef]

42. Kolev, N.G.; Ramsdell, T.K.; Tschudi, C. Temperature shift activates bloodstream VSG expression site promoters in Trypanosoma brucei. *Mol. Biochem. Parasitol.* **2018**, *226*, 20–23. [CrossRef]

43. Hertz-Fowler, C.; Figueiredo, L.M.; Quail, M.A.; Becker, M.; Jackson, A.; Bason, N.; Brooks, K.; Churcher, C.; Fahkro, S.; Goodhead, I.; et al. Telomeric expression sites are highly conserved in Trypanosoma brucei. *PLoS ONE* **2008**, *3*. [CrossRef]

44. Horn, D. Antigenic variation in African trypanosomes. *Mol. Biochem. Parasitol.* **2014**, *195*, 123–129. [CrossRef] [PubMed]

45. Pays, E.; Tebabi, P.; Pays, A.; Coquelet, H.; Revelard, P.; Salmon, D.; Steinert, M. The genes and transcripts of an antigen gene expression site from T. brucei. *Cell* **1989**, *57*, 835–845. [CrossRef]

46. Vanhamme, L.; Postiaux, S.; Poelvoorde, P.; Pays, E. Differential regulation of ESAG transcripts in Trypanosoma brucei. *Mol. Biochem. Parasitol.* **1999**, *102*, 35–42. [CrossRef]

47. McCulloch, R.; Horn, D. What has DNA sequencing revealed about the VSG expression sites of african trypanosomes? *Trends Parasitol.* **2009**, *25*, 359–363. [CrossRef]

48. Stockdale, C.; Swiderski, M.R.; Barry, J.D.; McCulloch, R. Antigenic variation in Trypanosoma brucei: Joining the DOTs. *PLoS Biol.* **2008**, *6*, 1386–1391. [CrossRef]

49. Borst, P.; Bitter, W.; Blundell, P.A.; Chaves, I.; Cross, M.; Gerrits, H.; Van Leeuwen, F.; McCulloch, R.; Taylor, M.; Rudenko, G. Control of VSG gene expression sites in Trypanosoma brucei. *Mol. Biochem. Parasitol.* **1998**, *91*, 67–76. [CrossRef]

50. Borst, P.; Fairlamb, A.H. Surface receptors and transporters of Trypanosoma brucei. *Annu. Rev. Microbiol.* **1998**, *52*, 745–778. [CrossRef]

51. Pays, E.; Lips, S.; Nolan, D.; Vanhamme, L.; Pérez-Morga, D. The VSG expression sites of Trypanosoma brucei: Multipurpose tools for the adaptation of the parasite to mammalian hosts. *Mol. Biochem. Parasitol.* **2001**, *114*, 1–16. [CrossRef]

52. Van Xong, H.; Vanhamme, L.; Chamekh, M.; Chimfwembe, C.E.; Van Den Abbeele, J.; Pays, A.; Van Melrvenne, N.; Hamers, R.; De Baetselier, P.; Pays, E. A VSG expression site-associated gene confers resistance to human serum in Trypanosoma rhodesiense. *Cell* **1998**, *95*, 839–846. [CrossRef]

53. Lips, S.; Revelard, P.; Pays, E. Identification of a new expression site-associated gene in the complete 30.5 kb sequence from the AnTat 1.3A variant surface protein gene expression site of Trypanosoma brucei. *Mol. Biochem. Parasitol.* **1993**, *62*, 135–137. [CrossRef]

54. Jackson, A.P.; Allison, H.C.; Barry, J.D.; Field, M.C.; Hertz-Fowler, C.; Berriman, M. A Cell-surface Phylome for African Trypanosomes. *PLoS Negl. Trop. Dis.* **2013**, *7*. [CrossRef] [PubMed]

55. Steverding, D. The significance of transferrin receptor variation in Trypanosoma brucei. *Trends Parasitol.* **2003**, *19*, 125–127. [CrossRef]

56. Nairz, M.; Dichtl, S.; Schroll, A.; Haschka, D.; Tymoszuk, P.; Theurl, I.; Weiss, G. Iron and innate antimicrobial immunity – Depriving the pathogen, defending the host. *J. Trace Elem. Med. Biol.* **2018**, *48*, 118–133. [CrossRef] [PubMed]

57. Steverding, D.; Stierhof, Y.D.; Fuchs, H.; Tauber, R.; Overath, P. Transferrin-binding protein complex is the receptor for transferrin uptake in Trypanosoma brucei. *J. Cell Biol.* **1995**, *131*, 1173–1182. [CrossRef]

58. Baral, T.N. Immunobiology of African trypanosomes: Need of alternative interventions. *J. Biomed. Biotechnol.* **2010**, *2010*. [CrossRef]

59. Pays, E. Regulation of antigen gene expression in Trypanosoma brucei. *Trends Parasitol.* **2005**, *21*, 517–520. [CrossRef]

60. Ansorge, I.; Steverding, D.; Melville, S.; Hartmann, C.; Clayton, C. Transcription of "inactive" expression sites in African trypanosomes leads to expression of multiple transferrin receptor RNAs in bloodstream forms. *Mol. Biochem. Parasitol.* **1999**, *101*, 81–94. [CrossRef]

61. Mussmann, R.; Engstler, M.; Gerrits, H.; Kieft, R.; Toaldo, C.B.; Onderwater, J.; Koerten, H.; Van Luenen, H.G.A.M.; Borst, P. Factors affecting the level and localization of the transferrin receptor in Trypanosoma brucei. *J. Biol. Chem.* **2004**, *279*, 40690–40698. [CrossRef]

62. Cully, D.F.; Ip, H.S.; Cross, G.A.M. Coordinate transcription of variant surface glycoprotein genes and an expression site associated gene family in Trypanosoma brucei. *Cell* **1985**, *42*, 173–182. [CrossRef]

63. Wilson, M.E.; Britigan, B.E. Iron acquisition by parasitic protozoa. *Parasitol. Today* **1998**, *14*, 348–353. [CrossRef]

64. Maier, A.; Steverding, D. Expression and purification of non-glycosylated Trypanosoma brucei transferrin receptor in insect cells. *Exp. Parasitol.* **2008**, *120*, 205–207. [CrossRef] [PubMed]

65. Salmon, D.; Geuskens, M.; Hanocq, F.; Hanocq-Quertier, J.; Nolan, D.; Ruben, L.; Pays, E. A novel heterodimeric transferrin receptor encoded by a pair of VSG expression site-associated genes in T. brucei. *Cell* **1994**, *78*, 75–86. [CrossRef]

66. Salmon, D.; Hanocq-Quertier, J.; Paturiaux-Hanocq, F.; Pays, A.; Tebabi, P.; Nolan, D.P.; Michel, A.; Pays, E. Characterization of the ligand-binding site of the transferrin receptor in *Trypanosoma brucei* demonstrates a structural relationship with the N-terminal domain of the variant surface glycoprotein. *EMBO J.* **1997**, *16*, 7272–7278. [CrossRef] [PubMed]

67. Gerrits, H.; Mußmann, R.; Bitter, W.; Kieft, R.; Borst, P. The physiological significance of transferrin receptor variations in Trypanosoma brucei. *Mol. Biochem. Parasitol.* **2002**, *119*, 237–247. [CrossRef]

68. Salmon, D.; Paturiaux-Hanocq, F.; Poelvoorde, P.; Vanhamme, L.; Pays, E. Trypanosoma brucei: Growth differences in different mammalian sera are not due to the species-specificity of transferrin. *Exp. Parasitol.* **2005**, *109*, 188–194. [CrossRef] [PubMed]

69. Bitter, W.; Gerrits, H.; Kieft, R.; Borst, P. The role of transferrin-receptor variation in the host range of Trypanosoma brucei. *Nature* **1998**, *391*, 499–502. [CrossRef]

70. Steverding, D. On the significance of host antibody response to the Trypanosoma brucei transferrin receptor during chronic infection. *Microbes Infect.* **2006**, *8*, 2777–2782. [CrossRef]

71. Mehlert, A.; Bond, C.S.; Ferguson, M.A.J. The glycoforms of a Trypanosoma brucei variant surface glycoprotein and molecular modeling of a glycosylated surface coat. *Glycobiology* **2002**, *12*, 607–612. [CrossRef]

72. Steverding, D.; Overath, P. Trypanosoma brucei with an active metacyclic variant surface gene expression site expresses a transferrin receptor derived from esag6 and esag7. *Mol. Biochem. Parasitol.* **1996**, *78*, 285–288. [CrossRef]

73. Jensen, R.E.; Simpson, L.; Englund, P.T. What happens when Trypanosoma brucei leaves Africa. *Trends Parasitol.* **2008**, *24*, 425–428. [CrossRef]

74. Mehlert, A.; Wormald, M.R.; Ferguson, M.A.J. Modeling of the N-glycosylated transferrin receptor suggests how transferrin binding can occur within the surface coat of trypanosoma brucei. *PLoS Pathog.* **2012**, *8*, e1002618. [CrossRef] [PubMed]

75. Benkert, P.; Biasini, M.; Schwede, T. Toward the estimation of the absolute quality of individual protein structure models. *Bioinformatics* **2011**, *27*, 343–350. [CrossRef] [PubMed]

76. Bienert, S.; Waterhouse, A.; De Beer, T.A.P.; Tauriello, G.; Studer, G.; Bordoli, L.; Schwede, T. The SWISS-MODEL Repository-new features and functionality. *Nucleic Acids Res.* **2017**, *45*, D313–D319. [CrossRef] [PubMed]

77. Waterhouse, A.; Bertoni, M.; Bienert, S.; Studer, G.; Tauriello, G.; Gumienny, R.; Heer, F.T.; De Beer, T.A.P.; Rempfer, C.; Bordoli, L.; et al. SWISS-MODEL: Homology modelling of protein structures and complexes. *Nucleic Acids Res.* **2018**, *46*, W296–W303. [CrossRef]

78. Bertoni, M.; Kiefer, F.; Biasini, M.; Bordoli, L.; Schwede, T. Modeling protein quaternary structure of homo- and hetero-oligomers beyond binary interactions by homology. *Sci. Rep.* **2017**, *7*, 10480. [CrossRef]

79. Guex, N.; Peitsch, M.C.; Schwede, T. Automated comparative protein structure modeling with SWISS-MODEL and Swiss-PdbViewer: A historical perspective. *Electrophoresis* **2009**, *30*, S162–S173. [CrossRef]
80. Blum, M.L.; Down, J.A.; Gurnett, A.M.; Carrington, M.; Turner, M.J.; Wiley, D.C. A structural motif in the variant surface glycoproteins of Trypanosoma brucei. *Nature* **1993**, *362*, 603–609. [CrossRef]
81. Bullen, J.J. The significance of iron in infection. *Rev. Infect. Dis.* **1981**, *3*, 1127–1138. [CrossRef]
82. Bullen, J.J.; Rogers, H.J.; Griffiths, E. Role of Iron in Bacterial Infection. *Curr. Top. Microbiol. Immunol.* **2012**, *80*, 1–35. [CrossRef]
83. Latunde-Dada, G.O. Iron metabolism: Microbes, mouse, and man. *BioEssays* **2009**, *31*, 1309–1317. [CrossRef]
84. Stijlemans, B.; Beschin, A.; Magez, S.; Van Ginderachter, J.A.; De Baetselier, P. Iron Homeostasis and Trypanosoma brucei Associated Immunopathogenicity Development: A Battle/Quest for Iron. *Biomed. Res. Int.* **2015**, *2015*, 1–15. [CrossRef] [PubMed]
85. Kořený, L.; Oborník, M.; Lukeš, J. Make It, Take It, or Leave It: Heme Metabolism of Parasites. *PLoS Pathog.* **2013**, *9*. [CrossRef] [PubMed]
86. Steverding, D. The transferrin receptor of Trypanosoma brucei. *Parasitol. Int.* **2000**, *48*, 191–198. [CrossRef]
87. Steverding, D.; Sexton, D.W.; Chrysochoidi, N.; Cao, F. Trypanosoma brucei transferrin receptor can bind C-lobe and N-lobe fragments of transferrin. *Mol. Biochem. Parasitol.* **2012**, *185*, 99–105. [CrossRef]
88. Coppens, I.; Opperdoes, F.R.; Courtoy, P.J.; Baudhuin, P. Receptor-Mediated Endocytosis in the Bloodstream Form of Trypanosoma brucei. *J. Protozool.* **1987**, *34*, 465–473. [CrossRef]
89. Kabiri, M.; Steverding, D. Studies on the recycling of the transferrin receptor in Trypanosoma brucei using an inducible gene expression system. *Eur. J. Biochem.* **2000**, *267*, 3309–3314. [CrossRef]
90. Higgins, M.K.; Lane-Serff, H.; MacGregor, P.; Carrington, A. Receptor's Tale: An Eon in the Life of a Trypanosome Receptor. *PLOS Pathog.* **2017**, *13*, e1006055. [CrossRef]
91. Gull, K. Host–parasite interactions and trypanosome morphogenesis: A flagellar pocketful of goodies. *Curr. Opin. Microbiol.* **2003**, *6*, 365–370. [CrossRef]
92. Landfear, S.M.; Ignatushchenko, M. The flagellum and flagellar pocket of trypanosomatids. *Mol. Biochem. Parasitol.* **2001**, *115*, 1–17. [CrossRef]
93. Perdomo, D.; Bonhivers, M.; Robinson, D.R. The Trypanosome Flagellar Pocket Collar and Its Ring Forming Protein-TbBILBO1. *Cells* **2016**, *5*, 9. [CrossRef]
94. Ligtenberg, M.J.; Bitter, W.; Kieft, R.; Steverding, D.; Janssen, H.; Calafat, J.; Borst, P. Reconstitution of a surface transferrin binding complex in insect form Trypanosoma brucei. *EMBO J.* **1994**, *13*, 2565–2573. [CrossRef] [PubMed]
95. Field, M.C.; Carrington, M. The trypanosome flagellar pocket. *Nat. Rev. Microbiol.* **2009**, *7*, 775–786. [CrossRef] [PubMed]
96. Allen, C.L.; Goulding, D.; Field, M.C. Clathrin-mediated endocytosis is essential in Trypanosoma brucei. *EMBO J.* **2003**, *22*, 4991–5002. [CrossRef] [PubMed]
97. Subramanya, S.; Mensa-Wilmot, K. Diacylglycerol-stimulated endocytosis of transferrin in trypanosomatids is dependent on tyrosine kinase activity. *PLoS ONE* **2010**, *5*, e8538. [CrossRef]
98. Subramanya, S.; Hardin, F.C.; Steverding, D.; Mensa-Wilmot, K. Glycosylphosphatidylinositol-specific phospholipase C regulates transferrin endocytosis in the African trypanosome. *Biochem. J.* **2009**, *417*, 685–694. [CrossRef]
99. Subramanya, S.; Mensa-Wilmot, K. Regulated cleavage of intracellular glycosylphosphatidylinositol in a trypanosome: Peroxisome-to-endoplasmic reticulum translocation of a phospholipase C. *FEBS J.* **2006**, *273*, 2110–2126. [CrossRef]
100. Mackey, Z.B.; O'Brien, T.C.; Greenbaum, D.C.; Blank, R.B.; McKerrow, J.H. A cathepsin B-like protease is required for host protein degradation in Trypanosoma brucei. *J. Biol. Chem.* **2004**, *279*, 48426–48433. [CrossRef]
101. O'Brien, T.C.; Mackey, Z.B.; Fetter, R.D.; Choe, Y.; O'Donoghue, A.J.; Zhou, M.; Craik, C.S.; Caffrey, C.R.; McKerrow, J.H. A parasite cysteine protease is key to host protein degradation and iron acquisition. *J. Biol. Chem.* **2008**, *283*, 28934–28943. [CrossRef]
102. Hall, B.S.; Smith, E.; Langer, W.; Jacobs, L.A.; Goulding, D.; Field, M.C. Developmental variation in Rab11-dependent trafficking in Trypanosoma brucei. *Eukaryot. Cell* **2005**, *4*, 971–980. [CrossRef]
103. Steverding, D. Bloodstream forms of Trypanosoma brucei require only small amounts of iron for growth. *Parasitol. Res.* **1998**, *84*, 59–62. [CrossRef]

104. Dautry-Varsat, A.; Ciechanover, A.; Lodish, H.F. pH and the recycling of transferrin during receptor-mediated endocytosis. *Proc. Natl. Acad. Sci. USA* **1983**, *80*, 2258–2262. [CrossRef] [PubMed]
105. Taylor, M.C.; Mclatchie, A.P.; Kelly, J.M. Evidence that transport of iron from the lysosome to the cytosol in African trypanosomes is mediated by a mucolipin orthologue. *Mol. Microbiol.* **2013**, *89*, 420–432. [CrossRef] [PubMed]
106. Basu, S.; Horáková, E.; Lukeš, J. Iron-associated biology of Trypanosoma brucei. *Biochim. Biophys. Acta Gen. Subj.* **2016**, *1860*, 363–370. [CrossRef] [PubMed]
107. Mußmann, R.; Janssen, H.; Calafat, J.; Engstler, M.; Ansorge, I.; Clayton, C.; Borst, P. The expression level determines the surface distribution of the transferrin receptor in Trypanosoma brucei. *Mol. Microbiol.* **2003**, *47*, 23–35. [CrossRef]
108. Van Luenen, H.G.A.M.; Kieft, R.; Mußmann, R.; Engstler, M.; Ter Riet, B.; Borst, P. Trypanosomes change their transferrin receptor expression to allow effective uptake of host transferrin. *Mol. Microbiol.* **2005**, *58*, 151–165. [CrossRef]
109. Benz, C.; Lo, W.; Fathallah, N.; Connor-Guscott, A.; Benns, H.J.; Urbaniak, M.D. Dynamic regulation of the Trypanosoma brucei transferrin receptor in response to iron starvation is mediated via the 3'UTR. *PLoS ONE* **2018**, 441931. [CrossRef]
110. Tiengwe, C.; Bush, P.J.; Bangs, J.D. Controlling transferrin receptor trafficking with GPI-valence in bloodstream stage African trypanosomes. *PLoS Pathog.* **2017**, *13*, e1006366. [CrossRef]
111. Stijlemans, B.; Brys, L.; Korf, H.; Bieniasz-Krzywiec, P.; Sparkes, A.; Vansintjan, L.; Leng, L.; Vanbekbergen, N.; Mazzone, M.; Caljon, G.; et al. MIF-Mediated Hemodilution Promotes Pathogenic Anemia in Experimental African Trypanosomosis. *PLOS Pathog.* **2016**, *12*, e1005862. [CrossRef]
112. Naessens, J. Bovine trypanotolerance: A natural ability to prevent severe anaemia and haemophagocytic syndrome? *Int. J. Parasitol.* **2006**, *36*, 521–528. [CrossRef]
113. Coffey, R.; Ganz, T. Iron homeostasis: An anthropocentric perspective. *J. Biol. Chem.* **2017**, *292*, 12727–12734. [CrossRef]
114. Taylor, M.C.; Kelly, J.M. Iron metabolism in trypanosomatids, and its crucial role in infection. *Parasitology* **2010**, *137*, 899–917. [CrossRef] [PubMed]
115. Ferrer, P.; Tripathi, A.K.; Clark, M.A.; Hand, C.C.; Rienhoff, H.Y.; Sullivan, D.J. Antimalarial iron chelator, FBS0701, shows asexual and gametocyte Plasmodium falciparum activity and single oral dose cure in a murine malaria model. *PLoS ONE* **2012**, *7*, e37171. [CrossRef] [PubMed]
116. Sarkar, S.; Siddiqui, A.A.; Saha, S.J.; De, R.; Mazumder, S.; Banerjee, C.; Iqbal, M.S.; Nag, S.; Adhikari, S.; Bandyopadhyay, U. Antimalarial activity of small-molecule benzothiazole hydrazones. *Antimicrob. Agents Chemother.* **2016**, *60*, 4217–4228. [CrossRef] [PubMed]
117. Gehrke, S.S.; Pinto, E.G.; Steverding, D.; Pleban, K.; Tempone, A.G.; Hider, R.C.; Wagner, G.K. Conjugation to 4-aminoquinoline improves the anti-trypanosomal activity of Deferiprone-type iron chelators. *Bioorganic Med. Chem.* **2013**, *21*, 805–813. [CrossRef]
118. Bergeron, R.J.; Wiegand, J.; Bharti, N.; McManis, J.S.; Singh, S. Desferrithiocin analogue iron chelators: Iron clearing efficiency, tissue distribution, and renal toxicity. *BioMetals* **2011**, *24*, 239–258. [CrossRef]
119. Rienhoff, H.Y.; Viprakasit, V.; Tay, L.; Harmatz, P.; Vichinsky, E.; Chirnomas, D.; Kwiatkowski, J.L.; Tapper, A.; Kramer, W.; Porter, J.B.; et al. A phase 1 dose-escalation study: Safety, tolerability, and pharmacokinetics of FBS0701, a novel oral iron chelator for the treatment of transfusional iron overload. *Haematologica* **2011**, *96*, 521–525. [CrossRef]
120. Merschjohann, K.; Steverding, D. In vitro growth inhibition of bloodstream forms of Trypanosoma brucei and Trypanosoma congolense by iron chelators. *Kinetoplastid Biol. Dis.* **2006**, *5*, 3. [CrossRef]
121. Tyler, K.M.; Higgs, P.G.; Matthews, K.R.; Gull, K. Limitation of Trypanosoma brucei parasitaemia results from density-dependent parasite differentiation and parasite killing by the host immune response. *Proc. R. Soc. B Biol. Sci.* **2001**, *268*, 2235–2243. [CrossRef]
122. Muyldermans, S.; Vincke, C. Structure and Function of Camelid VHH. *Encycl. Immunobiol.* **2016**, *2*, 153–159. [CrossRef]
123. Cortez-Retamozo, V.; Backmann, N.; Senter, P.D.; Wernery, U.; De Baetselier, P.; Muyldermans, S.; Revets, H. Efficient Cancer Therapy with a Nanobody-Based Conjugate. *Cancer Res.* **2004**, *64*, 2853–2857. [CrossRef]

124. Conrath, K.E.; Lauwereys, M.; Galleni, M.; Matagne, A.; Frere, J.M.; Kinne, J.; Wyns, L.; Muyldermans, S. Beta-Lactamase Inhibitors Derived from Single-Domain Antibody Fragments Elicited in the Camelidae. *Antimicrob. Agents Chemother.* **2001**, *45*, 2807–2812. [CrossRef] [PubMed]

125. Baral, T.N.; Magez, S.; Stijlemans, B.; Conrath, K.; Vanhollebeke, B.; Pays, E.; Muyldermans, S.; De Baetselier, P. Experimental therapy of African trypanosomiasis with a nanobody-conjugated human trypanolytic factor. *Nat. Med.* **2006**, *12*, 580–584. [CrossRef] [PubMed]

126. Stijlemans, B.; Conrath, K.; Cortez-Retamozo, V.; Van Xong, H.; Wyns, L.; Senter, P.; Revets, H.; De Baetselier, P.; Muyldermans, S.; Magez, S. Efficient Targeting of Conserved Cryptic Epitopes of Infectious Agents by Single Domain Antibodies: AFRICAN TRYPANOSOMES AS PARADIGM. *J. Biol. Chem.* **2004**, *279*, 1256–1261. [CrossRef] [PubMed]

127. Stijlemans, B.; Caljon, G.; Natesan, S.K.; Saerens, D.; Conrath, K.; Pérez-Morga, D.; Skepper, J.N.; Nikolaou, A.; Brys, L.; Pays, E.; et al. High affinity nanobodies against the Trypanosome brucei VSG are potent trypanolytic agents that block endocytosis. *PLoS Pathog.* **2011**, *7*, e1002072. [CrossRef] [PubMed]

128. Conrath, K.E.; Lauwereys, M.; Wyns, L.; Muyldermans, S. Camel Single-domain Antibodies as Modular Building Units in Bispecific and Bivalent Antibody Constructs. *J. Biol. Chem.* **2001**, *276*, 7346–7350. [CrossRef]

129. Cuesta, Á.M.; Sainz-Pastor, N.; Bonet, J.; Oliva, B.; Álvarez-Vallina, L. Multivalent antibodies: When design surpasses evolution. *Trends Biotechnol.* **2010**, *28*, 355–362. [CrossRef]

130. Hmila, I.; Abdallah R, B.A.B.; Saerens, D.; Benlasfar, Z.; Conrath, K.; El Ayeb, M.; Muyldermans, S.; Bouhaouala-Zahar, B. VHH, bivalent domains and chimeric Heavy chain-only antibodies with high neutralizing efficacy for scorpion toxin AahI'. *Mol. Immunol.* **2008**, *45*, 3847–3856. [CrossRef]

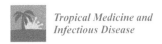

Tropical Medicine and Infectious Disease

Article

(+)-Spectaline and Iso-6-Spectaline Induce a Possible Cross-Talk between Autophagy and Apoptosis in *Trypanosoma brucei rhodesiense*

Kah Tee Lim [1], Chiann Ying Yeoh [2], Zafarina Zainuddin [1,3] and Mohd. Ilham Adenan [1,4,5,*]

[1] Malaysian Institute of Pharmaceuticals and Nutraceuticals (IPharm), National Institutes of Biotechnology Malaysia, Ministry of Science, Technology and Innovation, Blok 5-A, Halaman Bukit Gambir, Penang 11700, Malaysia
[2] Faculty of Medicine and Health Sciences, Universiti Putra Malaysia, UPM Serdang 43400, Selangor, Malaysia
[3] Analytical Biochemistry Research Centre (ABrC), Universiti Sains Malaysia, Penang 11800, Malaysia
[4] Faculty of Applied Sciences, Universiti Teknologi MARA, Shah Alam 40450, Selangor, Malaysia
[5] Universiti Teknologi MARA Pahang Campus, 26400 Bandar Tun Abdul Razak Jengka, Pahang, Malaysia
* Correspondence: mohdilham@puncakalam.uitm.edu.my; Tel.: +6019-292-2020

Received: 17 May 2019; Accepted: 27 June 2019; Published: 1 July 2019

Abstract: In our previous study, two known piperidine alkaloids (+)-spectaline (**1**) and iso-6-spectaline (**2**) were isolated from the leaves of *Senna spectabilis* and showed no toxic effect on L6 cells. In view of the potential use of piperidine alkaloids in *S. spectabilis* for the treatment of sleeping sickness, further investigation on the cell death actions of the parasite after treatment with compound **1** and **2** suggested that the treated parasites died by a process of autophagy based on the characteristic morphological alterations observed in intracellular *T. b. rhodesiense*. In search for apoptosis, interestingly, trypanosomes treated with high concentration of compound **1** and **2** after 72 h significantly induced an early apoptosis-like programmed cell death (PCD) such as phosphatidylserine (PS) exposure, loss of mitochondrial membrane potential and caspases activation. No DNA laddering discriminated late apoptosis event. Taken together, these findings demonstrated the potential of compound **1** and **2** as a natural chemotherapeutic capable of inducing a possible cross-talk between autophagy and apoptosis in *T. b. rhodesiense*.

Keywords: (+)-spectaline; iso-6-spectaline; *Trypanosoma brucei rhodesiense*; autophagy; apoptosis; cross-talk

---

1. Introduction

Human African Trypanosomiasis (HAT) also known as "sleeping sickness" is caused by two protozoan parasites, *Trypanosoma brucei rhodesiense* and *Trypanosoma brucei gambiense*. The trypanosomes are transmitted to humans by a bite of the infected *Glossina* spp. (tsetse fly) and multiply extracellularly in blood, lymph, and cerebrospinal fluid. The disease affects about 50 million people yearly in 36 sub-Saharan Africa, with an estimated incidence of about 30,000 cases per annum [1]. The disease has two distinct stages. In the early stage, trypanosomes reproduce in the hemolymphatic system of the patient, whereas in the second stage, trypanosomes cross the blood–brain barrier (BBB) to the central nervous system that results in a coma and finally, death of the patient if left untreated. Endemics are prevalent in rural regions where public health facilities needed for an effective treatment are absent. At present, there are only a few drugs registered for the treatment of HAT, such as suramin, pentamidine, melarsoprol, eflornithine, and nifurtimox. Except for eflornithine and nifurtimox, the other drugs were developed a half century ago [2,3]. Suramin and pentamidine are effective against the early stage of HAT, whereas the second stage of the disease can only be treated with melarsoprol and eflornithine. Drugs for the treatment of sleeping sickness are depending on the causative subspecies and their ability to cross the BBB. In addition, antigenic variation that protects the trypanosome to survive attack by the host's immune response poses difficulties in developing vaccines for the treatment of the disease [4].

Since trypanosomes have been recognized as human pathogens, HAT has been considered one of the most devastating health and economic development problems in sub-Saharan Africa. Current treatment for HAT is very limited and not ideal due to toxicity issues and impractical administration regimes, a situation that poses significant challenges in poorly equipped areas with inadequate medical facilities and resources. There are no other treatments available if the strains of trypanosome have evolved resistance to the limited drugs currently used in chemotherapy [5]. In addition, except for eflornithine, the mechanisms of action of the current drugs remain poorly understood. Many pharmaceutical companies are unwilling to develop drugs for HAT because developing an effective drug are expensive and require capital, and knowing that their target markets are the poorer countries—Asia, Latin America, and Sub-Saharan Africa [6]. All of these factors highlight the need to screen and discover new drug leads with a high activity and low toxicity effect against HAT for future drug development. To overcome the problems of the current treatment for HAT, plants and their derived products could be an interesting source of lead compounds with a strong activity and low cytotoxicity effect. Several studies have demonstrated the anti-trypanosomal activity of plant natural products. The toxicity and possible anti-trypanosomal properties of the plants collected from the Malaysian forest have been evaluated through an *in vitro* approach for the identification of anti-trypanosomal agents in our high-throughput screening campaign in searching for potential anti-trypanosomal agents. Elucidation of molecular events of programmed cell death (PCD) in *T. b. rhodesiense* may lead to the discovery of new targets for future chemotherapeutic drug development.

In 2016, our group had isolated two piperidine alkaloids, (+)-spectaline (**1**) and iso-6-spectaline (**2**) (Figure 1) from the leaves of *Senna spectabilis* [7]. These two compounds inhibited growth of *T. b. rhodesiense* without toxic effect on mammalian L6 cells. Thus, it can be considered a potential candidate for HAT early drug discovery. Subsequently, the ultrastructural alterations in the trypanosome induced by these compounds leading to PCD were characterized using electron microscopy. These alterations include an unusual amount of trypanosome at the dividing state, wrinkling of the trypanosome surface, alterations in the kinetoplast, swelling of the mitochondria, and the formation of autophagosomes. These findings provide evidence of a possible autophagic cell death in *T. b. rhodesiense*. Furthermore, the formation of autophagic vacuoles and mitochondrial damages through monodansylcadaverine and MitoTracker Red labeling agreed with the electron microscopy data. Interestingly, trypanosomes treated with IC_{90} of compound **1** and **2** after 72 h exhibited an effect that significantly induced an early apoptosis-like PCD, which included phosphatidylserine (PS) exposure, loss of mitochondrial membrane potential, and caspases activation. Taken together, these findings demonstrated the potential of compound **1** and **2** as a natural chemotherapeutic. capable of inducing a possible cross-talk between autophagy and apoptosis in *T. b. rhodesiense*. This is the first report on the ultrastructural and cellular aspects of these two piperidine alkaloids on *T. b. rhodesiense*.

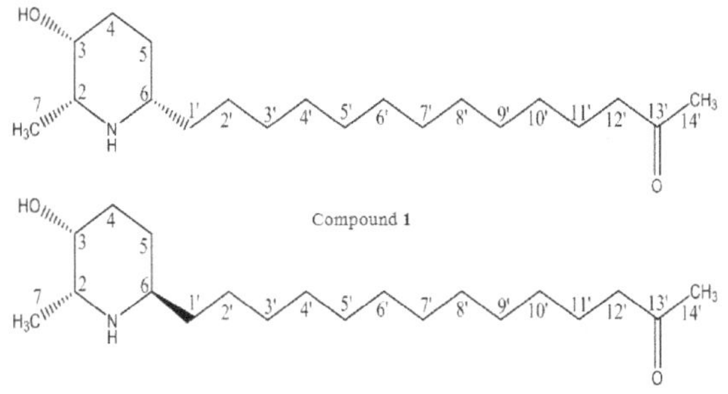

Figure 1. Chemical structure of piperidine alkaloids (+)-spectaline (**1**) and iso-6-spectaline (**2**) isolated from *S. spectabilis*.

2. Materials and Methods

2.1. General Experimental Procedures

Trypanosomes were treated with **1** and **2** at IC_{50} (0.41 and 0.83 µM, respectively) and IC_{90} (0.71 and 1.21 µM, respectively) for 72 h based on the inhibitory effects previously determined by [7] and examined with cytochemical methods to determine the mode of cell death action in *T. b. rhodesiense*. The trypanosomes were grown in a T25 vented cap flask and incubated at 37 °C under a humidified atmosphere of 5% CO2 in air. Untreated trypanosomes served as a control. Treated and untreated trypanosomes were harvested by centrifugation at 2700 rpm for 10 min, washed in phosphate buffer saline (PBS) pH 7.4, and resuspended in respective solution as indicated. Data acquisition was immediately carried out on a flow cytometer (10,000 events were read) and analyzed with the CellQuest software. In a parallel experiment, cells stained with detection reagents were microscopically viewed on a confocal microscope. All the results were averaged from duplicates over three independent experiments.

2.2. Measurement of Mitochondrial Membrane Potential

Mitochondrial damage of trypanosomes upon treatment with compound **1** and **2** were assessed by flow cytometry using a cell permeable dye MitoTracker Red CMXRos according to the manufacturer's instructions (Invitrogen). MitoTracker Red was passively diffused via the plasma membrane of viable cells and accumulated in active mitochondria. Briefly, treated and untreated trypanosomes were harvested, washed, and resuspended in 100 µL of 100 nM MitoTracker Red. The trypanosome suspension was incubated for 15 min at 37 °C. After incubation, 400 µL of PBS was added to the suspension. Immediately, the trypanosome solutions were analyzed using flow cytometer.

2.3. Detection of PS Exposure

The annexin V-FITC staining was performed with ApoDetect™ Annexin V-FITC Kit as per manufacturer's instructions (Invitrogen). Annexin V (a Ca^{2+}-dependent phospholipid binding protein) has a high affinity for PS and is useful for characterizing apoptotic cells with externalized PS. Concurrent application of the DNA binding dye propidium iodide (PI) and analysis of the stained trypanosomes by flow cytometry was used to discriminate the late apoptotic or necrotic cells from the early apoptotic cells. Briefly, the treated and untreated samples were harvested, washed, and resuspended in 100 µL of 1× binding buffer. After that, 5 µL of annexin V-FITC and PI were added to the trypanosome suspensions and incubated for 15 min in the dark at room temperature. After incubation, 400 µL of 1× binding buffer was added to the suspensions. Immediately, data acquisition was carried out on a flow cytometer. Quantitative analysis of FITC fluorescence was done to show the PS exposure.

2.4. DNA Fragmentation Analysis

The DNA fragmentation analysis was performed with Quick Apoptotic DNA Ladder Detection Kit as per manufacturer's instructions (Invitrogen). Treated and untreated trypanosomes were harvested, washed, and resuspended in 35 µL of Tris-EDTA lysis buffer. The mixture was incubated at 37 °C for 15 min in the presence of 5 µL of RNAase A. Next, 5 µL of proteinase K was added to the mixture and incubated at 60 °C for 30 min. After that, the solution was precipitated overnight at −20 °C with 5 µL of ammonium acetate solution and 100 µL of absolute alcohol. Following overnight incubation, the sample was centrifuged at 14,000 rpm for 10 min. The pellet was washed with 0.5 mL of 70% alcohol, air dried for 10 min, and resuspended in 50 µL DNA suspension buffer. DNA concentration was quantified at 260/280 nm on a spectrophotometer. DNA (10 µg/lane) was electrophoresed in 1.2% agarose gel containing 1× SYBR®Safe in 1× TAE buffer for 40 min at 70 V, visualized under UV light and photographed using gel documentation system.

2.5. Determination of Caspase-Like Protease Activity

Caspase-like protease activity was measured using caspase-3/7 green detection reagent according to the manufacturer's instructions (Invitrogen). The reagent is a novel substrate for activated caspases-3 and -7. Briefly, treated and untreated samples were harvested, washed, and resuspended in 100 µL of 5 µM detection reagent. The trypanosome suspensions were incubated for 15 min at 37 °C. Immediately, the trypanosome solution was analyzed using flow cytometer.

2.6. Autophagy Assay

To confirm the formation of autophagy vacuoles, the effect of these compounds in the autophagic cell death was evaluated by monodansylcadaverine (MDC) labeling. MDC reagent (Sigma) is an autophagolysosome marker that is particularly taken up by autophagic cells and stains autophagosome structures. The MDC labeling was performed according to the protocol described by [8]. Briefly, the treated and untreated trypanosomes were harvested, washed, and resuspended in 100 µL of 0.05 mM MDC in PBS. After incubation for 15 min at 37 °C, trypanosomes were washed and lysed in 10 mM Tris-HCl pH 8.0 containing 1% SDS. Intracellular MDC was measured on a Clariostar®microplate reader (excitation wavelength of 380 nm and emission wavelength of 525 nm). To normalize the measurements to the number of trypanosomes, ethidium bromide was added to a final concentration of 2 µM and total DNA fluorescence was quantified on the Clariostar®microplate reader (excitation wavelength of 530 nm and emission wavelength of 590 nm). Results were expressed as specific activity (% respect to the control). The specific activity is the ratio of the MDC signal divided by the DNA concentration of the MDC assay.

3. Results and Discussion

3.1. Measurement of Mitochondrial Membrane Potential

Alterations of the mitochondrial membrane potential ($\Delta\Psi$m) upon treatment with **1** and **2** for *T. b. rhodesiense* were assessed by flow cytometry using cell permeable dye, MitoTracker Red CMXRos. MitoTracker Red is a red-fluorescent dye that stains active mitochondria in healthy cells, which passively diffuse across the plasma membrane and reside in mitochondria with an active membrane potential. Spectrofluorometric data presented in Figure 2 shows a marked decrease in fluorescence intensity ($\Delta\Psi$m values), indicating depolarization of the membrane potential in cells following treatment with **1** at 0.41 and 0.83 µM and **2** at 0.71 and 1.21 µM. Trypanosomes treated with 0.41 and 0.83 µM of **1** resulted in a reduction of MitoTracker positive cells from 99.74 ± 0.11% (control) to 83.92 ± 2.68% and 58.31 ± 11.75%, respectively. On the other hand, treatment with **2** at 0.71 and 1.21 µM induced $\Delta\Psi$m reductions of 86.83 ± 8.19% and 54.65 ± 22.04%, respectively. As shown in Figure 2, there was virtually no difference between the control group and trypanosomes treated with 0.41 and 0.71 µM of **1** and **2**. In contrast to the trypanosomes treated with 0.41 and 0.71 µM, treatment with 0.83 and 1.21 µM of **1** and **2** exhibited significant depolarization of mitochondrial membrane potential (one-way ANOVA, $p < 0.05$) compared with untreated controls.

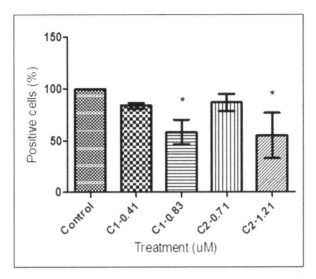

Figure 2. Quantitative analysis of mitochondrial membrane potential of *T. b. rhodesiense*. Treated and untreated trypanosomes were exposed to **1** at 0.41 and 0.83 μM, and **2** at 0.71 and 1.21 μM for 72 h, stained with potentiometric probe MitoTracker Red (100 nM) for 15 min and analyzed by flow cytometry. Trypanosomes treated with 0.41 and 0.83 μM of **1**, and 0.71 and 1.21 μM of **2** resulted in the reduction of MitoTracker Red positive cells from 99.74 ± 0.11% (control) to 83.92 ± 2.68%, 58.31 ± 11.75%, 86.83 ± 8.19%, and 54.65 ± 22.04%, respectively. Data are presented as means ± SD from triplicates over three other independent experiments. The asterisks indicate significant differences between the treated and untreated groups calculated by one-way ANOVA with Tukey post-test (* $p < 0.05$). C, compound.

3.2. Detection of PS Exposure

During the early stage of apoptosis, PS was translocated to the outer layer of the plasma membrane and was exposed on the external surface of the cells. PS externalization was studied by annexin V binding of trypanosomes following bio-active compounds treatment. Quantitative analysis showed an increased in annexin V-positive cells in treated trypanosomes compared with untreated controls. As shown in Figure 3, there was virtually no difference between control group and trypanosomes treated with **1** at 0.41 and 0.83 μM and **2** at 0.71 and 1.21 μM. In contrast to the trypanosomes treated with 0.41 and 0.71 μM, treatment with 0.83 and 1.21 μM of **1** and **2** exhibited significant increases in the percentage of trypanosomes positive to annexin V (one-way ANOVA, $p < 0.05$) compared with untreated controls.

3.3. DNA Fragmentation Analysis

PCD through apoptotic pathways is identified by biochemical and morphological changes that result from nucleases and proteases activities. Together with the formation of apoptotic bodies and chromatin condensation, DNA laddering in oligonucleosomal fractions is one of the last steps in the apoptotic process. Oligonucleosomal DNA fragmentation analysis of *T. b. rhodesiense* was carried out following treatment of the trypanosomes with **1** at 0.41 and 0.83 μM and **2** at 0.71 and 1.21 μM. DNA laddering profiles presented in Figure 4 clearly demonstrate no fragmentation of the genomic DNA of the trypanosomes following treatment with **1** and **2** for 72 h.

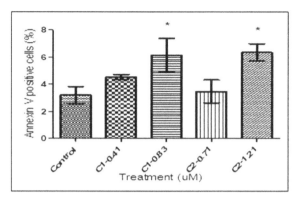

Figure 3. Fluorescence-activated cell sorting (FACS) analysis for PS exposure, measured by double staining with annexin V and PI in *T. b. rhodesiense*. Trypanosomes were treated with **1** at 0.41 and 0.83 μM and **2** at 0.71 and 1.21 μM for 72 h. An increased in annexin V-positive cells in treated trypanosomes (IC_{90}) compared with untreated controls. The bars represent the means ± SD of three independent experiments. The asterisks indicate significant differences between the treated and untreated groups calculated by one-way ANOVA with Tukey post-test (* $p < 0.05$). UL, upper left; UR, upper right; LL, lower left; LR, lower right; C, compound.

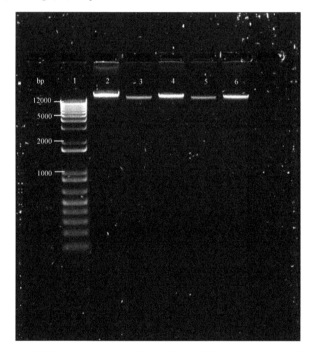

Figure 4. Analysis of DNA fragmentation in **1**- and **2**-treated *T. b. rhodesiense* for 72 h. Agarose gel represent the results of a typical experiment that produced similar results. Genomic DNA (10 μg/lane) from treated and untreated trypanosomes was resolved on a 1.2% agarose gel for 40 min at 70 V, then visualized under UV light. Lane 1, size marker 1 kb DNA ladder; lane 2, untreated trypanosomes; lane 3 and 4, DNA from trypanosomes treated with 0.41 and 0.83 μM of **1**; lane 5 and 6, DNA from trypanosomes treated with 0.71 and 1.21 μM of **2**. bp, base pair.

3.4. Determination of Caspase-Like Protease Activity

Caspases are activated to produce a controlled form of cell death. A fluorometric assay of caspase-3/7 was carried out using its specific cell-permeant substrate DEVD-peptide (Asp-Glu-Val-Asp) conjugated to a nucleic acid binding dye. This substrate is basically non-fluorescent because the DEVD-peptide inhibits the dye to bind to DNA. After the activation of caspase-3/7 in apoptotic cells, the substrate is cleaved by caspase-3/7 and the dye stains the nucleus to produce a bright green fluorescence. Trypanosomes treated with 0.41 and 0.83 μM of **1** resulted in an increment of caspase-3/7 positive cells from 1.35 ± 0.50% (control) to 3.70 ± 1.97% and 12.29 ± 4.59%, respectively. On the other hand, treatment with 0.71 and 1.21 μM of **2** induced increment of caspase-3/7 positive cells to 4.20 ± 2.70% and 11.64 ± 3.11%, respectively. As shown in Figure 5, there was virtually no difference between control group and trypanosomes treated with 0.41 and 0.71 μM of **1** and **2**. In contrast to the trypanosomes treated with 0.41 and 0.71 μM, treatment with 0.83 and 1.21 μM of **1** and **2** exhibited significant caspases-like activity (one-way ANOVA, $p < 0.05$) compared with untreated controls.

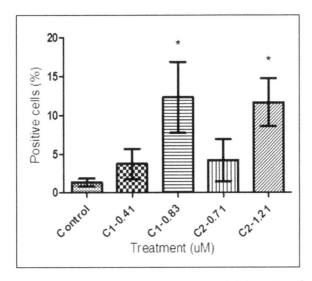

Figure 5. Quantitative analysis of caspase-like activity in *T. b. rhodesiense*. Treated and untreated trypanosomes were exposed to **1** at 0.41 and 0.83 μM, and **2** at 0.71 and 1.21 μM for 72 h, stained with caspase-3/7 green detection reagent (5 μM) for 15 min and analyzed by flow cytometry. Trypanosomes treated with 0.41 and 0.83 μM of **1**, and 0.71 and 1.21 μM of **2** resulted in an increment of caspase-3/7 positive cells from 1.35 ± 0.50% (control) to 3.70 ± 1.97%, 12.29 ± 4.59%, 4.20 ± 2.70%, and 11.64 ± 3.11%, respectively. Data presented as means ± SD from triplicates over three other independent experiments. The asterisks indicate significant differences between the treated and untreated groups calculated by one-way ANOVA with Tukey post-test (* $p < 0.05$). C, compound.

3.5. Autophagy Assay

To confirm the formation of autophagic vacuoles in *T. b. rhodesiense* after 72 h treatment with **1** and **2**, the effect of these compounds in the autophagic cell death was evaluated. As shown in Figure 6, the percentage of autophagic cells positive to MDC staining was increased from 56.21 ± 20.85% in untreated cells (control) to 90.40 ± 10.02%, 85.01 ± 27.94%, 90.29 ± 20.00%, and 77.39 ± 17.26% following treatment with 0.41 and 0.83 μM of **1** and 0.71 and 1.21 μM of **2**, respectively. Using MDC staining, a significant staining difference between control cells and treated trypanosomes was observed by one-way ANOVA analysis followed by Tukey's multiple comparison tests.

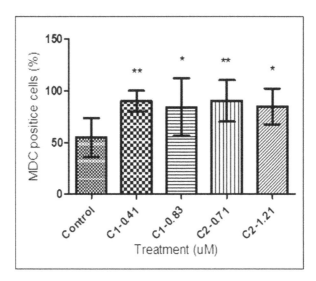

Figure 6. MDC labeling quantification of 1- and 2-treated *T. b. rhodesiense*. Treated and untreated trypanosomes were exposed to **1** at 0.41 and 0.83 μM and **2** at 0.71 and 1.21 μM for 72 h, stained with MDC (0.05 mM) for 10 min, normalized by staining with EtBr. The fluorescence signal was measured on a fluorometer. Trypanosomes treated with 0.41 and 0.83 μM of **1** resulted in increment of MDC positive cells from 56.21 ± 20.85% (control) to 90.40 ± 10.02% and 85.01 ± 27.94%, respectively. On the other hand, treatment with 0.71 and 1.21 μM of **2** induced increment of MDC positive cells to 90.29 ± 20.00% and 77.39 ± 17.25%, respectively. Data are presented as means ± SD from triplicates over three other independent experiments. The asterisks indicate significant differences between the treated and untreated groups, calculated by one-way ANOVA with Tukey post-test (* $p < 0.05$, ** $p < 0.01$). C, compound.

[9] have found that not all alkaloids induced PCD. In addition, the literature reports most tropane, quinolizidine, piperine, pyridine, purine, steroidal, and diterpene alkaloids were inactive up to a concentration of 100 μM. Therefore, the piperidine alkaloids **1** and **2** in this study represent interesting lead structures for potential anti-trypanosomal drugs. In our previous study, the observed changes are too small to provide evidence for apoptosis- or necrosis- like PCD suggesting an autophagic cell death due to compound **1** and **2** treatments, as there were no late apoptotic features shown by the parasites which include membrane blebbing, DNA laddering, cellular shrinkage, and the formation of apoptotic bodies [7]. Interestingly, compound **1** and **2** were also found to induce early apoptosis-like PCD in *T. b. rhodesiense*. Externalization of PS in the outer surface of the plasma membrane and caspases-like activity led to a dose-dependent increase of early apoptotic-like PCD in trypanosomes treated with **1** and **2** were evidently stronger at 0.83 and 1.21 μM. Taken together, these findings demonstrated the potential of compound **1** and **2** as a natural chemotherapeutic capable of inducing a possible cross-talk between autophagy and apoptosis in *T. b. rhodesiense*. Fungi, plant, and protozoa express metacaspases because they lack caspases. Although metacaspases have some similarity to the multicellular caspases, literature data do not give any evidence regarding the direct involvement of *T. brucei* metacaspases in apoptosis [10]. However, in a recent study, [11] proposed that metacaspases in kinetoplastid parasites such as *L. major* plays a vital role in the apoptosis and in the autophagy pathway. Therefore, in the context of these recent findings on trypanosomes, the caspase-like activity reported earlier needs to be examined. It is not uncommon for the cross-talk between autophagy and apoptosis to happen in kinetoplastids such as *T. cruzi* [12] and *L. major* [11]. To the best of our knowledge, this is the first report on the cellular aspects of these compounds in *T. b. rhodesiense*.

Trop. Med. Infect. Dis. **2019**, *4*, 98

4. Conclusions

In view of the potential use of piperidine alkaloids in *S. spectabilis* for the treatment of sleeping sickness, further investigation into the cell death actions of the parasite after treatment with compound **1** and **2** suggested that the treated parasites died by a process of autophagy based on the characteristic morphological alterations observed in intracellular *T. b. rhodesiense*. In the search for apoptosis, interestingly, the trypanosomes treated with a high concentration (IC_{90}) of compound **1** and **2** after 72 h significantly induced an early apoptosis-like PCD. No DNA laddering discriminated against a late apoptosis event. Taken together, these findings demonstrated the potential of compound **1** and **2** as a natural chemotherapeutic capable of inducing a possible cross-talk between autophagy and apoptosis in *T. b. rhodesiense*. Further clarification of the molecular events related to the cross-talk for PCD that was induced in *T. b. rhodesiense* by compound **1** and **2** is of great interest as the full elucidation of the mechanism of cell death would help to identify new possible targets for the chemotherapeutic intervention in trypanosomiasis. Due to the promising results obtained, in vivo studies are suggested to confirm the therapeutic potential of both active piperidine alkaloids. Besides that, continued investigation of cross-talk between autophagy and apoptosis is necessary to elucidate the mechanisms controlling the balance between survival and death in stress response conditions caused by chemotherapeutic natural products. Understanding of mechanisms that regulate the cross-talk for PCD is important for discovery of therapeutic tools in combating the disease.

Author Contributions: K.T.L.; Designed and performed experiments, analysed data and wrote the paper. C.Y.Y.; Aided in interpreting the results and co-wrote the paper. Z.Z.; Proofread the paper. M.I.A.; Supervised the research. All authors discussed the results and commented on the manuscript.

Funding: This research was supported by grants from the Ministry of Science, Technology and Innovation (MOSTI) of Malaysia (grant number: 02-05-20-SF0005). We thank Swiss Tropical and Public Health Institute (Swiss TPH), Basel for providing the strain of *T. b. rhodesiense* STIB 900 used in this study.

Conflicts of Interest: We wish to confirm that there are no known conflicts of interest associated with this publication.

References

1. Bowling, T.; Mercer, L.; Don, R.; Jacobs, R.; Nare, B. Application of a resazurin-based high-throughput screening assay for the identification and progression of new treatments for human African trypanosomiasis. *Int. J. Parasitol. Drugs Drug Resist.* **2012**, *2*, 262–270. [CrossRef] [PubMed]
2. Phillips, E.A.; Sexton, D.W.; Steverding, D. Bitter melon extract inhibits proliferation of Trypanosoma brucei bloodstream forms in vitro. *Exp. Parasitol.* **2013**, *133*, 353–356. [CrossRef] [PubMed]
3. Steverding, D. The development of drugs for treatment of sleeping sickness: A historical review. *Parasit. Vectors* **2010**, *3*, 15. [CrossRef] [PubMed]
4. Bacchi, C.J. Chemotherapy of human African trypanosomiasis. *Interdiscip. Perspect. Infect. Dis.* **2009**, *2009*, 1–5. [CrossRef] [PubMed]
5. Gehrig, S.; Efferth, T. Development of drug resistance in Trypanosoma brucei rhodesiense and Trypanosoma brucei gambiense. Treatment of human African trypanosomiasis with natural products (Review). *Int. J. Mol. Med.* **2008**, *22*, 411–419. [PubMed]
6. Martyn, D.C.; Jones, D.C.; Fairlamb, A.H.; Clardy, J. High-throughput screening affords novel and selective trypanothione reductase inhibitors with anti-trypanosomal activity. Bioorg. *Med. Chem. Lett.* **2007**, *17*, 1280–1283. [CrossRef] [PubMed]
7. Lim, K.T.; Amanah, A.; Chear, N.J.; Zahari, Z.; Zainuddin, Z.; Adenan, M.I. Inhibitory effects of (+)-spectaline and iso-6-spectaline from Senna spectabilis on the growth and ultrastructure of human-infective species Trypanosoma brucei rhodesiense bloodstream form. *Exp. Parasitol.* **2018**, *184*, 57–66. [CrossRef] [PubMed]
8. Jimenez, V.; Paredes, R.; Sosa, M.A.; Galanti, N. Natural programmed cell death in T. cruzi epimastigotes maintained in axenic cultures. *J. Cell Biochem.* **2008**, *105*, 688–698. [CrossRef] [PubMed]
9. Rosenkranz, V.; Wink, M. Alkaloids Induce Programmed Cell Death in Bloodstream Forms of Trypanosomes (Trypanosoma b. brucei). *Molecules* **2008**, *13*, 2462–2473. [CrossRef] [PubMed]

10. Helms, M.J.; Ambit, A.; Appleton, P.; Tetley, L.; Coombs, G.H.; Mottram, J.C. Bloodstream form Trypanosoma brucei depend upon multiple metacaspases associated with RAB11-positive endosomes. *J. Cell Sci.* **2006**, *119*, 1105–1117. [CrossRef]

11. Casanova, M.; Gonzalez, I.J.; Sprissler, C.; Zalila, H.; Dacher, M.; Basmaciyan, L.; Späth, G.F.; Azas, N.; Fasel, N. Implication of different domains of the Leishmania major metacaspase in cell death and autophagy. *Cell Death Dis.* **2015**, *6*, e1933. [CrossRef]

12. Menna-Barreto, R.F.S.; Salomão, K.; Dantas, A.P.; Santa-Rita, R.M.; Soares, M.J.; Barbosa, H.S.; de Castro, S.L. Different cell death pathways induced by drugs in *Trypanosoma cruzi*: An ultrastructural study. *Micron* **2009**, *40*, 157–168. [CrossRef] [PubMed]

MDPI

St. Alban-Anlage 66

4052 Basel

Switzerland

Tel. +41 61 683 77 34

Fax +41 61 302 89 18

www.mdpi.com

Tropical Medicine and Infectious Disease Editorial Office

E-mail: tropicalmed@mdpi.com

www.mdpi.com/journal/tropicalmed

Lightning Source UK Ltd.
Milton Keynes UK
UKHW050631120123
415065UK00011B/165